Raymond Adams

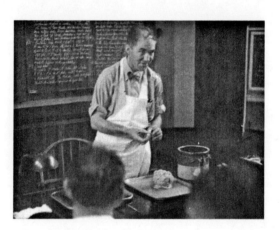

Raymond D. Adams at brain cutting conference in the Mallory Institute of Pathology at Boston City Hospital.

April 23, 2010

Raymond Adams

A Life of Mind and Muscle

ROBERT LAURENO, MD

For Edwina Fowler,

In appreciation of your fine work for the Washington Hospital Center and with admiration for your grace under fire.

With all best wishes,
Robert Laureno

OXFORD
UNIVERSITY PRESS

2009

OXFORD
UNIVERSITY PRESS

Oxford University Press, Inc., publishes works that further
Oxford University's objective of excellence
in research, scholarship, and education.

Oxford   New York
Auckland   Cape Town   Dar es Salaam   Hong Kong   Karachi
Kuala Lumpur   Madrid   Melbourne   Mexico City   Nairobi
New Delhi   Shanghai   Taipei   Toronto

With offices in
Argentina   Austria   Brazil   Chile   Czech Republic   France   Greece
Guatemala   Hungary   Italy   Japan   Poland   Portugal   Singapore
South Korea   Switzerland   Thailand   Turkey   Ukraine   Vietnam

Published by Oxford University Press, Inc.
198 Madison Avenue, New York, New York 10016

www.oup.com

Oxford is a registered trademark of Oxford University Press

Library of Congress Cataloging-in-Publication Data

Laureno, Robert.
Raymond Adams : a life of mind and muscle / Robert Laureno.
    p.   ;   cm.
Includes index.
ISBN 978-0-19-537908-2
1. Adams, Raymond D. (Raymond Delacy), 1911–   2. Neurologists—Massachusetts—
Boston—Biography.   I. Title.
[DNLM: 1. Adams, Raymond D. (Raymond Delacy), 1911–
2. Physicians—United States—Biography.   3. Physicians—United States—
Interview.   4. History, 20th Century—United States—Biography.   5. History, 20th
Century—United States—Interview.   6. Neurology—United States—Biography.
7. Neurology—United States—Interview.
WZ 100 A2145L 2009]
RC339.52.A33L38 2009
616.80092—dc22
[B]
2008049514

9 8 7 6 5 4 3 2

Printed in the United States of America
on acid-free paper

For Alison D. Laureno and Reva G. Laureno

CONTENTS

PREFACE

I FIRST BEGAN TO APPRECIATE RAYMOND D. ADAMS' unusual stature in 2000, when I interviewed Dr Maurice Victor for the historical record. The discussion quickly turned to the subject of Raymond Adams. Although I had always known that Raymond Adams was an important figure in neurology, I was surprised to hear Victor, an impressive and eloquent neurologist, unequivocally express deference to Dr Adams. In 2002, a Maurice Victor Memorial Symposium was held at the Allen Memorial Medical Library in Cleveland, Ohio. Between sessions I visited with Allan Ropper, a very bright and accomplished neurologist. In the course of our conversation, Dr Ropper similarly deferred to Raymond Adams to an extent that I found remarkable.

Because these two distinguished neurologists had such esteem for Raymond Adams, I realized that his story deserved attention. I became interested in studying and documenting his career. I wondered whether this Boston neurologist was from the famous Adams family of Massachusetts. (He was not.) I wondered about the process of his becoming, as many would argue, the greatest neurologist of his time.

Fortunately, Raymond Adams was alive and clear-minded. Allan Ropper kindly arranged the initial contact. I began to interview Ray Adams in person and by telephone. There were approximately fifty interview sessions, which took place primarily in the years 2002 through 2003. Phone calls and visits to his study continued with some frequency during 2004–2005. He reviewed and corrected the transcriptions for grammar, clarity, and content. I have annotated the interviews. I also have interviewed many of his former colleagues, residents, and fellows, and these interviews have continued through 2008. I have interviewed members of his family and I have studied his family archives. I have familiarized myself with Adams' writings and their historical context. The following chapters have emerged from these investigations.

There are several major divisions of this book. Chapter 1 describes Ray Adams as a person and as a professional. There follows a section of interviews about the phases of his life; these provide information about his early years, his childhood, his college experience, and his medical school, and postgraduate education. Admixed are his thoughts about his memories and experiences. His many interesting teachers are portrayed, as are his encounters with the cultures and institutions of North Carolina and Boston. There are interviews on the phases of his professional career, especially his years at Boston City Hospital and Massachusetts General Hospital. The third section, interviews on Adams' investigative work, puts some emphasis on the circumstances or events which led to his entering into each area of study. His personal life is discussed only in its relationship to his neurological career. Chapter 7 discusses the impact of his institution building, educational endeavors, original studies, and published books. Many of the specifics about his most important investigative works are described in Chapter 5. The appendices will aid the reader in understanding and appreciating Raymond Adams; the interview with Maurice Victor is most illuminating. From the book as a whole, I hope that the reader will begin to grasp the magnitude of Adams' contributions to medicine.

Raymond Adams' career was long and his interests broad. His recollections include important experiences in the fields of internal medicine, pediatrics, psychiatry, and pathology. Hence this book is as much a contribution to the history of twentieth-century American medicine as it is a neurological record. Naturally, the book is focused on the history of Ray Adams' life in medicine. However, neurologists, psychiatrists, neurosurgeons, and others involved in the clinical neurosciences may be interested in concepts and ideas that Dr Adams has expressed herein. I hope that some of these readers will be stimulated by Dr Adams' comments to pursue new areas of research. Clearly Ray Adams was brilliant; most of us are not so gifted. However, this book amply demonstrates that hard work played a big part in Adams' success. Thus, I hope that the medical student or the recent graduate will find encouragement in these pages that, through industry, he or she can also make original contributions to medical knowledge and thereby advance the profession.

ACKNOWLEDGMENTS

I THANK THOSE WHO AGREED TO BE INTERVIEWED FOR THIS BOOK. Listed here are the professionals whose interviews were most extensive or helpful. Many of these people provided documents or photographs. One of the positions attained is listed for each person:

Jay Angevine, PhD,
Professor of Anatomy
University of Arizona College of Medicine

Arthur Asbury, MD
Professor and Chairman
Department of Neurology
University of Pennsylvania School of Medicine

Betty Banker, MD
Professor of Neurology and Neuropathology
Case Western University
School of Medicine
Cleveland Metropolitan General Hospital

J. R. Baringer, MD
Professor and Chairman
Department of Neurology
University of Utah

Ivan Brown, MD
Professor of Surgery
Duke University School of Medicine
Duke University

George Collins, MD
Professor of Neuropathology
State University of New York
College of Medicine and Health Science Center

John P. Conomy, MD
Chairman
Department of Neurology
Cleveland Clinic

Robert Cook
Professor and Chairman
Department of Pediatrics
Johns Hopkins University School of Medicine

S. Allen Counter
Director
Harvard Foundation

Robert DeLong, MD
Professor of Pediatrics
Duke University School of Medicine

Darryl DeVivo, MD
Professor of Neurology
College of Physicians and Surgeons
Columbia University

Philip Dodge, MD
Professor and Chairman
Department of Pediatrics
Washington University School of Medicine

C. Miller Fisher, MD
Professor of Neurology
Harvard Medical School
Massachusetts General Hospital

Joseph Foley, MD
Professor and Chairman
Department of Neurology
Case Western Reserve University School of Medicine

William Glass, MD
Hartford, Connecticut

Mark Hallett, MD
Clinical Director
National Institute of Neurological
Disorders and Stroke
National Institutes of Health

Donald Harter, MD
Professor and Chairman
Department of Neurology
Northwestern University

Fred Hochberg
Associate Professor of Neurology
Harvard Medical School

Johnathan Horton, MD, PhD
Professor of Ophthalmology, Neurology, and Physiology
University of California, San Francisco

Richard Johnson, MD
Professor and Chairman
Department of Neurology
Johns Hopkins University
School of Medicine

Herbert Karp, MD
Professor and Chairman
Department of Neurology
Emory University

Walter Koroshetz, MD
Deputy Director
National Institute of Neurological Disorders and Stroke

Harvey Levy, MD
Professor of Pediatrics
Harvard Medical School

Elliot Mancall, MD
Director
Division of Neurology
Hahnemann Medical College

Joseph Martin, MD
Dean
Harvard Medical School

Richard Mayer, MD
Professor of Neurology
University of Maryland School of Medicine

Paul McHugh, MD
Professor and Director of the Department of Psychiatry and
Behavioral Sciences
Johns Hopkins University School of Medicine

Guy McKhann, MD
Professor and Chairman
Department of Neurology
Johns Hopkins University School of Medicine

Hugo Moser, MD
Professor of Neurology and Pediatrics
Johns Hopkins University School of Medicine

Nancy Newman, MD
Professor of Ophthalmology and Neurology
Emory University School of Medicine

Bruce Price, MD
Chief
Department of Neurology
McLean Hospital

Allan Ropper, MD
Executive Vice Chair
Department of Neurology
Brigham and Women's Hospital
Lecturer in Neurology
Harvard Medical School

Martin Samuels, MD
Professor of Neurology
Harvard Medical School
Neurologist-in-Chief
Brigham and Women's Hospital

Herbert Schaumburg, MD
Professor and Chairman
Department of Neurology
Albert Einstein College of Medicine

Eunice Kennedy Shriver
Executive Vice-President
The Joseph P. Kennedy, Jr. Foundation

Eli Shuter, MD
Assistant Professor of Clinical Neurology
Washington University School of Medicine

Murray Sidman, PhD
Professor of Psychology
Northeastern University

Richard Sidman, MD
Bullard Professor of Neuropathology (Neuroscience)
Harvard Medical School

Eugene Streicher, PhD
Director, Division of Fundamental Neurosciences
Extramural Program
National Institute of Neurologic Disease and Stroke

Roy Swank, MD
Head
Division of Neurology
University of Oregon Medical School

Maurice Victor, MD
Professor of Neurology
Case Western Reserve University
Director, Neurology Service
Cleveland Metropolitan General Hospital

Byron Waksman, MD
Chairman
Department of Microbiology
Yale University, School of Medicine

Henry Webster, MD
Chief
Laboratory of Experimental Neuropathology
National Institute of Neurological Diseases and Stroke

Many thanks to these Adams family members for sharing information, records, photos, and insights:
Mary Elinor Adams Dudley
John William Adams
Carol Adams Still
Sarah Ellen Adams Aldrich
Nina Salam
Alden Woodbury Dudley Jr. MD

Thanks to the following for providing information and materials:
Heather Briston
Archivist Special Collections
University of Oregon

Russell S. Koonts
Director
Duke University Medical Center Archives

Jack Eckert
Reference Librarian, Rare Books and Special Collections
Francis A Countway Library of Medicine

Arnulf Koeppen, MD
Professor of Neurology and Pathology, Albany Medical College
Chief, Neurology Service, VA Medical Center, Albany, NY

Ms Sue Smyth
The Joseph P. Kennedy, Jr. Foundation
   I greatly appreciate the hospitality of Ms Antonina (Nina) Salam and Jadwiga (Iga) Zabnienska during my visits to Dr Adams in Chestnut Hill, Massachusetts.
   Thanks to Ms Jennifer Wood for library research. Thanks to the library staff of the William B. Glew Health Sciences Library of the Washington Hospital Center, especially Ms Nina Brown, and also to:

Ms Brooke Henley
Ms Layla Heimlich
Ms Ernestine McCoy
Mr Frederick King
Mr Douglas Sloane
Ms Sharon Williams-Martinez
Ms Lynne Siemers

   Thanks to Mr Peter Brandt for assistance with photographic reproduction. For providing photographs I thank Dr Adams' friends, family, former residents, and former fellows. For photographs I also thank various libraries and Oxford University Press publications; other sources of photographs are specified in the figures. Thanks to Dr Mark Lin, my colleague, for technical assistance and wise counsel. Many thanks to Mrs Louella Baterna for preparation of the manuscript and for decades of faithful support of every kind.
   I thank my editor Craig Allen Panner for his guidance and his assistant David D'Addona for his help. I also thank the production editor, Karen Harmon.

CHRONOLOGIC HIGHLIGHTS

1911	Birth on February 13 in Portland, Oregon
1933	AB University of Oregon, AM (Psychology) University of Oregon
1937	MD Duke University
1937–1938	Intern and Assistant Resident in Medicine, Duke University
1938–1939	Resident in Neurology, Massachusetts General Hospital (Rockefeller fellow)
1939–1940	Assistant in Psychiatry, Massachusetts General Hospital (Rockefeller fellow)
1940–1941	Fellow in Psychiatry, Yale University (Rockefeller fellow)
1941–1951	Neurologist, Boston City Hospital, and Neuropathologist, Mallory Institute of Pathology with final ranks of Assistant Pathologist and Assistant Professor of Neurology (Harvard Medical School). (During these years he was also on the Tufts Medical School faculty (1944–1951) and was Chief, Neurological and Psychiatric Service, New England Center Hospital (1949–1951)
1951–1978	Chief, Neurology Service, and Neuropathology, Massachusetts General Hospital
1954–1978	Bullard Professor of Neuropathology, Harvard Medical School

1955	President, American Association of Neuropathologists
1967	President, American Neurological Association
1985	Hower Award in Pediatric Neurology (selected by the Child Neurology Society)
2008	Death on October 18 in Boston, Massachusetts

Raymond Adams

1

THE PHENOMENON OF
RAYMOND D. ADAMS

Calm, indefatigable, knowledgeable beyond human expectation, and completely devoted to teaching and demonstration...his extemporaneous presentations flowed in perfectly arranged sentences, clear, concise, and authoritative, often to the amazement of his audience...he was the ablest neurologist of his time...Truly, Adams ranks with the giants of neurology.[1]

C. Miller Fisher

IN SCIENCE, it has long been said that proper method is more important than genius. Accordingly, Raymond Adams' accomplishment derived as much from his systematic approach to studying disease as from his brilliance. A third factor, industry, was equally responsible for his success. After studying this man, I came to understand that Adams' career exemplifies William Osler's dictum: "the master-word is Work."[2]

The Man

Writing this book required me to interview many distinguished physicians. Nothing astonished me more than my encounter with Dr Joseph Foley. His awe was evident as he mused about the "phenomenon of Raymond Adams"—the incessant work, the energy, the concentration, the intellect, and the motivation. Recalling Adams at the Boston City Hospital, he seemed amazed, "I couldn't have worked that hard. I didn't want to work that hard. My wife wouldn't have let me work that hard." Betty Banker, one of Adams' fellows at Massachusetts

General Hospital (MGH), remembered the experience, "Work, work, work. Even at an airport, I never saw him look at a newspaper. He was always writing."

Work flowed from Ray Adams long before he turned to scholarly undertakings. There was always work: assembling newspapers, swabbing decks, digging ditches, scrubbing kitchens, or chopping ice. Work flowed from him before the sun rose. Work flowed from him as midnight passed. Like his father, he never had an idle moment. An inclination to hard work was in his nature.

His energy and concentration were such that he could work continuously. Because he remained focused, all of the hours spent were productive. As a high school and college student he juggled multiple jobs and his schoolwork. He finished high school six months early. At the university he acquired an undergraduate degree, a master's degree, and all courses needed for a PhD in four years. At medical school he would be up before dawn to lift 50-pound ice blocks from the icehouse. He would chop them and deliver the ice to ward kitchens and to urinals throughout the hospital. (Before the invention of air conditioning, ice was used in urinals to cut the odor.) All this was done before classes began. He finished his required medical school courses in three years by meeting requirements in the summer.

Adams had such stamina, C. Miller Fisher remembers, that "he could drive all night and work as well as on any other day." At Boston City Hospital, Philip Dodge recalls Adams working for over 80 hours a week; Joseph Foley remembers seeing him regularly at 1 a.m. in the Mallory Institute of Pathology. He would often arise by 5:30 a.m. and clean the stables before going to work. At MGH, Richard Johnson recalls his "incredible" hours of work, from early morning until late at night.

Although his industry was remarkable, it was Adams' intellectual capacities and remarkable power of language that struck people the most about him. By all accounts his memory was extraordinary. He practically memorized Fulton's treatise on neurophysiology. In discussing a current case, Adams would spontaneously discuss the details of the microscopic pathology of a similar case that he had seen years earlier. Later his secretary, Miss G, would track down the autopsy report. According to Richard Johnson, "The name was wrong, the year was wrong but the morphology he had remembered exactly ... amazing." Similarly he would remember the clinical details of an old case, which enabled him to compare it to a patient under discussion. It was the same with his memory for the literature. His son-in-law, Dr A.W. Dudley, had received an interesting brain from a Minnesota neurologist—the substantia nigra was pale but there had been no sign of Parkinson disease. Dudley had found an obscure article by two Japanese authors about a similar case. Suspecting that this Minnesota patient might be the first case of this type recognized in a Caucasian, he told Ray Adams about this brain. Off the cuff, Adams mentioned that those Japanese doctors had been fellows at the Mayo Clinic. It turned out that Dudley's case was from the same family as the patient described by the Japanese decades earlier. According to Dudley, this incident was typical; if Ray Adams read something, he never forgot it. (Ray's memory was inherited by at least one of his grandchildren, Raymond Adams Dudley, a professor of internal medicine in San Francisco.)

This exceptional memory was only one component of his prodigious intellect. Most remarkable was his ability to organize information. He was able to develop classifications of disease that might be important conceptually and/or useful clinically. He could synthesize the temporal features, clinical manifestations, and pathologic aspects of a disease in a meaningful way. Naturally, his memory enhanced his ability to do all this.

Traits other than industry and intellect were important to Ray Adams' success. He was a confident, competitive, and ambitious man. As a young neurologist at Boston City Hospital, he did not back down from disagreement with the famous Derek Denny-Brown. Once, a resident witnessed Denny-Brown storm off after exploding, "You don't know everything, Ray!" Joseph Foley, a fellow at the city hospital, remembers an occasional wry smile, which he took to mean that Ray knew that what was being said was incorrect. (Once, when I interviewed him, I corrected him on the pronunciation of the name of one of his former residents. The faint smile on his lips, I learned, indicated that he knew that I was wrong. I was.) Foley had no doubt that Ray was going places, and that Ray knew that he was on the way up. At tennis Adams always played to win. He was so quiet, his daughter states, that he did not seem to be competitive—he simply seemed to be doing his best. He was an "interesting driver" according to Darryl DeVivo; he drove fast and was highly competitive on the highway. Over coffee one night, Adams told Herbert Schaumburg that he wanted to be the best in his profession. His daughters Sarah and Carol feel that he had always wanted to be recognized and remembered.

All of this competitiveness and confidence was evident in action, not in open emotion. There was no bombast. His manner was reserved and respectful. "He never said a bad word about anybody." If the pronouncement of a visiting professor was wrong, he would politely disagree by saying, "This has not been part of our experience."

Adams was reserved and formal. People who were not well known to him found him to be reticent. He might look down on being introduced to somebody from outside his circle. I had this experience during a brief introduction to him, years before I thought of writing this book. His daughter confirms that he was shy in social settings, especially with unfamiliar people. Adams told the author that he "never adapted very easily into social groups." Although he was friendly to those he knew, he would not be interested in gossip. At work conversation would be sustained only when it related to neurology.

Despite his apparent shyness Adams did well with very personal relationships. Kind, he was a person, from whom a close friend, such as Maurice Victor or Mandel Cohen, could get personal advice. He was very loyal to his friends.

His respected colleague and protégé, Robert DeLong, was fired from MGH during the years after Adams had retired as chair. DeLong had been allowed to remain in an office at the hospital during the years 1985–1987 but was no longer employed. As DeLong prepared to depart to head pediatric neurology at Duke, he learned that he owed MGH $50,000 for office rental and related expenses. He mentioned this to Adams. Shortly thereafter Ray told DeLong that the debt had been wiped off the books. Two decades later it occurred to DeLong that Ray Adams might have paid it for him.

There was a strong personality behind the outer calm. This confident, competitive, reserved man was very independent. Family lore holds that the young Ray Adams once found a streetcar parked at a station: the conductor had stepped off for a moment. Ray, who had always wanted to drive a streetcar, jumped on and took it for a short ride. The outraged conductor came to the Adams' home to protest. As a Rockefeller fellow he did not feel the need to endear himself to those who were supporting him (see Appendix C, D). Furthermore the aim of the three-year fellowship, to develop him as a psychiatrist to return to Duke, was in the end avoided—he was able to become a neurologist and to stay in Boston.

Later, at MGH, Ray did not easily fall into line. When there was sub-optimal neurosurgical performance, he sent patients elsewhere. When the psychiatry department provided an inadequate experience for neurology residents, he pulled them out and sent them to another hospital for education in psychiatry. Having separated from his wife, he lived with his wife-to-be for many years until he finally obtained a divorce. At that time, such an arrangement was quite unconventional in puritanical Boston. Having developed professional relationships in Lausanne, he decided to spend the summer months there every year. He did not ask for permission to do this. Other chairmen at the MGH, unbeknownst to Ray, resented his long absences. He was oblivious to their jealousy. Joseph Martin recalls that Adams, no longer chairman, would not hesitate to walk out of a boring lecture by a visiting neurologist. One has the impression that he simply followed his own inclination, unconcerned about, even tone-deaf to the approval or disapproval of professional associates.

C. Miller Fisher found him to be very levelheaded. Even when he was angry, he remained calm. "I never saw him lose his temper no matter what the circumstance." The author found two accounts of Adams being flushed with anger but there was no indication of loss of composure in either case. Both instances occurred when his important plans for developing faculty and programs were thwarted by someone else. Once he interviewed an alcoholic patient at Grand Rounds. In a state of withdrawal, the patient greeted Adams with an expletive exclamation, never uttered in the professional circles of mid-century Boston. Adams turned to the audience and said, "A loss of propriety is characteristic of this disorder." He revealed that he was perturbed only after the conference, when he told the residents that they should never again present an alcohol withdrawal patient at Grand Rounds.

Not only did Ray Adams show little emotional range, but also, at the peak of his career, he was rather ordinary in appearance. "He looked like a street car driver," said one ex-fellow, who revered him. He had simple tastes in food and cars. At the American Neurological Association meeting in Atlantic City he did not stay at the Claridge Hotel with everyone else. He would stay around the corner at the very modest Florida Hotel, recalls Dick Johnson. His daughter Carol could not remember seeing him in a restaurant except for one Chinese establishment, which the family patronized during her childhood. In those days he always ate the same meals, cereal and fruit for breakfast, soup for lunch, and hamburger for dinner. He was extravagant only in spending for the education of his children and grandchildren.

Money was of little motivation to him. Hugo Moser recalls that patients would come from New York to Boston to see him; Adams' fee was so small that the patient's total expense for the trip was less than what the consultation would have cost had the person seen a neurologist in Manhattan. He was motivated by his intellectual pursuits. It was science that made him tick.

His daughter Carol felt that Ray was so immersed in medicine as to be "not realistic." She has no memory of ever seeing him in a grocery store, for example. When he was in his eighth decade, she took him to a hardware store. He was intrigued by an automatic paint-mixing machine. Although such machines had been commonplace for sometime, Ray had never heard of one let alone seen one. She feels that he lived in his medical world so much of the time that he was not aware of the everyday world as much as the average person was.

When Adams turned his intellect to introspection at my request, he described himself as "somewhat eccentric in my reactions." He viewed himself in retrospect, as "individualistic and irrationally opinionated." Reflecting on his youth, he said "I was late in maturing intellectually." Although nobody noticed, he admits that, "I was always aware of my deficiencies, when I was working with people from the Eastern universities."

Although Ray Adams was a serious man, he was not humorless. One Sunday night in the 1950s, a resident overheard him in a disagreement with C. Miller Fisher. Ray Adams was contending that Fisher's note in a chart was illegible. When the resident appeared, Adams called him over and asked him to read the note aloud. As the resident struggled and fumbled unsuccessfully, a smile began to faintly show on the face of Ray Adams. In the 1980s, a retirement celebration was held for his former fellows, Maurice Victor and Betty Banker. Although they had long since moved to positions in Cleveland, the gathering was held at the MGH on the occasion of the American Neurological Association meeting in Boston. Adams introduced the special scientific session in the Ether Dome. I remember how he reminisced about the difficulty that Victor had encountered in convincing Betty Banker to marry him. "And to this day," reflected

Adams, as he showed the curriculum vitae of one and then of the other, "I see that Dr Victor considers this marriage one of his accomplishments . . . and that Dr Banker does not."

His family seemed unaware but many sophisticated professional observers state that Ray Adams had a minor tic. When he was irritated, frustrated, or angry, he would turn his head, tug on his collar, and show some facial movement. This may have been a familial trait because one of his daughters Sarah reports that she has had throat-clearing tics.

Tennis was his passion, second only to neurology. With natural gifts and hard work he had become an excellent player. His strengths were anticipation and beautiful ground strokes. A natural teacher, he would constantly correct the play of his partner, whether it was his son or a resident: "Your back hand is a little early." As always, hard work was the solution for all problems. "Harry", he told one resident, "there isn't a single aspect of your game that would not improve, if you hit a million tennis balls."

The Neurologist

As a clinical neurologist Ray Adams was "magisterial." He brought a certain grace to the bedside when he entered a patient's room. He was official and pleasant, and always in charge. He relied very much on the history; he would do a focused examination to supplement the exam reported by the resident. Although he was cool, the patients were in awe of him, according to Mark Hallett. Richard Johnson considered him an "extraordinary" bedside clinician. Once, a patient screamed, "Am I going to die?" Jay Angevine witnessed Ray cradle her head, as he mentioned from memory the names of all of her children. There was an electrifying effect on all in the room. As a visiting professor at Peter Bent Brigham Hospital, he was shown a puzzling patient, a ten-year-old with episodes of spasmodic jaw opening. Adams observed these episodes and suddenly commanded, "Don't do that again!" The patient never did it again. He knew exactly what questions were appropriate to ask a patient in order to bring out the person's capacity. According to Richard Mayer, Adams frequently asked patients about the current batting average of Ted Williams, Boston's baseball hero. Hugo Moser presented a patient, who had performed poorly on tests of cognitive ability. Adams went to the bedside and asked, "How do you assemble a motor?" The patient's answer, which Adams recognized to be complete and correct, convinced him that the man was fine. Moser stated that Adams' life experience was so rich that he could draw on it to relate to any kind of patient. Patients would come from all over the world. According to Miller Fisher, "he had a manner about him" which made the patient feel he couldn't do better. He would write out his analysis of an inpatient case in about one-third of a page.

The Teacher and Chairman

In the 1970s, Allen Ropper found him a "stupendous" teacher. Martin Samuels compared him to a skilled athlete or ballet dancer, who makes a perfect performance appear effortless. Walter Koroshetz, a resident in the 1980s, recalled that Adams might be hard on himself; he would mention a prior mistake, if it were relevant to the case at hand. His "incredibly organized thought process continually amazed" Richard Baringer in the 1960s. Compared to what he observed at other academic institutions, Baringer found Adams unique in his intellectual curiosity. Always he said, "What is this patient trying to teach us?" Arthur Asbury also found it refreshing. Many other neurology programs took an empirical approach, he said, but Adams always would ask, "How did this come about?" In this way he helped people grow. Asbury still looks puzzled when he explains how Adams would ask in the 1960's, "What is your concept of this disease?" He was not asking for the cause or the physical findings or the treatment; he was asking Asbury to go beyond. As eras changed, Adams remained a model—attentive, thorough, thoughtful, thinking of the unusual, and enunciating a textbook-like presentation of the issues of a case under discussion. "For Adams," says C. Miller Fisher, "teaching was as natural as breathing."

Most but not all of his faculty were grateful to him. Jay Angevine was visibly cold during his first two winters in the department. With two children he was barely getting by on his small salary. Adams noticed, inquired about his situation, and arranged for a raise in pay. Adams would pick good people and let them work. After he hired psychologist Murray Sidman, he asked, "Can you work out ways to communicate with retarded patients?" This question triggered Sidman's years of research on this topic. During Adams' long collaboration with Byron Waksman, they regularly reviewed slides from their experimental studies. "Every time he sat down with me, he would sneak in a slide and say, 'what do you think of that?' He might show anything to do with myelin." Thereby he was not only helping Waksman to grow as a microscopist but also looking for ideas, mining Waksman's mind. When Hugo Moser failed to get a promotion he was encouraged by Ray, "Don't worry about it. Write some more papers. Everything will be okay." Many felt that he did not attend to promotions of his faculty and suspected that he delegated some responsibility for handling promotions to his secretary! As in any department, some members of the faculty were not enamored of the chairman. When a faculty member would provocatively disagree at Grand Rounds, Adams would answer, "Thank you."

He built a department by choosing people and letting them try to accomplish something. As Ray was preparing to move to MGH to assume the neurology chair, he approached Philip Dodge, a resident, in the Boston City Hospital's parking lot. "He asked me if I would develop child neurology at

Massachusetts General Hospital." Dodge answered, "I'd love to." When Hugo Moser was a resident at MGH, Adams approached him at an elevator and suggested that he develop a neurochemistry research arm for the department after he finished his residency. Moser accepted the offer and proceeded to build a program to study leukodystrophies. Robert DeLong, approaching the end of his second year of residency, was stunned by Adams' suggestion that he assume the vacated position of chief of child neurology at MGH. DeLong's subsequent outstanding contributions to the study of cretinism justified Adam's faith in him. In sum, Ray Adams was very effective in choosing people and in getting them to reach their potential. He had the capacity to instill direction. By granting responsibility and opportunity, he made young neurologists feel that they could achieve. Harry Webster calls him "one of the best farmers of the human vegetable."

Ray could be very directive in such matters: "Alex, now you should go to Hahneman and spend a year in neurophysiology with Fuller." Many complied. Richard Johnson was spending a year of study in virology in Australia when he received a letter: "Dear Richard, Byron Waksman has accepted a job at Yale. It is very important. You will be able to assume the position as head of those labs." He instructed Johnson to truncate his stay in Australia and to return to MGH promptly. He did not ask whether Johnson would like to do this. Johnson was one who knew his own goals; he declined. Paul McHugh credits Adams for an "amazing and instrumental change in my life. . .he had a capacity in broad vision and individual direction."

Selection of residents was a simple matter during the early days at the MGH. He was known to warn an applicant, "You know, neurology is a lot of work." Richard Mayer had no interview. He simply received a letter of acceptance. As the number of applicants increased, the process became more formal. At some point, certainly by the early 1970s, a "star chamber" interview process was initiated. Applicants, packed into a hallway, waited to be called. Those not forewarned were startled to find themselves with Adams at the head of a long table. Neurology faculty lined the table and the walls. Residents and staff would explain to Adams that this was an intimidating and undesirable interview method. He refused to change the efficient procedure, which allowed him and his faculty to see all of the applicants in one day.

Adams did not pay much attention to the application process. His office was in one building; his secretary's office was in another. The reportedly prejudiced Miss G was a power because Adams left her to organize the routine departmental affairs including residency applications. She did not like English or Canadian applicants. In the presence of Richard Johnson she glanced at an application and thrust it into her bottom drawer, saying: "We don't need any more Canadians." Guy McKhann, frustrated because he had never received a response to his inquiry about residency, traveled to Boston and walked into Adams' office, "Oh, I thought we had accepted you," was Adams' response.

Ed Kolodny could not get accepted due to Miss G's handling of his application, until Charles Kubik intervened to help him.

The power of this untethered secretary extended beyond the application process. Richard Johnson, as a resident, arranged, through Adams, a sixth-month exchange with John Walton. Johnson would go to New Castle and Walton to MGH. Each was to be paid by his home institution. Miss G told Johnson, "Don't go! Don't do this!" When Johnson reached New Castle, no paycheck followed. In desperation, he was borrowing money. Finally he called Ruth Symonds, another departmental secretary, who arranged for him to get his pay.

Although Adams did not deal with such day-to-day administrative affairs, he did not neglect leading and building his department. He led by example. The faculty emulated him and tried to work as hard as he did. He took care of business at lunch or when on an elevator. Robert DeLong found this style "wonderfully non-bureaucratic." In 1951, Adams had come to a department, where Charles Kubik was the only full-time neurologist. By 1966, when Harry Webster left for a position in Miami, there were 130 people in the department. The numbers alone indicate that Ray Adams was a "doer," a spectacular success as a department leader.

All this was accomplished by a man, who despised politics. His influence at the hospital was due to his being respected as a great figure in medicine and a great builder of his department. He would avoid meetings at the hospital. At a national level he participated little in neurological organizations. A frequently heard joke was that Ray Adams did not go to the meeting of any group, unless he was the president.

The structure of the residency program was regimented. Some academic hospitals were known as intern's hospitals, where the fundamental responsibility went to the least experienced doctor. Adams' program was controlled from the top. The attending neurologist told the resident exactly what to do.

Work seemed normal to Ray Adams. Furthermore, he had entered medicine via the grueling Hopkins' style medicine at Duke. Hence it is no surprise that the program for his residents in the 1950s was physically demanding. Richard Johnson recalls his schedule: first year, no vacation; second year, one-month vacation; and third year, no vacation. The consult service was very hard work. Adams would meet the consult resident at 7 a.m. in the stairwell and then run to the top of the hospital with the resident trailing behind. They would then see patients as they walked down floor by floor. In order for the resident to be ready to report at 7 a.m., he would have to pre-round at 6:30. Johnson thinks that Adams ran up the stairs neither for exercise nor due to elevator claustrophobia; he believes that Adams simply considered it the proper way to do things.

Ray Adams envisioned neurology as the equal of medicine and surgery. A neurology resident was assigned to the emergency room, where neurology was a primary triage service. By the 1970s a patient would get a color-coded tag indicating the primary triage service. Once a patient was tagged, the patient was the responsibility of the neurology service. By the 1980s the neurology resident thought of himself as the "gatekeeper" for the CT scanner, a very busy and important person in the emergency room.

The residents would "slog day and night for him," according to Miller Fisher, because they knew that, when he came, he would "give." Work came naturally from him and the residents emulated him. Herbert Schaumburg gave up his position as assistant professor of neurology at Albert Einstein and came to be a fellow at the MGH. "I cranked out thirteen papers. I worked like an animal like everyone else there did. Adams, Richardson, and especially C. Miller Fisher never seemed to leave the building. I heard somebody once came to Adams to say that he was very depressed. Adams said that depression was the most common disease at Mass. General and there was only one cure for it. Adams said it was hard work."

This work ethic epitomized by Adams and Fisher was actually part of the hospital ethos. Herbert Schaumburg: "I think that everybody at that hospital developed the delusion, that if they missed a day of work or didn't really work hard, the whole place would fall apart. I think that was part of the mystique of the hospital. People who got to their position were obviously the very best in the business. I will never forget—we had a terrible blizzard once and Mass. General had the lowest absentee rate of any institution in the city. One guy, who had broken his leg, had his neighbors drag him there on a sled. This was somebody who worked in admissions! And Adams was part of that." (My first appointment to interview Dr Adams was made two months in advance. There was a December blizzard which made car travel perilous, nearly impossible. I arrived 10 minutes late. He did not comment on the weather, but I sensed that I gained credibility by being undeterred and little delayed by the weather.) When Schaumburg was about to leave MGH, Adams advised him that, "it's okay to work 75% of two jobs but don't work 100% of two jobs" (being a neurologist and being a neuropathologist). About work he taught George Collins, "if you are going to be a neuropathologist, you have to sit at the microscope for endless hours."

Grand Rounds consisted of a case presentation, demonstration of the patient, and discussion by Ray Adams. He used no notes, no slides, and no blackboard. When the case for presentation would be selected late on the night before the conference, the clinical exposition was no less extraordinary. The case selection was by Adams and the chief resident. One observer was "floored by his skills." In a phenomenal way he would discuss the symptoms and one by one explain why various possible diagnoses had to be excluded before coming to the final possibility and correct diagnosis. In this process he was remarkably parsimonious in his use of words.

Brain cutting conference had a different format. Everyone, starting with the junior resident, had a say. He would not criticize mistaken commentary. He would thank each person for his remarks. At the end he would make his own lucid analysis of the case. Roy Swank remembers how Adams simplified everything. Swank, in his long career in Montreal and Oregon, never saw these conferences surpassed in quality.

At the microscopic pathology conference, all in attendance would study the microscopic slides of unknown cases selected by E.P. Richardson and staff. After a time, Adams would say, "Well has everyone seen enough?" Then he would call on people to comment. Adams, recalls Guy McKhann, would ask, "What did you see?" and "What do you think the disease is?" Many found these sessions the most exciting of all the conferences. By looking at the slides Adams would predict the signs, symptoms, and clinical course in an instructive way. Only then were the actual clinical events revealed. Due to his own vast experience he would teach about ideas that others would "discover" decades later. Richard Sidman remembers Adams' teaching that Alzheimer disease was not simply a presenile dementia; the same pathology underlay senile dementia. Katzman and Terry publicized this concept in an influential paper over ten years later.

Ray seldom gave formal lectures at MGH. When he lectured to medical students or at other institutions, the talks were erudite, very well organized, and beautifully delivered. Such lectures were distinguished by their scholarship; there was no charisma or showiness. In the 1970s, I attended such a lecture in Cleveland; there was no hint of humor but I was absorbed by the content. Every sentence was dense with information and every sentence was logically connected to the next.

On rounds with residents he was formal. There were no jokes. He tolerated no silliness. "Let's get serious," he sometimes had to command a jolly resident. He was always demanding, in a quiet way, of completeness and excellence. Eli Shuter recalls that Adams was unmatched for his extemporaneous discussions of patients at the bedside. He showed how one works to observe a patient and to draw things together inductively. C. Miller Fisher recalls, "other attendings would be puzzled" by a patient, and Adams "would come and give a spontaneous lecture on the case. I had never seen anything like it."

When a resident had made an error, Adams was encouraging, not critical. "He helped me over the small obstacles of my mistakes without crushing me," says Paul McHugh. In the emergency room (ER), McHugh had seen a fifty-year-old who could not walk; tendon reflexes were intact; and McHugh referred the patient to psychiatry. Three hours later the patient returned to the ER with cyanosis and areflexia. The patient, now on respirator, was presented to Ray Adams. McHugh said, "I thought she was hysterical; I'm embarrassed." Adams' response: "Don't be embarrassed—I made that mistake myself once. It's interesting; early Guillain Barre can do this." When McHugh made another error in not recognizing a case of Wernicke aphasia, Adams reassured him that it was a "common mistake." Herbert Schaumburg remembers, "one chap missed a subdural once and was just crushed at the autopsy table, and I heard Ray take him aside and explain how difficult it was. That was quite good of him."

When a resident had done a remarkably good job he would encourage him. Not in front of others but off to the side he might discretely whisper an appropriate comment like, "You're on your way!" By finding a moment to give a compliment in privacy, Adams spared the other residents any discouragement in seeing a colleague recognized for a level of excellence, to which they had not risen.

Adams was known to be very loyal to his residents and faculty. In the middle of his first year of residency, Richard Baringer was crestfallen to learn that he had been drafted for the cold war crisis in Berlin. Adams told him, "Don't worry. When you finish we will do whatever is necessary. You can resume your residency." Two years later Baringer was released from the military in the middle of an academic year. Adams allowed him to resume his residency immediately.

Adams was not judgmental about people's behavior. Hugo Moser remembers that Ray would accept "deviations" in people whom he thought were able. He supported a resident who had been "kicked out" of a rotation at another hospital for behavior disrespectful to the administrator. At times Ray's tolerance was a problem; more than one of his trainees felt that Ray was not good at recognizing mental illness in his own residents and faculty. When Adams was informed that a first-year resident was having a mental breakdown, Ray told the chief to give the resident more work; that would solve the problem. He would refer to the "demonic urges" of a faculty member, when everyone else knew that the man had bipolar illness.

One problem residents faced was Ray's difficulty with remembering names. The residents had no way of knowing that this problem was a familial trait. Daughter Mary would call her son by one name after another including that of the dog; she couldn't get it right. His son, Bill, has the same problem. Some of Adams' now eminent residents were called by the wrong but consistent first names through their training. Out of respect, many would not correct him. Others learned that they had to make sure that he got the name right during the initial weeks, in order to avoid three years of being called Peter instead of Bob. Sometimes he would not recognize a first-year resident as being a neurology resident at all. On such an occasion he expressed his regret to a senior resident, confessing his trouble.

Adams did not limit his teaching to the facts and methods of neurology. He spoke to the residents about the dignity of medicine and service to people, and none of this teaching was preachy or contrived. He taught about proper dress and behavior and about ways to enhance productivity. Jay Angevine was invited to rounds with Adams. On one occasion a resident had behaved inappropriately in a patient's presence. Outside the room Adams "excoriated him" firmly but not sadistically: "I am sure you will remember this!" Then he invited the resident to resume rounds with the group. When Richard Mayer visited the Adams' home in Milton, Ray took him to his study. He explained that by taking brief naps in the easy chair one could be productive in writing for many hours at night. A resident, accustomed to the casual dress of doctors on the West coast, encountered Adams on the first day of his neurology residency. Adams addressed him as "son," as he politely but firmly suggested that he leave to get a dress shirt and tie. He many times advised George Collins that "at the end of the day, start something new. That means that, when you come to work on the next morning, you will already have momentum."

Adams would promote the advancement of residents and fellows by giving them opportunities for co-authorship. For example, Adams encouraged Henry Webster to write a chapter on brain tumors for Harrison's *Principles of Internal Medicine*. After many drafts, Webster recalls, "Harry wasn't getting it." The deadline was approaching. One day Adams said to Webster, "Look what I jotted down." It was a perfect chapter on brain tumors with Webster as the first author. "Dr Adams I did not write a word of this!" Adams answered, "Harry, you worked hard. You learned a lot. In science you have to write; it has to be clear." Webster at age eighty reflects that he has never again seen a teacher so generously help his students by enhancing their bibliographies and by teaching them to write well. Webster states that Adams helped enormous numbers of residents and fellows in this way. For example, Richard Sidman, Adams' co-author of *Introduction to Neuropathology*, states that it was basically Adams' book.

Many residents from the 1950s use words like "revered," "father figure," and "friend" in speaking of Ray Adams. In the 1980s some of a new generation remember "fearing" him, while still recognizing him as a brilliant neurologist and teacher. He was as formal and serious as ever in a new era. He seemed out of date to some residents. Joseph Martin, his successor as chairman, was on an elevator with Ray. A resident stepped in and said, "Hello Dr Adams. Hello Joe." After the resident stepped out on the seventh floor, Ray Adams responded in disbelief, "You don't permit the residents call you by your first name, do you?" Ray Adams remained a "clean cut, conservative, quiet, intellectual" in an age when residents would grow beards and would worry about political and societal problems that might affect their patients. As always, Adams said whatever he thought. For example, he would say that women are better for pediatric neurology—it's natural. He would mention, matter of factly, that intelligence was inherited. He was either oblivious to or did not care about the sensitivities of a generation of residents, who had been told, at the universities, that there was gender discrimination and that the environment was important in determining intelligence and other traits. If he referred to a patient as a "Jewess," as he must have for decades, residents, who considered the term pejorative, were offended. These residents had no idea that his best friends, Mandel Cohen and Maurice Victor, were Jewish, that the two faculty members he hired at Tufts in the 1940s were Jewish and black, that he wrote papers with an African-American fellow in the 1940s, and that he had helped African-American students with special summer programs at Shriver Center. His serious demeanor, unmodern vocabulary, and age caused some residents to assume that he was a rich Boston Brahmin, a ridiculous notion to anyone who knew his life story. (He came from a family of uneducated farmers.) Despite such mistaken impressions, when residents from this skeptical generation reminisce, they use words like "genius" to describe him and attribute to him their academic success, rigor, and critical approach to literature. In this new era, there was continued respect but lessened reverence.

Some residents, certainly in the 1970s, sensed that the department at MGH had a sense of superiority, a belief that it was better than other places. Outsiders were sensitive. On a National Institutes of Health site visit in the 1960s, a PhD sensed that an unsmiling but courteous Ray Adams felt imposed upon by the visit. In the 1970s, a site visitor found Adams' concise summary of his department's activity the "most arrogant presentation I have ever seen." A professor, who had invited Adams to his hospital to lecture, found him aloof and disdainful. Such perceptions declined after he retired as chairman.

With medical students he was friendly but cool and serious. A student presenting a case might become flustered by the formality of his questions. He was especially serious about the neuropathology course for second-year medical students.

Ray Adams took over direction of this course from Stanley Cobb. It was the introduction to neurology for the Harvard medical students. Adams was devoted to the course and, as always, aimed for excellence. Gradually the syllabus grew to be the size of a telephone book. The neurology residents working in neuropathology and the neuropathology fellows served as instructors for the small group microscopy sessions. For the fellows, attending the lectures by Adams and Denny-Brown and directing small laboratory sessions were memorable experiences. Elliot Mancall, after half a century, recalls it: "amazing. I still have the notes; I still refer to them occasionally." Henry Webster, as a resident, was "for the first time impressed with Harvard University." Betty Banker, a fellow, said the course was "excellent...superb...absolutely superb...beautifully done."

Some students immersed themselves in the course. As a second-year student Robert DeLong found the course impressive. He was very much "into it." Harry Webster remembers that one year two students in his class wrote essay exams so outstanding that they were publishable. He remembers the students being quizzed about microscopic unknowns with the questions: "What is the tissue?...From where in the CNS is the tissue?...What is the disease?" Most students did not appreciate the course, did not realize what they were getting. They thought that there was too much information and too much work.

The instructors tended to agree. Each year there was a "post mortem" session, when the course faculty members gathered. All of the instructors believed that the course was too hard, that there was too much work. They urged Adams to simplify things. Each year he disagreed. He did not want to dilute; he wanted to maintain excellence.

This situation reached a crisis in 1968, when Ray Adams published *Introduction to Neuropathology*, a book of some 600 pages. It was an enhanced version of the syllabus with carefully selected illustrations. Restive students of the 1960s did not want to pay to buy the book and did not want to do the work. From their point of view the course was an impossible burden; imagine every subspecialty in pathology or medicine with its own book and such heavy demands. A student headed toward dermatology or obstetrics could not see the sense in struggling through the material. Adams' point of view was that he had devoted himself to developing an outstanding course. He could not see that many people lacked his stamina and capacity for work. The students, supported by the dean, gave up a unique experience, the opportunity to be taught and stretched by great men. Adams refused to participate in a watered-down replacement course. He never taught at the medical school again.

This confrontation in academe was not simply a matter of Adams' drive for excellence and his unwillingness to compromise. It was, in part, a manifestation of the time. This clash of the professor and students is one example of the campus tensions of the late 1960s. For example, failure of the university to adequately discipline rebellious students led to the resignation of irreplaceable government department faculty at Cornell University. Academics suffered as a result of administrative weakness.

Unwillingness to settle for mediocrity and striving for excellence were two related characteristics of Raymond Adams. Confidence and social shyness like competitiveness and soft-spokenness were interesting complexities of his personality. Added to these traits were brilliance, intellectual integrity, industry, concentration, and motivation—a formidable combination—the fruit of which is documented in the following pages.

Raymond Adams may have been the only man of his generation to have extensive training in psychology, internal medicine, neurology, psychiatry, and neuropathology. That he advanced all of these fields and all of the realms of neurology, from higher cortical to peripheral, is a remarkable achievement and the primary subject of this book.

Notes

1. Castleman B, Crockett DC, Sutton SB. *The Massachusetts General Hospital 1955–1980*. Little Brown and Company, Boston, pp 163–164, 1983.

2. Bliss M. *William Osler: A Life in Medicine*. Oxford University Press, New York, pp 299–300, 1999.

2

EDUCATION AND PROFESSIONAL ENDEAVORS

A Boy in Oregon

Raymond D. Adams descended from soldiers of the Indian and Civil Wars and from pioneers who crossed the Great Divide. His father had built the home, where Ray was born in 1911. There he lived his early years without gaslight or electricity. Hard work and self-reliance came naturally to Ray Adams. These inborn traits were reinforced by his parents' example and expectations.

RL: *What is your earliest memory?*
RA: I have a few scattered memories of my first ten years of life. I remember going to my grandfather's house, picking pears and Italian prunes. I remember sitting on the back of my grandfather's lumber wagon. I remember a particular cherry tree in the backyard that I used to climb; my grandfather planted it when I was born. When you are in late years, early memories fade.
RL: *Tell me about him, your mother's father.*
RA: My grandfather fought in the Civil War; he was a Yankee. I several times marched with him on the fourth of July.
RL: *Did he put on his uniform?*
RA: Yes. He was very proud of how many Southerners he killed.
RL: *Please tell me more about your family.*
RA: My origins were from families of farmers out in Oregon. None of the family, as far as I know, had ever gone to high school. They were farm families, relatively uneducated.

RL: *Were your parents readers?*

RA: They did very little reading. We had few if any books in the house.

RL: *Where was your father's family?*

RA: Near Rochester, New York; Churchviile was the name of the place. My father was forced, at a young age, to take over the family farm. He did all of the work himself. His brothers were lazy and he was fed up with supporting them. I think his mother had died. So he suddenly packed his bag and left; he never contacted them again in his life. He just left—tragic for him. He went to California and then to Oregon, where he married my mother.

RL: *Did you ever meet anybody from his side of the family?*

RA: No.

RL: *Did any of your mother's siblings or their children practice medicine?*

RA: There were a number of them. Some became farmers. Two of her brothers were butchers, I think. And their children were not outstanding.

RL: *Did you inherit any particular traits?*

RA: No. My mother was well organized and competent in everything she did.

    She ran a house and, in order to defray the expenses of me and my sister at the University of Oregon, she worked for years as a sales clerk in a bakery at the same time. She was highly efficient. She probably was fairly smart.

    My father was quick with figures; he had an agile mind. He was clever. He built the home, that I was born in, by himself, and he could repair almost anything. He could manage animals very well. I would guess that he had a good intelligence, but I don't know how to extrapolate from things like that.

RL: *Tell me about your father.*

RA: He was a good farmer and a very energetic fellow. I never saw anyone more honest. He was very supportive but worked all the time. Whenever he had an idle moment, he'd be doing something around the house or orchards or chicken coops. He loved music; he liked the Battle Hymn of the Republic. He was capable of hard physical work for long periods.

RL: *What was your father's occupation?*

RA: He worked for Standard Oil Company. He distributed oil to Clackamas in Multanomah County; it was very close to Portland . . . just south. We had a pleasant house. There were storage tanks in the back where they delivered the oil. He used a tank wagon, pulled by horses, to deliver the oil to gas stations and businesses that used it for heating.

RL: *How did you heat your own house?*

RA: We had a furnace in the basement. My father would buy about 20 cords of wood. He would buy logs. We didn't have a saw of any kind. So he would hire someone later to come and saw them to 12- or 15-inch lengths. And my job was to throw it through the basement window and stack it. It would last all through the winter and spring. And there was a wood stove, which burned kindling and small pieces. We got the house quite warm that way. Of course, in Oregon, it isn't very cold, west of the Sierra Nevada Mountains. It's kept warm by the Japanese current along the coast. It's only over the mountains, inland, that one encounters a continental, very cold climate.

RL: *How did you light the house?*

RA: We only had oil lamps for every room. We had to be awfully careful about fire, of course. But that was the standard method, at that time, of illumination.

RL: *Do you mean that you had no electricity in your home for much of your childhood?*

RA: That's right. It was a great event when gaslight was available.

RL: *Tell me about your Christmases.*

RA: My mother did everything possible to make them very pleasant. I always was given the assignment of finding a Christmas tree. I would ride my bike out into the endless forest, not too far from our home, find a tree some place. You never had to worry about whether it was on someone's property because there were so many trees.

RL: *So you would chop down a tree and bring it home on your bicycle?*

RA: Yes. A full size tree, and my mother would have my sister and me help in the trimming. We used candles because there was no electricity. And we had only a few bulbs on the tree because they were too expensive. So she would make strings of popcorn and decorate the tree. We always had our Christmas gifts on morning of Christmas day. Also I would earn money by selling trees. I would go out everyday and get one or two.

RL: *Did you take orders or did you go door to door?*

RA: Door to door. Sell them for 50 or 75 cents.

RL: *What else can you tell me about your family?*

RA: My other closest relative was my mother's youngest brother, and he took it upon himself to teach me a number of things that a father would ordinarily teach. He taught me to swim and look after myself in the woods, things like that. He was a bisexual I think—never sure about that. He married late, and his son was a homosexual. My sister's son was homosexual.

RL: *Do you think that there is a genetic component to homosexuality?*

RA: Oh, sure—no question I think. There's some very good genealogy on homosexuality. Have you seen those?

RL: *No.*

RA: There's one that came out in Lancet years ago.

RL: *Tell me about your sister.*

RA: We were five years different in age. We always got along amicably—never any dispute or rivalry of any kind.

RL: *Did you have a religious upbringing?*

RA: My mother was a fairly devout Baptist. My father was essentially an agnostic or atheist. He would, in deference to my mother, attend church occasionally, but it constituted no part of his existence. She was insistent that I attend Sunday school and that I adhere to the usual restrictions of the Baptist faith, no alcohol and no playing on Sundays. I had to wear my good clothes all day on Sunday. I was baptized about age 12 in a baptismal chamber, where I was submerged. During late adolescence and adult years I came to reject the main tenets of the church as based on faith and imagination and not subject to proof. My sister retained her religion.

RL: *Did your religious training have any lasting effect on you?*

RA: I dislike blasphemy and vulgar language. I suppose that would be an effect. My father would curse and that would upset my mother very much.

RL: *Did you go to public elementary school?*

RA: Yes, we walked about a mile to get to school.

RL: *Do you have any early recollection of being interested in the brain or the nervous system?*

RA: Not at all. I didn't know the first thing about it, and I was a rather mediocre student in high school. I would always pass easily, but I didn't make any great effort. The children that I grew up with disdained scholarship and study.

RL: *Where did you and your friends direct your energy?*

RA: We were involved endlessly in sports, baseball, basketball, and football. I was not big enough to make first team. So I was not very successful along those lines, although I was well coordinated.

RL: *Did you practice a lot?*

RA: Oh, a lot, yes. We spent hours. I caught on quickly on how to throw a curve as an adolescent, and I could strike out a lot of my contraires.

RL: *You told me that you had an early memory of riding on the lumber wagon with your grandfather. Was that a horse-drawn wagon?*

RA: Yes. We never had a car until, oh, I must have been twelve or fifteen years old. We couldn't afford one. By then my father was working for the railway and we had no horses. So he bought a Chevrolet. I remember he never really learned how to drive it well. He could handle four horses with ease, but he never figured out how to back the Chevrolet into the driveway.

　　I was always very envious of people who had cars, when they first came out. And I remember one of my classmates and I were able to buy, for $10, an old Ford. We took the motor apart and got it running again. And I learned to drive on my car.

RL: *How did you get to high school?*

RA: I took a streetcar for 5 cents.

RL: *When you were in high school, were you much of a reader?*

RA: No. Not to any great extent. On weekends and summers I was very much encouraged by my parents to earn money at various types of work. So there was little time to study outside of the classroom. And I made little effort to do so, probably diverted by these other activities.

RL: *Your high school yearbook says you were "rarely talkative."*

RA: I never would fit in with my classmates particularly. I was never in afterschool activities; I was always working.

RL: *What did you do with the money you earned?*

RA: My mother made me save a good part of it.

RL: *At what jobs did you work at during high school?*

RA: Oh, I had all kinds of jobs. I set type at a printing company after school. But for the last two years in high school I not only delivered papers from four to six in the morning, but on weekends I would work from three in the afternoon on Friday until midnight and then from noon of Saturday until two to three in the morning on Sunday and would get almost a week's pay that way. I was just putting together the *Oregonian*, which was the leading newspaper, a large multi-section paper. The sections would be thrown together by hand; I was one of several compositors that did that. It paid quite well by the standards of that day, and it enabled me to have enough money to pay for part of my first year at the University of Oregon.

RL: *On the Washington High School Commencement program you are not included in the top quarter of the class on the honor roll.*

RA: My performance was less than it could have been. I did well enough to pass any tests that I took . . . C's and B's, but I didn't excel.

RL: *Did you at some point become aware that you had cognitive talents that were way above average?*

RA: Not really. I knew that I could do well when I tried. Not having money or good clothes, that sort of thing, I was rather eliminated by cliques of students who were from wealthy families. That was a source of envy, as would be expected, I suppose.

RL: *Despite this background, you went to the University of Oregon?*

RA: Well my parents were persuaded that one had to be educated to make a mark in life, and they were very supportive. They were quite insistent. And so I matriculated at the University of Oregon without the slightest idea of what I should study.

The University of Oregon: Finding His Game

Having finished his high school requirements early, Ray Adams sought experience away from home. His parents finally conceded to his demands. For $30 a month he signed on to the S.S. Moffett, an oil tanker which sailed from Alaska to San Diego to El Salvador and back. As an ordinary seaman, he scrubbed decks, stood watch, and did other jobs on board. After nine months exposure to this "rather seamy side of life," he returned to Oregon to enter college.

RL: *What was it like to be a university student in Eugene, Oregon?*

RA: I think I was just slow in finding things that interested me and also in avoiding distractions, many of which were more interesting than the course work. I tried out for baseball and I tried out for track. I was not very good at either one. I had played tennis since I was eleven or twelve, never had any instruction, and was able to make the tennis team, which had one or two outstanding tennis players. The coach was more interested in the outstanding ones, Sidney B. Wood, who won at Wimbledon, and Harrison, who won the national amateur championship in the States. I practiced a lot without very good instruction, and I did play competitive tennis. And

I tried golf. Also my mother encouraged me toward music, and I played, for a while, in the band at the University of Oregon. Again, I had all sorts of distraction during that first and second, even into my third year. As a young person who had no particular guidance, I was just trying out everything.

RL: *What were your academic goals?*

RA: At the university, my faculty adviser was inept, I think. I didn't know what I wanted to study or what profession I wanted to enter, if any. And so he was just having me take general courses. I signed up for economics, political science, and chemistry, not a program that was necessarily designed for anything. So I would say that I wasted a good bit of time at the university.

RL: *Where did you live after freshman year?*

RA: I was living in a fraternity house, Alpha Upsilon. They let me live there for doing odd jobs. I'd clean up the kitchen and work around the house—whatever the housekeeper assigned. So I became a member of the fraternity that way, but it was a second rate fraternity, not one of the big ones. And the members were from ordinary families. There were a lot of communists and radical thinkers. A number of them were gamblers. There was a card game going almost continually, poker or pinochle. A couple of them were from Coos Bay, a lumber producing area in southern Oregon—wanted to get a little polish by going to college; they were not interested in studying at all.

RL: *Was communism popular in those days?*

RA: Oh, yes! During the Depression people were starving, and the government was dumping carloads of potatoes in the ocean. Much bad feeling. And so, amongst the young people, communism was rife.

RL: *Were you attracted?*

RA: I never got involved in political things. I always had so many other problems. My family was nonpolitical.

RL: *Was your family affected by the Great Depression?*

RA: My father lost his job. Eventually he found work as a baggage handler for the railroad. My father had trouble making ends meet. I think his salary, when he was working for the railroad, was something like $80 or $90 a month.

RL: *How did you pay for the university?*

RA: I did odd jobs around the university. I worked at the fraternity house for my food; I worked at a library at odd hours. One could get by on very little.

RL: *When did you become aware that you had exceptional ability to organize your thoughts and to verbally express them?*

RA: When I was in my third and fourth years, I began to take physiology and psychology, and courses like that. I found that I made A's in all of them.

RL: *At some point did you feel an urge to accomplish something in your profession or to do something important?*

RA: I wanted to excel then. And I was stimulated, to some extent, by the performance of my future wife, who was very scholarly. And I obtained enjoyment in being able to achieve a good grasp of the material of these courses. So, from that point on, my studies were always easy and stimulating.

RL: *It sounds like you finally stumbled on a subject, which interested you enough, that you were motivated to achieve.*

RA: Yes, essentially that.

RL: *Tell me about your future wife, Margaret Elinor Clark.*

RA: She was brought up on a farm in eastern Oregon. Her parents died when she and her sister were children. And they were raised very strictly by her paternal grandparents and three aunts, who were high school teachers. Their father left them each some amount of money for their education, and Margaret Elinor matriculated in the Monmouth Teachers' College. She went there for, I think, two years and got a teaching certificate. And it was at the completion of that course of study that we met, one summer, when I was working on a construction crew in Monmouth.

RL: *What were your responsibilities on that crew?*

RA: I was digging ditches and doing labor. She took a teaching position at a nearby village for $80 a month, half of which had to be spent in the town. And she had all eight grades in one room. So she had quite a lot of experience in teaching everything in grammar school. I became enamored. At the end of the year, with some persuasion on my part, she entered the University of Oregon. She was an excellent student, made high grades and was elected Phi Beta Kappa in her senior year. She was a person who was very strict in her behavior, very loyal.

RL: *How did you meet?*

RA: We met at some social function during the summer at the Monmouth College, where I used to play tennis in the evenings. I think we met on a number of occasions there and finally developed a very close relationship, always nonsexual.

RL: *How did you turn to psychology?*

RA: I became interested through a general course in psychology. And I took other courses, one in physiological psychology with Crosland. He taught about sensation and sense organs and the physiology of perception and probably influenced me very much toward medicine. Then I took a course in abnormal psychology with Conklin,[1] who was chairman of the department. He discussed in his lectures, at some length, psychiatric entities such as hysteria and schizophrenia. He used to go to an insane asylum near Eugene, where he interviewed patients. He was an isolated, eccentric individualist; he lectured beautifully. He wrote very, very well and was an impressive scholar. He certainly impressed me.

RL: *I gather that these two men attracted you to the field.*

RA: Yes.

RL: *Did you use any books that made a lasting impression?*

RA: I think Conklin's book on abnormal psychology was quite influential. It was very objective and was based on his wide reading of German and American psychology. I treasure Conklin's book.[2]

RL: *Had psychoanalysis affected the psychology department at Oregon?*

RA: Well it was being taught, and I had two or three courses in psychoanalysis; all the main principles were reviewed by Conklin. (He was a student of Allen, a very important personality at Clark University, who brought Freud to America for the first time in 1906 or so.) Psychoanalysis was well known throughout the United States, and we were quite familiar with its main premises.

RL: *What did your parents think of your decision to study psychology?*

RA: They, being uneducated people, couldn't guide me at all. My parents just figured that, if I was at the university and could graduate from it—that was enough. That was more than they ever expected for themselves at least.

RL: *Tell me more about your study of psychology.*

RA: By taking courses during the summer, I condensed the four years of college to three. And then I went into a master's degree program. I was taking graduate courses in 1932–1933.

RL: *Tell me about your graduate studies.*

RA: I was able to finish that master's program in about a year and a half. I was assigned to do my master's thesis under Robert Seashore,[3] [see Figure 7] a young member of the faculty. I wrote a thesis on studying various tests of tremor and ataxia as an aid in the selection of workers for factories. At that time there was a movement toward industrial psychology, whereby the methods of physiologists and psychologists could be applied to workers to search out certain skills and to eliminate individuals who lacked them. That was a movement strongly supported by Robert Seashore. I was indoctrinated by Seashore in the scientific method, the importance of measurement and documentation, and the development of and the testing of a hypothesis. The importance of control material was instilled in me by Seashore.

The master's thesis was entitled the Importance of "Steadiness" in Marksmanship and several other Practical Skills.[4] Five tests of steadiness were performed on military students, pianists, draftsmen, athletes, and the rifle team. As the latter group did better than the others, the possibility was raised that such tests could be used to screen applicants for sharpshooter positions. The thesis contained a long discussion of literature on tremor and postural steadiness drawn from neurological sources. Adams referred to an article on paralysis agitans in Brain, to the *Textbook of Nervous Diseases* by Dana, and to *Studies on Neurology* by Henry Head. He also referred to an 1886 article on steadiness and equilibrium by a Boston neurologist, W.N. Bullard. Ray Adams would not have known that Bullard and his family had established, at Harvard Medical School, the Bullard Professorship of Neuropathology, an appointment Adams would receive thirty years later.

RL: *How did you succeed in your psychology studies?*

RA: I failed to make Phi Beta Kappa because of my mediocre first year. I was elected to Sigma Xi, the honorary fraternity for science, in the fourth year.

RL: *Prior to your college commencement you and Margaret Elinor married.*

RA: Yes.

RL: *How long had you been engaged?*

RA: Two years.

RL: *Who attended your wedding?*

RA: Only a friend and his wife. We were married at their home by a local clergyman. Margaret Elinor's three aunts were opposed to the wedding.

RL: *After graduation you stayed in Eugene to complete the master's thesis.*

RA: Yes but she went immediately to Friborg, Switzerland, for a year of scholarship at a French speaking, Catholic University.

It was that summer that I really became dissatisfied with the way psychology was trending. I saw, more and more, the weakness of psychology in general and the difficulty in doing experimental work. I assume that must have influenced my decision to get a sound grounding in anatomy, physiology, and pharmacology of the nervous system and to get my doctorate degree in medicine rather than finish up my psychology doctorate degree.

RL: *Were you influenced by peers going off to medical school?*

RA: No, I was mainly influenced by my course work at the university. On a chance, really, I happened to see a catalogue, during the summer, that Duke University was accepting applicants for medical school. So, in July, after my wife had gone to Switzerland, I sent an application in to Wilburt Davidson, the dean, and told him my background and that I wanted to study medicine in order to find out more about the nervous system. And he said, "Come along." And so I was accepted with his letter. Of course that would never happen now.

RL: *You just happened to find a catalogue?*

RA: Yes, I just happened to be in a library, and it was thrown on a library table.

RL: *Were you looking at a shelf of medical school catalogues?*

RA: No, it was the only one I applied to.

RL: *Did you write to Duke before or after your July oral examination for the master's degree?*

RA: After.

RL: *From your account, I have the impression that the dean handpicked the class by himself without a committee.*

RA: That's right. And that was true at Harvard too. Hale, who was dean in charge of admissions, just made the choice himself. He would look at these fellows and, if he liked their looks and the way they responded to questions, he would take them on the spot. It wasn't until later on that a committee was in charge of admissions.

RL: *I also have the impression that you did not have to provide a letter of recommendation or transcripts when you applied to Duke Medical School.*

RA: No. I was not asked to submit letters. Things were very different in that period of time.

RL: *I gather that your plan to pursue a PhD had been serious.*

RA: As a graduate student I had all the course work done for my doctor degree, but I would have had to stay on for three more years on a thesis. Through Robert Seashore's contacts I was offered small scholarships at Iowa and at Brown to complete the PhD. The $300–$400 yearly stipend was not enough to support myself.

RL: *Was Seashore disappointed that you did not continue on to complete the PhD?*

RA: I don't know. He was away for the summer; I left a letter for him on his desk. It was a rather spur of the moment decision.

RL: *Were you ever in touch with him after that?*

RA: No, I don't think so.

The telegram of medical school acceptance was dated September 12, 1933. Less than two weeks later Ray Adams was in Durham, North Carolina.

Notes

1. Seashore RH, Davis RG, Kantor JR. Edmund Smith Conklin 1884–1942. *Science* V97, pp 393–394, 1943.

2. Conklin, Edmund S. *Principles of Abnormal Psychology*. Henry Holt and Company, New York 1927, p 457.

3. Lindsley D. Robert Holmes Seashore 1902–1951. *Am J Psychol* V65, pp 114–116, 1951.

4. Adams RD. *The Importance of "Steadiness" in Marksmanship and Several Other Practical Skills*. A Thesis Presented to the Faculty of the Graduate School of the University of Oregon, June 1933. University of Oregon.

In All the Splendor: The Study of Medicine at Duke University

As the son of a railroad baggage handler, Ray Adams was able to travel free of charge from Portland, Oregon, to North Carolina. He sat up all the way for the three-day train ride to Richmond, Virginia. From there he took a train to a small town in North Carolina. The last leg of his trip to Durham was on a one-car freight train, which had a few seats at one end of a baggage car. He had enough money to pay for one year of medical school tuition, but he had no money for room and board. There are surviving Duke students, who remember him from medical school. "We all deferred to him," said one classmate. Another Duke student remembers him as "outstanding intellectually." "He was so poor," said another contemporary, "that he used to eat peanuts and milk for supper." Puzzled by Adams' poverty, a classmate said, "Where was he from—West Virginia?" His mother preserved the following letter describing his arrival in Durham for medical school. The exhausted Ray Adams wrote in pencil on YMCA stationery. The postmark was September 25, 1933. [see Figure 8]

Dearest Mother:

Well at last I arrived in Durham in all the splendor of the commonest tramp. I had to walk around Richmond from 6 P.M. until 3 A.M. before I could get a train here. Altho it cost $6 we rode until 6 P.M. and after they transferred the only two passengers going towards Durham to an 1890 modelled coach which was hitched on back of a one-horse freight train. The old coach was a shabby model with oil lamps, heating stove, and straight backed seats.

Durham is a nice place altho it smells about like the inside of a tobacco can. It is a town of about 40,000 and is a manufacturing center for cigarettes. The University is as pretty as any I have seen. It consists of the east and west campus which is about 2 miles apart and connected by bus. The grounds are immense and beautifully planned. West campus consists of a huge Gothic Chapel that faces a long half-mile drive bordered by fountains right up to its steps. The Chapel is about 200 ft. long, 100 high inside and about 100 wide and studded with exquisite displays of rose glass etc. From each side of it extends and is connected to it a huge wing each of which are about four city blocks squared altho there are no lots here, just undeveloped, forested country. In the left wing is the library, law school, and medicine. The medical school and hospital are all one and are about the size of the Portland Sanatarium. It has 5 or six floors, modern elevator, and each floor has a different subject on it. For instance the second floor is the center for biochemistry and physiology and all the members of the faculty, which teaches the subject, have their offices on this floor. Each man has a three or four room suite of modernistic offices and research rooms and in order to see even an assistant professor you must have an appointment and be admitted and introduced by his secretary. This laboratory was just built in 1929 as was all the West campus. The other wing is all dormitory and contains everything under one roof from barber shops, post office, to a first national bank.

The East campus is on a hill and is equally as beautiful altho it had so many large building that I lost track of them. The women live here altho only about 500 attend.

It is a peculiar thing that I was the last student admitted this year in medicine. I was no. 60 for which several students were applying.*

As to job, I have walked about 15 miles today—3 times to and from the campus—2 miles each way and my feet feel like they are worn off at the ankles. I haven't been able to get more than about 2 hours sleep a night and none last night so I am kinda tired now.

First I went to the campus Y.M.C.A. and dormitories and was told I didn't have a chance. Then I walked back to town and tried everything from saloons to churches. As a result I had three job offered me. The first

---

*Of the 60 first year students only 44 graduated.

was washing dishes which I couldn't accept because I have classes everyday at 1:30—they lunch at 1 P.M. here. The second was in a butcher shop and he wanted me the worst way but couldn't use me unless I worked Friday afternoon and all day Saturday which I couldn't do. The third is a job with the A.P. chain stores as grocery clerk. It looks very promising. The manager said he'd try and arrange schedule so that I could work from 4–6 everyday and 12–7 Saturday. I'll know in a day or two.

I know I had classes until 5 every day so I went back to school and was introduced to Dr. Heatherington who will be my assistant professor of anatomy and histology. He said I might try it and see how it went. I told him I had some knowledge of psych. and statistics. So he send it to me Dr. Rhine a young comparative psychologist. He thought my psych. and medicine should make a good combination and invited me to attend some evening seminars conducted by himself, Mac Dougall, & Dr. Adams, a young animal & child psychology professor. Also he sent me to see the head nurse who had previously mentioned that she wanted someone to talk to her nursing students on intelligence testing. I haven't seen her yet nor two educational psychologists whom he thot might have some stat. work. He told me to drop in and see him when I felt like it. I almost suggested that I stay and sleep on his big davenport.

A Methodist preacher is going to try & get me a tutoring job & two Italians told me to come back later & I might get on washing dishes. I also applied as part time caretaker for the cemetery but no soap. I am staying at Y.M. tonite but I will move tomorrow because it costs too much. I think I have spotted a place for board & room in an old southern home about 1 mile from school for $30.00 per month. I'll take it if I get the grocery job.

That is the sum total of my first days efforts. Everyone I met was congenial, lazy, and friendly.

Today was about as warm as July in Oregon.

Perhaps you had better take $50.00 more out of bank & sent it to me. I spent $150 tuition today and still have $55.00 left but I'll have to make a down payment on a microscope and can't tell what else might come up.

Your loving son,

Ray

P.S. Send it to me c/o Duke Medical School, Durham, N.C.

Ray Adams could not afford to live in the dormitory with the other medical students. He lived in a janitor's closet under the auditorium. This room and $1 a day were his pay for delivering ice (vide infra). He learned that, across from a knitting mill, a woman made her living by serving a large dish of Brunswick stew for only 10 cents. There Ray Adams often dined with the mill workers for his evening meal. Thus began the medical education of the man, who would return to Duke as awardee in 1969, when Duke initiated a tradition of honoring distinguished medical alumni.

RL: *So you entered Duke Medical School...*

RA: The professor of biochemistry was very upset because I had not had organic chemistry. He wanted me to take a year off and study chemistry after I got to Duke. That was a blow because I didn't have the money to do that. Davidson talked him out of that, gave me a book on organic chemistry that I read during the month of September. I satisfied Perlzweig, the professor of biochemistry, that I knew enough to go on to medical school. I remember reading through the Bodansky book on organic chemistry. I tried to remember all I could. I sat out under a tree and read the blasted thing all day long and was able to squeak through the exam. The amusing part was that, when I took the biochemical part of the national boards, I had one of the highest scores in the country, which showed that the questions didn't really test organic chemistry at all. It was physiology largely. I don't know any organic chemistry now; I never did.

RL: *How long did you study organic chemistry before being examined?*

RA: A couple of weeks.

RL: *Tell me about the dean, Wilburt Davidson.*

RA: I found that he was really a remarkable man. He was a Princeton graduate, Rhodes scholar, later Hopkins, and he was on the faculty at Hopkins for a number of years and later was selected by the Duke family to establish a medical school. And he hired the entire faculty at the medical school, mostly from Hopkins. (Some were very good; there were a few that were quite pedestrian.)

He was a large and rather gruff-man—office always open. And he was a professor of pediatrics, wrote a pediatric manual that was quite popular. He was a real scholar and a very effective organizer; put the hospital staff together; opened the hospital. What he said went.

RL: *At some point along the way you evidently had become a serious student.*

RA: Well, I did well in medical school; I was always well up in the class, from my first month. I was AOA*.

RL: *How old was the medical school when you entered?*

RA: I was in the third class at Duke, and it was a rather rum bunch of students. There was a minister who had decided that he wanted to study medicine. There was a fellow that had periodic paralysis due to hypokalemia, and there was a psychopath, who got arrested for stealing a clock out of the home of the president of the Southern Railway. There were several good students. So the competition was not very great and the teaching was irregular. There were good teachers, inspiring teachers, and mediocre teachers on the clinical side because they had a free hand in engaging in private practice, being seemingly more interested in that than in the students. By and large I got an adequate medical education. I did it in three years by going to summer school.

---

*AOA = Alpha Omega Alpha.

RL: *What exposure to neurology did you get during medical school?*

RA: We had a three-month course in neuroanatomy. I found it appealing.

RL: *Did you ever deviate from your interest in studying the nervous system?*

RA: No, although the medical school teaching of the neurology and psychiatry was mediocre. I was quite interested even when I graduated in 1936* and did internal medicine until 1938. I was much more interested in neurological internal medicine than in general internal medicine. And I came under the influence of Robert Graves, a gifted man. He was bright. (He had taken a PhD in meteorology before entering medicine.) He was given training under Penfield and Kinnier-Wilson and Ramón y Cajal. He came back to Duke in the Department of Neurology. He got me interested in the histology of the nervous system; he was using the Cajal technique to study the cerebellum and tried to teach me some of the methodology. And he taught me how to do a meticulous neurological exam, more complete than I'd ever seen. (He was almost compulsively thorough in his exam and notes.) And I worked up all the cases, that I could, that he was going to see. He'd see cases at night but was teaching neuroanatomy in the daytime. Graves was one of the best clinicians I have ever seen. I learned more clinical neurology during that year than at any other time. He was only an instructor or an assistant professor at the time. Since nobody else in my class was interested in neurology, he was delighted to have me as a student. My clinical teaching was modeled after Graves' method. He had a great influence on me. [see Figure 12]

RL: *Did Graves publish any important findings?*

RA: Yes. He wrote a number of papers on the histology of the cerebellum and the embryology of the cerebellum. He never generated enough drive to follow a program of detailed research. He was a superb analyst of clinical phenomena.

RL: *Did Robert Graves refer you to any neurology book?*

RA: He introduced me to Ramón y Cajal's two volumes on the histology of the nervous system. And I referred to that, when I was trying to learn newer staining techniques for the study of the cerebellum.

RL: *Did you stay in touch with Graves at all?*

RA: Years later, when I was presenting a paper on the protoplasmic astrocyte reactions in liver disease at the Association for Research in Nervous and Mental Disease, he was in the audience. He came up to say hello. By then he had left Duke and gone to Albany as professor of neurology. That was the last I ever saw of him. He died sometime after that. An ignominious end; I think alcohol did him in.

RL: *Can you tell me anything about the racial situation that you encountered when you were at Duke?*

RA: Yes. Of course I was unfamiliar with Southern society. I enjoyed the Negro population as patients. On a colored ward (they always had them segregated) there would always be a choral group singing their old songs. They were delightful patients, always very respectful of the doctors. The white people were not so.

---

*The degree was formally granted in 1937.

And we had a maid looking after my daughter all day long; we paid her $4 a week. She would work for $4 a week if she didn't tote. She would work for $3 if she was permitted to tote, meaning she could take any extra food home at the end of the day. A very warm, friendly, young woman who had two or three children of her own.

RL: *Was the care given to the Negro population equivalent to the care given to the white population?*

RA: Yes, I think so. They were treated very well.

RL: *Was there any prejudice on the medical staff?*

RA: Yes, I think they were looked upon as being a breed unto themselves. I remember seeing one fellow brought in, who was just slashed from head to foot. And I tried to find out who did this, and he said he wouldn't tell me. And I said, "Well you ought to." And he said, "Oh doc, he didn't mean to—he was just mad." So he had no grudge against him. And if one Negro killed another at the time, they might put him in jail for a year or two. They had a different standard of criminality for the Negro than they did for whites.

RL: *Your wife was in Switzerland when you enrolled in medical school.*

RA: When she finished her year in Switzerland, she returned to Durham, North Carolina, and we finally found a one-room apartment, over in Chapel Hill, which cost, I think, $10 a month. And she went to graduate school at the University of North Carolina and did her MA in Romance languages and then became a French teacher in Durham public high school.

RL: *How did you spend summers during medical school?*

RA: I spent two summers with Dr Yoder, a Quaker, at a tuberculosis sanitarium in Winston Salem. I stayed at his house. He and his wife had no children; he showered upon me all of his attention and care. Basically I had free room and board beyond my stipend as a so-called intern. I had an old beaten up Ford. Widely known in the community, he arranged for me to trade that Ford into a used car dealer for a second hand Pontiac.

Yoder was extremely attentive to my inadequacies as a student and did everything he could to teach me to be a doctor. I had excellent training in chest auscultation. I did chest fluoroscopy, having patients turn their head to cough so I could watch the movement of a lesion up and down. If the lesion was healing, the lesion would get smaller over time. Pneumothorax was a common treatment for unilateral tuberculosis. They lined the patients up three or four at a time. The plan was to inject air into the pulmonary cavity. I was taught to do this.

At the end of one summer I gave myself a Mantoux tuberculosis skin test, and my arm virtually sloughed off, a huge ulcer. My lungs were clear on X-ray; there was no treatment.

RL: *Did you stay in touch with Dr Yoder after completion of medical school?*

RA: I lost contact with him after I left Duke. I should have written to him.

RL: *Did you have other jobs during your medical school years?*

RA: From the beginning I had to find work to pay for board and room. I had various jobs in the library and making deliveries.

Later Tom Kinney and I shared a job delivering ice cubes to all the wards in the hospital. I would push the wagon of ice and scoop it out on each ward into the kitchen, from which food was distributed.

RL: *At what time of day did you do this?*

RA: We had to get to the hospital before 6 a.m.

RL: *What happened to Tom Kinney?*

RA: He had narcolepsy. So I took lecture notes for him. He became a pathology resident at Boston City Hospital, pathologist at Peter Bent Brigham, and eventually chairman of pathology at Duke.

RL: *Did all of your jobs allow you to pay the bills?*

RA: I had to borrow for my last year.

RL: *What was your night call schedule when you were a medical intern a Duke?*

RA: We were on every night. We were supposed to have one night a week off, provided the assistant resident would take our call. It was a full-time job. It was in that period of time when you were supposed to take care of your patients 24 hours a day. No one thought much about it. The pay was zero—parking, meals, uniforms, and a room in the hospital were all free.

RL: *Did you see hyperthermia used as a treatment?*

RA: They did have hyperthermia at Duke, and that was used for Syndenham's chorea. My recollection is quite vivid because of the difficulty in keeping the patient's blood pressure and vital functions stable with a temperature around 104 or 105, even up to 106 for 6, 8 hours. They had to be sedated; you had to use very low dose of sedative, phenobarbital, I think it was.

RL: *How would you induce the hyperthermia?*

RA: They were put in a hot box, and the temperature was raised gradually.

RL: *What was the source of the heat?*

RA: It was a lamp I think. It did no good, whatsoever, as far as you could tell.

Ray Adams applied to a single neurology residency, Dr Ayer's program at Massachusetts General Hospital. There survives a letter of recommendation which was submitted to support his application:

Forsyth County Sanatorium for the Treatment of Tuberculosis
R.F.D. No. 1
Winston-Salem, N.C.
Office of the Superintendent
May 1, 1937

Dr. J. B. Ayers
Mass. General Hospital
Boston, Mass.

Dear Dr. Ayers,

I am informed that Dr. R. D. Adams, a graduate of the Duke University Medical School, has applied to you for an appointment at the Massachusetts General.

Dr. Adams worked with us here at the Forsyth County Sanatorium during the summer vacation between his third and fourth years of medicine, and following the completion of his medical course at Duke University was here as Assistant Physician for several months while awaiting his Internship appointment. I have had opportunity, therefore, to study him closely and am delighted to recommend him to you most highly in every way.

He is a most unusual young man, and apparently combines exceptional intelligence with a very high degree of practical common sense. He is sober, industrious, conscientious, dependable, studious, and in fact I do not know of a single point about him that is not most desirable.

I feel that he is destined to go far in his chosen work.

Yours very sincerely,

P.A. Yoder, M.D.
Supt. & Med. Director

RL: *Why didn't you finish your assistant residency in medicine at Duke?*

RA: I was released early for the neurology residency at Mass. General. I did well enough as an internist to impress Hanes, the chairman of the department of medicine that I might be someone that they could recruit for the psychiatry department at Duke in the future.

RL: *I have here a series of letters from Frederick Hanes, recommending you to Ayer.*

RA: He was part of the Hanes family that owned knitting mills and the Wachovia National banks, an extraordinarily rich man, lived in a palace. Somehow or other he took an interest in recommending me for one of the Rockefeller fellowships set up to give training to promising young people. So I had one of them, the only fellowship available that paid a living stipend.

RL: *It was Hanes who arranged this fellowship for you.*

RA: Yes. And he obtained a life insurance policy for me. He thought I ought to have some sort of insurance, when I went off to Mass. General. He paid the premiums for the three years that I was a Rockefeller fellow.

RL: *You had a child by then?*

RA: Yes.

RL: *Were you surprised when he bought this policy for you?*

RA: Indeed.

Neurology Residency: Massachusetts General Hospital

During the first half of the twentieth century, it was the Rockefeller foundation that advanced public health and medical research more than any institution in the world. Its grants nourished medical institutions in China, Europe, Canada, and the United States. In the mid-1930s, Rockefeller fellowships were limited to psychiatry, a field of special interest to Alan Gregg, director of the foundation's Division of Medical Sciences. As alternative sources of support were limited, the awards were highly prized. Through the intervention of Dr Hanes at Duke, Ray Adams was granted a three-year Rockefeller fellowship. It was understood that Adams would return to Duke as a psychiatrist, after he completed the fellowship. Because Adams had already arranged a one-year neurology residency at Massachusetts General Hospital, the Rockefeller Foundation allowed him to spend the first year of his psychiatry fellowship in neurology.

RL: *How did you select the Massachusetts General Hospital for neurology training?*

RA: It was one of the few residencies available, and Boston medicine was already receiving acclaim. I can't recall more than that, except that it seemed a good choice. At any rate, I knew they had a residency there. I had applied for it and received it, even before I had received the Rockefeller fellowship.

RL: *Here is a letter from Dr Ayer dated June 30, 1937, telling you that you had been accepted as a neurology resident at Mass. General.*

RA: Yes this is for August 1938.

RL: *Did you make an easy transition from Duke to MGH?*

RA: It was an interesting period—took a lot of adjustment on my part. The Duke Hospital was new and not as entrenched in its ways as the MGH, where they had wards with sixteen beds around a circle. I hadn't seen such big wards before; I was not accustomed to doing consultations without privacy. They had a little trolley, a wagon on wheels, that they would use to take nonambulatory patients to the bathroom. I had never seen anything like that before.

I was one of two residents on the service under James Ayer, Chief of Neurology.[1] And he was very supportive. The residency had been in existence about six years before I came. In fact, they only had one resident in neurology up until shortly before I came. Ayer, a very wealthy person, paid half my salary out of his pocket; the Rockefeller Foundation paid half the stipend. He was part-time but full professor. And he was an impressive figure, unpretentious and honest. Ayer was not with the residents very much. He visited only one month a year, when he would go around seeing cases for only 1½ hours in the mornings. He had an office, near the medical school, where he spent the afternoons.

There was a neurology ward that Dr James Ayer had set up. (His predecessors, E. Willis Taylor and J.J. Putnam had been consultants without their own ward.) He established the first EEG lab in a general hospital in the country. He also established a laboratory for testing cerebrospinal fluid.

There were other people who visited on the wards. Henry Viets set up the myasthenia gravis clinic. Schwab set up an epilepsy clinic. McDonald, who was a neurologist in Providence, was a kind of sleuth. He delighted in making the diagnosis without the patient speaking. He could tell the patient's handedness by the way the shoes were tied—kind of a Sherlock Holmes. Carner was a famous tennis player—a meticulous, unimaginative neurologist. But they would visit for a month or visit in the outpatient clinic in order to keep a hospital appointment. Nobody on the staff received pay except for Ayer and Kubik. The visiting people were not outstanding at the time except for Viets. They were competent people, uninspiring in any way. I suppose Schwab was the most original of the group.

RL: *Tell me about Ayer?*

RA: During WWI Ayer worked with Weed, who developed much of our information on cerebrospinal fluid (CSF) dynamics and started protein measurement in CSF. Ayer was a clever fellow. He always downplayed his role. He developed the CSF manometer that we use even today. (Houston Merritt persuaded Ayer to give him the data that he had collected on spinal fluid, which was considerable.[2]) Ayer never published much of anything; he'd publish an occasional paper. He was very careful in selecting cases for the weekly Ether Dome conference; the cases would illustrate an anatomical point.

RL: *How did you first meet Charles Kubik?*[3]

RA: Actually I met him the first month I came as a resident in neurology at the Massachusetts General Hospital. He was the visiting neurologist for that month. He was a consultant as well as being head of neuropathology. And I found him really quite exasperating. I remember I was full of energy and ideas and keen on finding solutions to every case. He would come and make rounds, and I would present a case to him. He would examine the patient carefully and stop and think, and he had a curious way of sniffing, and then he would turn and walk off without saying anything. And I was eager to learn and find out something, and he would say, "Well, I'll examine the patient again tomorrow and meantime let's do this and this." Then comes tomorrow...

RL: *So you would bring him back the second time and all he would do is sniff and walk off again?*

RA: Yes, and after about a week or so of this, I was quite irritated, and he said, "Well, I think we'll find out in a month or two what this disease is. I don't know now." And he thought that just by studying and following a case, you would eventually get the solution. You'd find out what the course of this disease was. That was an approach that was quite novel to a young physician from where I'd come.

And I found out later that, if you would stop him in the corridor and ask a question about sciatica, it would probably be worth about 30 minutes of your time, for him to question you and ask exactly what you wanted to know and for you to listen to his experience with that sort of thing. And I came to have an enormous respect for him as one of the more astute minds in neurology at the time. He was certainly not a spectacular person. The same way with neuropathology; he would get a tumor that he couldn't classify and he kept setting it aside and going back to look at it again. He drove the pathology department mad by the fact that he had so many cases, that he wouldn't sign out, because he couldn't make a diagnosis.

RL: *You seem to have had more access to Kubik than the other neurologists.*

RA: Charles Kubik was there full time. Whenever I had a problem I would go over to his lab in another building on Allen Street and tell him about the case. He would always have some wise suggestion.

RL: *What was his approach to the study of a brain?*

RA: Very, very careful. Yes, and he would sometimes go back and re-cut the material; he did a lot of this. When he first went to the Mass. General Hospital, he did all the Nissl stains and Cajal stains and microtome work himself at night. He had no technician. He was an excellent technician, and he was superb at dissection. He would open a cranium and, if necessary, take out a brain with the entire dura intact, without a nick in it. He kept careful notes on his findings.

RL: *Did Kubik write much?*

RA: Kubik had ideas about everything from his own experience in pathology, but he never wrote papers. However, he wrote with admirable clarity. From him I learned about careful observation, precise description and the separation of fact from artifact.

RL: *What was his background?*

RA: American of Czechoslovakian descent. Trained in neuropathology by Greenfield— he was Greenfield's first fellow—and in neurology at the National Hospital. Kubik was critical of Greenfield as being loose in his concepts. He came to work with Southard at the Boston Psychopathic Hospital. Ayer met him and hired him as neuropathologist for Mass. General in 1926.

RL: *Tell me more about the residency experience.*

RA: We didn't have much supervision because none of the senior neurologists would be around in the afternoon or night or weekend. Rarely we would call Dr Ayer. We were quite independent, in a way, and we made decisions that we probably were not prepared to make. More senior people were available to help at Duke. There was no one like that at Mass. General, which was a little frightening at first. We were on alternate nights; we were on every other weekend. We had a bed between us.

RL: *What kind of cases did you see at MGH?*

RA: I tried to keep track of what I had seen. I made cards on all of the interesting cases. I learned a lot on my own. We would go to the emergency room; I saw some interesting things at odd times during the residency. I saw several cases of tetanus, and a couple of them I remember being fatal.

RL: *How did you treat tetanus?*

RA: Well, we gave them antitoxin and respiratory support.

RL: *Did you give sedation?*

RA: Yes, certainly to a variable extent. I got into a rather amusing incident. When I was a resident, the first case of tetanus I saw at the Mass. General was during the early hours, two or three in the morning. I asked that the patient be given chloroform to suppress the spasms, and within an hour the professor of anesthesiology and the professor of neurology and several of the staff members were in there, wildly excited; chloroform had never been used at the Mass. General and it never would be! I was naïve enough to point out that down south they used chloroform. Chloroform had been effective in Alabama and was recommended in the South.

RL: *Why were they reluctant to use it?*

RA: Because ether was the thing to use. Ether was the Mass. General anesthetic; at MGH ether had replaced chloroform. The ether dome was where we had our conferences, and they thought it was a travesty to even think of using chloroform. The patient was given ether to quiet the spasms, but the patient died anyhow. We never did use the chloroform.

RL: *When you were a resident at Mass. General Hospital, were there female medical students?*

RA: No.

RL: *What else can you tell me about your year of neurology residency?*

RA: We were issued a lumbar puncture needle with a whetstone. We were to keep the needle sharpened and sterile. If a needle were lost or broken, one had to go to Baker, assistant superintendent of the hospital, in an obsequious manner. The food was terrible. There was mumbling continually. The superintendent, Washburn, told us that if we didn't like it, we could get out—it was easier to hire residents than cooks. We accepted these inconveniences as part of the residency.

Notes

1. Denny-Brown D, Viets H, Adams R, et al. James Bourne Ayer, MD 1882–1963. *Arch Neurol, Chicago* V11, pp 449–451, 1964.
2. Merritt HH, Fremont-Smith F. *The Cerebrospinal Fluid.* W.B. Saunders, Philadelphia, 1938.
3. Richardson Jr, EP, Astrom KE, Kleihus P. The Development of Neuropathology at the Massachusetts General Hospital and Harvard Medical School. *Brain Pathol* V4, pp 181–195, 1994.

A letter from Ray Adams' wife, Elinor, to Ray Adams' mother:

Dr. Ayer told Ray that the last group of students Ray has been teaching at the hospital were so enthusiastic about Ray that they came to Ayer and asked if he couldn't arrange it for Ray to spend more time with them. Ayer says this proves Ray's ability as a teacher for it is rare to find anyone who can correlate neurology, chemistry, pathology and anatomy as well as Ray does. Ayer seemed *very* pleased. He was the next person to work with these students and said he had never found a group who knew so much and knew how to go about things so well—that they were trained better than any he had ever seen there. Isn't that splendid? I guess Hanes will be getting a better teacher than he realizes.

Psychiatry Fellowship: Massachusetts General Hospital

Having finished a year in neurology training, Ray Adams remained at Massachusetts General, in Stanley Cobb's department of psychiatry. Alan Gregg of the Rockefeller Foundation had supported the neurology research unit of Stanley Cobb,[1-2] at Boston City Hospital. With continued Rockefeller funding, Cobb had left the field of neurology and taken his Bullard Professorship of Neuropathology (a Harvard appointment) to Massachusetts General Hospital. There he developed the psychiatry department, where Ray Adams spent the second year of his Rockefeller Fellowship.

RL: *Tell me about your year in the psychiatry department at Massachusetts General Hospital.*

RA: I was a supernumerary. I didn't have any particular assignment. Research activity was virtually nil. I was permitted to share a room with a medical student and Jurgen Reousch, a Swiss psychiatrist. I became quite friendly with both of them. Reousch was indoctrinated in the Bleuler method of psychiatry and in Jungian and Adlerian principles. He was very astute and taught me classic psychiatry. He taught me how to do a Rohrschach Test, which was much in vogue in Switzerland at the time. That and thematic apperception were two tests being used to explore the subconscious. He later went to the University of California and became the chairman.

　　I attended weekly staff conference and heard the views of the psychiatrists; five or six of them were psychoanalysts. They would present a case. Cobb would talk to the patient briefly; then the patient would be taken away. Cobb would present his viewpoint. Various explanations were discussed. The medical and neurologic side were neglected. I didn't find the conferences particularly informative. Mandel Cohen, Cobb's assistant, tried to introduce nonpsychoanalytic views, but he was not given much of an audience.

　　One patient caused great excitement. There was a psychological problem and there was pain in the flank. The psychoanalysts were fascinated because the flank pain occurred in the same week that the patient's wife had gone into labor—the pain had been synchronized in some way, in his subconscious, with his wife's suffering— the pain had been transferred. Mandel Cohen, after 2 hours of discussion, stood up and asked, "Why don't you get an X-ray to see if there is kidney stone?" They ignored him. A day or two after that, the resident called the urologist. There was a stone and they removed it.

RL: *Can you comment further on psychoanalysis?*

RA: Well, I think that most of what they said with reference to the sexual drive, being a major determinant of human behavior and mental illness, has never been verified.

RL: *It's just an idea.*

RA: It's just an idea, yes. And that was why I was inclined to reject it from the time I was on Cobb's service.

RL: *Did you have clinical responsibilities as a psychiatry fellow?*

RA: There were times when I went with a resident when he did consultations. I did try to fulfill my obligation to psychiatry by attending the clinic once a week for 1 or 2 hours with Erich Lindemann. He was bright and alert, but I was discouraged. I would tell him what the patient had said, and he would tell me what the patient would say next week, on the basis of analytical theory. It was a one-sided exposure—no psychotic patients. One of the patients, I had seen two or three times, committed suicide. I lost my faith in myself as a psychiatrist and in Lindemann as a supervisor. He found me critical and resistant and probably lost interest in me as a potential scholar.

So I took the easy route. I just continued my interest in the neurology service and did what I thought was enough psychiatry to satisfy the purpose of my fellowship. The thing that saved the year for me was my being able to go to the ether dome neurology conferences and to do neuropathology with Charles Kubik. I spent half of my time in neuropathology with Kubik. He was my most influential pathology teacher. Also, I was instructing medical students. I was not terribly busy. I had time to read neuropathology and neurology.

RL: *Did you work on a specific project with Kubik during that year?*

RA: We started the work on subdural empyema.

RL: *How did this project get started?*

RA: I was in Kubiks' lab every day. I realized that we were able to make the diagnosis from the clinical records although the clinicians had not. I started putting these cases together. Kubik never took the trouble to put together, in writing, material like this.

RL: *You mentioned Cobb's assistant, Mandel Cohen.*

RA: I became very friendly with Mandel Cohen.[3,4] He taught the neurology residents the essentials of psychiatry, enough so that, when I took my boards in neurology, I had done so well on the psychiatry part of it that they just put me down for that too. He was opposed to the analytic interpretations and to some of the wild speculation about the genesis of psychosomatic diseases.

Cobb had taken Cohen on as a research fellow on anxiety states and neurocirculatory asthenia. That work went very well, largely through Mandel's insistence that strict methods of science be applied. Mandel wrote some very good papers with Paul Dudley White and Stanley Cobb on anxiety states and showed with Ruggles Gates that it was a Mendelian dominant. That work was the first indication that anxiety states had a biological basis; it is lost sight of. He also made the observation that lactic acid was elevated in the serum of patients with neurocirculatory asthenia. He was a hard-headed scientist. He was interested in whether anxiety could be regarded the equivalent of fear. I remember he would bring patients into the laboratory and unexpectedly fire a gun under the laboratory bench to try to compare their response with their anxiety. (Some psychoanalysts had claimed that fear and anxiety were the same.)

RL: *Did he draw a conclusion?*

RA: He thought they were different. He thought you could do research in psychiatry that would measure up to the best standards in medicine. So he was an influence on many of us there. The relationship of Cobb and Cohen began to fall apart, when Mandel was critical of Cobb's departure from physiology, at which he excelled, and his adoption of a psychoanalytic approach. Cohen worked up Cobb's admissions to the private service, and it was about such cases that differences in interpretation frequently arose. Cobb just couldn't stand the criticism, and, after a few years, he had little to do with Mandel Cohen. Mandel knew the field of psychiatry as well as anyone I've ever known. [see Figure 14]

RL: *Did the term psychosomatic medicine exist before there was the idea of psychoanalysis?*

RA: No. It came after. I think Cobb and a woman by the name of Dunbar[5] were the two figures that had most to do with the concept. They got the idea that one's psychological status would influence either the cause or the perpetuation of those diseases, such as migraine and hayfever, that had no pathology or where the pathology was known but the cause was not. Of course, the leading example was peptic ulcer. There was a famous case, where the stomach was exposed. They found that, if the person got upset, there was an increase in acid formation from his stomach. An elaboration of that idea into other diseases of unknown cause, like hypertension, was the basis of the whole concept of psychosomatic disease, which Cobb made the focus of his laboratory at Mass. General. Since he had a number of collaborators that were analysts, it was no large step to bring them into the realm of psychosomatic disease. They had concocted theories about how certain experiences could foster the development of these diseases. Cobb was appointing young people as fellows, who would work with him on ulcers, colitis, mucous colitis and things of that sort. They did find out that these patients did not have any of the conventional psychiatric illnesses, such as anxiety states or depression.

They persuaded a number of the internists that they had a lead to the major diseases in their division. And quite a number underwent psychoanalysis. There was a swing very strongly toward psychoanalysis during that period. For example, Chester Jones, head of gastrointestinal medicine, was quite persuaded that mucous colitis was due to tension or nervousness. So, if you couldn't understand why someone had a GI disorder, he would call it psychosomatic, offer psychological treatment. I think that it wasn't too long before these internists, who were quite sensible people, realized that nothing was happening to the patients, when they were treated psychologically. So they went back to their old practices. This swing to psychoanalysis really represented a phase in the development of medicine in Boston.

RL: *Did all students of psychosomatic disease have a psychoanalytic approach?*

RA: There was a strong overlap. There were exceptions like Harold Woolf, in New York, who, I think, was never much influenced by psychoanalysis.

RL: *Tell me about Stanley Cobb.*

RA: Stanley Cobb was a real charmer. I admired him as a person. He was a gentleman with a wide range of interests. He was an excellent physiologist, and he was an ornithologist. He had his way of saying things, with a stutter that everyone liked. He would accept anything, that was not understood, as psychogenic in cause. I had a patient with torticollis and another with spastic dysphonia, and he was certain that each could be cured by psychoanalysis, by looking at his early life. This was a psychiatric approach that was unscientific and speculative.

RL: *Was Cobb properly considered a neuropsychiatrist?*

RA: Yes. Cobb was that, really, because he had been trained in physiology. He then spent a year with Adolph Meyer, then became Bullard professor of Neuropathology and then spent two years in England and Europe under Kinnier-Wilson and Walter Spielmeyer in Munich. But he never really mastered neuropathology. He was a bit of a dilettante in that respect but with a broad orientation. His weakness was that he let psychoanalysis dominate his department. You really couldn't see a consultation without having an analyst come along to see it. "The asthmatic had fallen into a cesspool when he was a baby" or something like that. It all got to be rather ridiculous.

RL: *Didn't psychoanalysis dominate much of American psychiatry at the time?*

RA: Cobb was strongly favoring psychoanalytic training for his residents. Years later it became apparent that all of them were just drifting into private practice. Frank Fremont Smith decided that they should bring together at Ithaca, New York the leaders in psychiatry and ask them why there were no young faculty members in psychiatry. The reason was that they were being psychoanalyzed; they had invested so much money and time and thought in that field that they thought it best to practice psychoanalysis, and there was no way to do that and be a faculty member at the same time. I mention this because, when Cobb retired in 1954, I went over to his office on his last day. He said that he was fed up with young psychoanalysts. He was disappointed in the generation of young psychiatrists he had trained. They had not done research, and he had been research oriented throughout his life. I asked, if he were going into medicine today and was interested in psychiatry, what he would study. He thought for a while and said that he would prepare himself by studying endocrinology. (Steroid psychosis had excited great interest on the part of Stanley Cobb.) I thought it was rather interesting, coming from a man who lived in supporting psychoanalysis during most of his late professional life.

Finesinger[6] was his leading associate. He had been psychoanalyzed by Freud. He was enough of a scientist to recognize that it was not a promising field. He discouraged me from undergoing psychoanalysis. I visited Finesinger, after he had moved to the University of Maryland. He was president of the American

Psychoanalytical Association. He thought that psychoanalysis was a dead end. He was very discouraged about it. When he circulated a questionnaire to psychoanalysts, asking how many patients they had treated with different psychiatric illnesses and the results of treatment, he got little data in the responses.

RL: *You mentioned that Cobb suffered with stuttering.*[7]

RA: He still stuttered despite two psychoanalyses. He was able to speak slowly and cover it up, but even at the age of sixty he still stuttered. Most mild stutterers tend to lose their stutter with further maturation of the brain. There are very few that are greatly handicapped by it in adult life.

RL: *You mentioned that he was ambidextrous . . .*

RA: Yes. He was very artistic. He both wrote well and drew well. He could simultaneously draw with both hands. And the students marveled at his drawings on the black board.

RL: *Is there any possibility that the ambidexterity and the stuttering were related?*

RA: Oh, they seem to be. Stutterers are often left handed and ambidextrous; these relations are widely accepted.

RL: *What else can you say about Cobb?*

RA: Fine human being, open minded. I think his downfall really was that he committed himself so fully to the analytic approach to mental illness and to psychosomatic disease. I always felt contrite about my failure to have a warmer, more understanding relationship to him; but I only knew him at a time, when he had departed from neurology so completely.

RL: *Who were some of his successful neurology residents?*

RA: Houston Merritt, Charles Aring, Harold Woolf.

RL: *Somebody wrote a biography of Cobb.*

RA: I think his name was White.[8] He never mentioned neurology in the book except that there was a fellow by the name of Ray Adams, who was hostile to psychiatry, which was not true at all. I was just hostile to this wild kind of speculation.

RL: *At that time were there any methods of treatment used for schizophrenia?*

RA: Nothing I remember for schizophrenia. Kurt Lindemann, who had come from Iowa, had started to use sodium amytal. I believe that was the first chemotherapy for depression. Dexedrine and sodium amytal, were the standard treatment for depression at MGH for many years. It definitely was beneficial.

RL: *Is there anything else you can say about this year?*

RA: It was during that year that I started going out regularly at night to Paul Yakovlev's[9] neuroanatomical discussions at Fernald School. He would, one night a week, for two or three months, put on a display. He had whole brains in serial sections. He would display sections of thalamus, discussing thalamic connections. On another week he would concentrate his discussion on another part. He would start at 9 p.m. and would go on until 3 or 4 a.m., if you would stay. He was a night owl; time meant nothing to him. He would go into great detail. He was a fine influence for all of us. He was a wonderful lecturer, with his curious dialect, a delightful companion. We became very good friends.

He always had a lot to say about Russian, French, Swiss and German neuroanatomy. He was colorful and very amusing. An eccentric personality, at the age of sixty to seventy, he took up motorcycle driving for locomotion. And was a hopeless driver of an automobile, always gesturing and not watching where he was going. He was not a histopathologist in the strict sense of the word. He was an anatomist who liked to see things on a global scale.

He had his own ideas, about how the nervous system was organized into three spheres. He felt that the inner third of the whole neuraxis was devoted to automatic reflex affairs. The outer layers were involved in learned activities and cognitive functions, and so on. And the intermediate third serving as connections between the two. It was an interesting theory that had some truth in it, just another way of looking at the nervous system.

RL: *It sounds like this year of "psychiatry" fellowship turned out to be a good educational year.*

RA: Yes, I had an instructive year, but it covered a lot of things that were not psychiatry. It was a rather mixed up year.

RL: *Perhaps you were already thinking that you shouldn't go into psychiatry.*

RA: I probably was. I was so much more attracted to neurology.

Notes

1. Adams RD. Stanley Cobb 1887–1968. *Trans Am Neurol Assoc.* V82, pp 28–31, 1969.

2. Adams RD, Binger CA, Castle WB, et al. Stanley Cobb (1887–1968). *J Neurol Sci* V10, pp 197–199, 1970.

3. Healy D. Mandel Cohen and the Origins of the Diagnostic and Statistical Manual of Mental Disorders, Third Edition: DSM III. *Hist Psychiatry* V13, pp 209–230, 2002.

4. Cohen AH. In Memoriam—Mandel E. Cohen, MD (March 8, 1907–March 19, 2000). *Ann Clin Psych* V15, pp 149–159, 2003.

5. Dunbar F. *Emotions and Bodily Changes* (3rd ed.). Columbia University Press, New York, 1946, 604 pp.

6. Cobb S. Jacob Ellis Finesinger 1902–1959. *J Nerv Ment Dis* V129, pp 115–116, 1959.

7. Cobb S, Cole E. Stuttering. *Physiol Rev* V19, pp 14–62, 1939.

8. White B. *Stanley Cobb a Builder of Modern Neurosciences.* The Francis A Countway Library of Medicine, Boston, 1984.

9. Kemper T. Paul Ivan Yakovlev. *Arch Neurol* V41, pp 536–540, 1984.

Psychiatry Fellowship: A Year with Eugen Kahn at Yale

Year three of the Rockefeller Foundation fellowship was to be spent in psychiatry. Whereas American psychiatry had come under the sway of psychoanalysis, European psychiatry had not. At Massachusetts General Hospital, Ray Adams had seen that psychoanalysis and related ideas about psychosomatic medicine dominated psychiatric thinking. His third fellowship year offered the potential for a different exposure. The hope was that he would work under Adolf Meyer, the Swiss neurologist who chaired the psychiatry department at Johns

Hopkins. His application to Meyer ended with a failed interview. Instead he went to work with the German neurologist–psychiatrist at Yale. Other departments at Yale offered special opportunities for enrichment. Most important were his experiences with Arnold Gesell of the Institute for Human Relations and his attendance at the neurophysiology department of John Fulton.

RL: *You were to spend a third year of fellowship with the famous psychiatrist, Adolf Meyer, before you were to join the faculty at Duke.*

RA: Lambert, who was supervising the fellowship for the Rockefeller Foundation, urged that I go to Johns Hopkins. I didn't know anything about Hopkins. So I went down and was interviewed. Dr Richards had just been appointed Chairman of Psychiatry at Duke, and he was interested that I spend a year with Meyer at Hopkins before my return to Duke. Richards took me into Adolf Meyer's office for an interview, which was a disaster. Meyer quizzed me fiercely and trapped me in all kinds of ways, partly my fault. I found myself deficient in the things he was interested in. He would ask me what books I'd read in psychiatry, when I was with Stanley Cobb, and I would reply. He'd ask me to describe a case I'd seen. He would make me define every word I'd use and explain the origins of each term and its connotations. I did not distinguish myself. And, after about an hour of this, he discharged me. And he sent his male secretary out afterwards: if I wanted to come to Hopkins, I could read in their library. Richards was mad as hops.

RL: *On that trip to Hopkins, did you see Frank Ford, the pediatric neurologist?*

RA: I'm not sure I ever met Ford. I have great respect for Ford, and I used his book regularly. I had probably the first edition—outstanding.[1] But he was mostly writing about children. (He was not highly regarded in the echelon of physicians at Hopkins. I don't know why. He was sort of outclassed by Adolf Meyer, who was a very important figure, and by Dandy). American neurologists in general had a favorable opinion on Ford.

RL: *Speaking of Walter Dandy,[2] did you see the famous Hopkins neurosurgeon, while you were at Johns Hopkins?*

RA: I went to watch Walter Dandy operate. There were two things that stood out. One was how disagreeable he was. He cursed everyone, nurses, residents; "Get the hell out of my way, you god damned fools." He would make them go over and stand in the corner some place. He was part of that whole generation of neurosurgeons, who were ill mannered. If it was a brain tumor, he'd stick his finger in and ream it out. My God! I had never seen such rough handling of the brain. He was the outstanding neurosurgeon at Hopkins. A good many of his residents were famous.

RL: *On this trip to Baltimore, Meyer rejected you, in effect.*

RA: Richards was very upset. And Lambert was as mad as could be; he called on the spur of the moment to Eugen Kahn at Yale and asked if he would take me on as a fellow. Kahn accepted me at once. That's how I happened to go to Yale.

RL: *Tell me about your year at Yale.*

RA: It turned out to be an extremely valuable year. My exposure to psychiatry at Massachusetts General Hospital was so much dominated by psychoanalysis that it wasn't very valuable. At New Haven, I came under the influence of Eugen Kahn,[3] who was a pupil of Kraeplin. [see Figure 15]

RL: *Was Kahn your supervisor?*

RA: I was assigned to his department. He had me work up his private outpatients and admissions, and he would go over each of them with me. And he also would speak to me regularly about a few of the cases that I had been assigned to take care of.

It was a wonderful association that I had with Kahn because he knew so much neurology and psychiatry. He was a superb teacher, a conventional psychiatrist, gave wonderful, very well-organized conferences. And some of his associates, who did all the consultative work, were very helpful. They had no neurology service there. Occasionally we would see a neurological case.

RL: *Would he bring the patient in to the conference?*

RA: Yes, and he would demonstrate cases with admirable skill. He would talk to the patients and draw out their main psychiatric symptoms, really superb. He was one of the best functioning psychiatrists that I'd ever seen.

RL: *What was Kahn's approach to psychiatric diagnosis?*

RA: He would just look for the symptoms of delusions, hallucinations and altered thinking and mood change.

RL: *So it was very much a medical approach?*

RA: Conventional psychiatry.

RL: *What was Kahn's original work?*

RA: Well he had a rather elaborate view of constitutional types.[4] He thought that a lot of the temperaments of humans were genetically ingrained; he referred to these as psychopathies. (The terminology never caught on.)

For example, one of his types was the "asthenic psychopath," who, all his life, was delicate, vulnerable to disease, physically inept, lacking in energy, lacking in drive, unable to compete in society; any of life's problems were liable to floor him. Psychologists, Kagan and Birch of a later generation, referred to this as timidity. These are very sound ideas. Kahn's concepts survive with neuropsychologists. The group down at Einstein has shown that you can separate babies on the basis of one or another of these traits, like activity level, and they're the same at six months as they're at five years. Kagan at Harvard finds that timidity, as a trait, persists from six months on. Although Kagan probably doesn't realize it, this corresponds to Kahn's "asthenia." There are other such traits being identified. With Kahn's work being in German and his terminology being weird, he is not remembered.

RL: *Kahn's idea, that personality traits can be inborn, is consistent with my personal experience.*

RA: Yes, and mine too. So that was, I suppose, his main contribution. By and large he felt that a lot of human behavior was ingrained and the part of the psychiatrist would be to seek out these traits and to help the individuals and their families to cope with them, to make allowance for the asthenic person or the timid person. You wouldn't change it but you could help them contend with it.

RL: *Less ambitious but more realistic.*

RA: Yes. I learned from Kahn that you have to recognize the patient's personality traits and treat the patient appropriately. Good doctors recognize the peculiarities of people and know that one has to be managed differently from another. Good doctors recognize this and work around it all the time without phrasing it in such terms, and Kahn was surrounded by people like that. I got instruction from Katherine Miles, a psychometrist; she taught me how to do standard psychological testing. I went to the laboratory of Evelyn Mann, a biochemist who studied the blood of manic-depressive patients. Ed Gildea was Kahn's first assistant, a jolly general psychiatrist; we would talk about his views of psychoses. I would go on rounds with Fred Pugh, a Kahn type psychiatrist. I got a much better view of conventional psychiatry. Kahn was really what you would call an organic psychiatrist.

RL: *And I gather that he was the biggest influence on you during that year.*

RA: Oh yes, by far. He had enormous experience. I remember a case of a student, gone beserk, ran naked up and down the campus, set fire. At conference they would all decide the disease was a major psychosis. But Kahn would conclude that he wasn't sure what it was, and that, based on what he had seen with other students, that boy would be back in school next year. (It was probably hypomania.) The implication was that, in order to decide what the condition was, you had to see the subsequent course. He was very shrewd. He knew what he knew.

RL: *Did you get exposure to other departments at Yale?*

RA: I was urged by Kahn to attend meetings of the staff of the Institute of Human Relations, a group of scholars, brought together, who were supposed to be renowned in their fields of psychology and social science: Bruno Malinowsky, Robert Yerkes, Arnold Gesell, John Dollard, Walter Miles, Clark Hull (head of the institute)...

It was quite an illustrious group of thinkers, but they were all older, had their set ways of thinking. They didn't cooperate. So the institute was not a great success.

RL: *How did this exposure benefit you?*

RA: I used to go to Gesell's lectures; he was superb.[5] I was most impressed with his developmental testing of normal children. He tried to work out ways of testing babies of different ages, pincer grasp, hand grasp. These tests are now a standard part of child neurology. He tried to document everything he said. A good observer, he wrote well.[6] As an aside, pediatrics at Yale was taken over by a pediatrician who had been trained in psychoanalysis. He turned on Gesell and attacked him viciously on the basis that his material was biased and unreliable, that his studies were on the children of faculty members, and that any conclusions that could be drawn from faculty children would be biased. The whole thing should be rejected. And he refused to let his pediatric staff to have anything to do with Gesell. Strangely pernicious influence of psychoanalysis during that period.

RL: *What else can you tell me about the Institute?*

RA: Kahn thought the whole business of psychoanalysis was fraudulent. Dollard and another sociologist at the institute were analysts. They thought that Kahn was an antiquated Kraeplinian. They criticized everything he did, as based on a bunch of flimsy premises, unreliable data. That led me, even when I was at the fellowship stage, to reject psychoanalysis as a legitimate field of endeavor.

RL: *What else did you do at Yale?*

RA: I went frequently to the magnificent department of neurophysiology. John Fulton had used generous support from Yale and his wife's fortune to enlarge his neurophysiology department into one of the leading laboratories in the world. Fulton was near retirement and had a problem with alcohol. Warren McCulloch and others gave regular meetings, which I enjoyed. McCulloch was later professor of neurophysiology at M.I.T.[7]

RL: *Comment on Fulton's neurophysiology textbook.*[8]

RA: A masterpiece. I memorized it practically because it was such an instructive reference.

RL: *What methods of psychiatric therapy did you encounter at Yale?*

RA: I think they just talked to patients, kept them more or less confined to the hospital for a time. For depression, at the time, they were still using protracted immersion in a tub of cold water. It was used to calm a patient with mania or mixed manic-depressive states.

RL: *Did you keep in touch with Kahn after you left Yale?*

RA: I sent a number of neurology residents to work with Kahn. I suggested Fritz Redlich.[9] Kahn turned Redlich down because he was a Jew. I said I never thought about whether he was or he wasn't. I asked Redlich whether he was Jew, and he said he wasn't. So Kahn took him!

RL: *I thought Kahn was Jewish.*

RA: He was. Kahn was being criticized by Dollard and others in the institute as being a Jew, bringing in a bunch of Jewish psychiatrists.

In those days there was in academic medicine an undercurrent of anti-Semitism. At Harvard Medical School there was a quota of 15% in the 1920s and 1930s. Dean Burwell was pushing a bill in the Massachusetts House of Representatives to eliminate the quota. The only Jewish professor he could find at Harvard was at Beth Israel Hospital!

RL: *Do you think you lost anything by taking the fellowship with Kahn at Yale rather than studying psychiatry with Meyer at Hopkins?*

RA: I think I was for better off having gone to New Haven. Meyer subscribed to the idea that early childhood experience could influence the development of an individual. This view was an acceptance of Freud's idea about early life experience, though Meyer rejected the sexual emphasis of the Freudians.

Kahn's perception of personality and character and psychogenesis of psychiatric illness was more consistent with modern concepts and more appropriate to the neurologist's scheme of brain disease. He was a neurologist, in a sense, himself. He would do a neurologic exam. He had a series of Alzheimer cases that he biopsied; he was interested in disease of the nervous system. Kahn was very influential in my career and steered me strongly away from psychiatry, even though I qualified in the field. He thought the future of psychiatry was not in psychiatry, as it was being promoted and practiced in the U.S. And his antagonism toward psychoanalysis, I think, must have influenced me or reinforced my own skepticism.

RL: *Do you remember any patients you saw with Kahn?*

RA: I remember blunders that I made, looking after patients. I had one patient who was a professor from Smith College. She came in because of "psychogenic diar-rhea." Being from a more medical background, I felt, well my goodness, I'd better get some bowel function tests on her, and Kahn said, "No, no . . . don't do that. She's been worked up at Massachusetts General Hospital, where Chester Jones, head of gastroenterology, had concluded that she's psychogenic." Well, it turned out that Chester Jones had been psychoanalyzed by someone or had been influenced by them. She had been with him for a few weeks at the Mass. General, and they could find nothing wrong with her. They decided that it was mucous colitis and all psychogenic. Her diarrhea worsened, and someone at Yale got a stool examination—full of fat. She had sprue, steatorrhea from malabsorption. We put her on a banana diet at home, and she was cured. And I was mortified that I had been treating her psychiatrically.

We let her illness slip through our fingers. And Chester Jones, whom I came to know later, when I went back to the Mass. General, was taken in worse than anyone because he had her in for study and didn't catch on. This was just at the time that psychoanalysis was going full force at the Mass. General. Also, at Beth Israel Hospital, psychoanalysis was blithely accepted.

RL: *Do you remember any other experience with Kahn?*

RA: I remember an obnoxious young patient, who kicked me in the rump, as I was leaving her room. Kahn laughed. He said, "You're never a full fledged psychiatrist until you've been kicked a few times. Never turn your back on a hypomaniac."

Notes

1. Ford, Frank R. *Diseases of the Nervous System in Infancy, Childhood and Adolescence.* Charles C. Thomas, Springfield, IL/Baltimore, 1937.

2. Horwitz, N. Walter E. Dandy 1886–1946. *Neurosurgery* V40, pp 642–646, 1997.

3. Pokorny, AD. In Memoriam. Eugene Kahn 1887–1973. *Am J Psychiatry* V130, pp 7, 822, July 1973.

4. Kahn, Eugen. *Psychopathic Personalities.* Yale University Press, New Haven, 1931, 521 p.

5. Obituary Arnold L. Gesell. *Br Med J* V1(5240), p 1689, June 10, 1961.

6. Gesell A, Amatruda CS. *Developmental Diagnosis: Normal and Abnormal Child Development, 2nd ed.* Hoeber-Harper, New York, 1954.

7. Perkel, DH. Logical Neurons: The Enigmatic Legacy of Warren McCulloch. *Trends Neurosci* V11, No.1, pp 9–12, 1988.

8. Fulton, John F. *Physiology of the Nervous System*. Oxford University Press, New York, 1938.

9. Lavietes S. Dr Frederick C. Redlich, 93, Biographer of Hitler. *The New York Times*, November 6, 2007.

Boston City Hospital: 1941–1951

After his third year of Rockefeller fellowship at Yale, Ray Adams was scheduled to join the psychiatry department at Duke. This prospect did not appeal to him because he was more attracted to neurology and neuropathology than to psychiatry. Thus, when Adams received an invitation from Houston Merritt to join him in the neurological research unit at Boston City Hospital, he accepted promptly. He requested the approval of Frederick Hanes, who released him from his obligation to Duke. At the chaotic Boston City Hospital he would work not only with Merritt but also with Derek Denny-Brown.

RL: *Tell me about Boston City Hospital.*

RA: It was huge, about 1,800 beds more or less; many buildings, poorly managed, dirty. Workers were lazy and disrespectful; you came to tolerate that and to make special arrangements to get anything done. Many were drunk a good part of the time. The autopsy rooms were filthy and contaminated. The amount of food stolen was unbelievable. Some residents fed their families on stolen food. I don't suppose you'd find a more corrupt hospital. It was run by Irish politicians. The budget was twice what was spent on the hospital, and no one knew where the rest of the money went. The mayor, Curley,[1] finally was arrested, after he had become a congressman, and he spent part of his term in jail. We all put up with it because we were free to do what we wanted.

The sixty patients on our neurological unit had very good care. We could admit them for as long as we wanted. It was ideal. If you wanted to study someone for three months, you could. We were consultants to the rest of the hospital. The clinical material was vast; in one month we saw 300 head injury cases in consultation. One third of all medical admissions were alcoholic. So, nutritional and metabolic diseases were abundant. Everything could be found there.

RL: *When you accepted Merritt's offer, I gather that you envisioned coming to work as a clinical neurologist and teacher at Boston City Hospital.* [see Figure 19]

RA: That's right.

RL: *Not long after you came to Boston City Hospital you found that you would have to take a position in pathology instead of the clinical job you had expected.*

RA: That happened in a rather strange fashion because Derek Denny-Brown of London and Oxford had been chosen as chairman of the department of neurology at Boston City Hospital in the summer of 1939. But he was an officer in the British army and could not be released, since England had gone to war against Germany in September. Therefore, Merritt was alone at the Boston City Hospital and needed help. My invitation was the consequence of that situation. I came to the City Hospital on July 1, 1941.

However, President Conant of Harvard University made some arrangement with the Churchillian government to suddenly release Denny-Brown in October of that year. Denny, as we called him, came to Boston City Hospital in either October or November. There was a salary for two people—that would be for Houston Merritt and Denny-Brown, and my salary was taken away within six months. They then decided that, in order to keep me on the staff, they would send me over to the Mallory Institute of Pathology, where I could do the neuropathology for the hospital. I would continue working part time in neurology. So my career from that point on was divided, maturing in neurology but mainly in neuropathology.

RL: *And that happened because they needed to find a way to fund your salary?*

RA: That's right. The salary was only $3,500 a year, $300 more than my Rockefeller fellowship, and I needed that to support my family.

RL: *Did you feel reluctant to change positions?*

RA: Well, I had no choice. I had given up my possibility of going back to Duke. So, I would either accept it or not have a job.

When I went over into the Mallory Institute of Pathology, I just sat back and thought about what I could do that might be in any way different than what was going on in neuropathology in this country. And one of the things, I thought, would be to take a look at the impact of all disease on the brain. That would entail looking at all specimens that would pass through an institute of pathology (800–900 brains a year) to see what the pathology of the nervous system was in these cases. Denny-Brown was very much opposed to this. He thought it was a waste of time, though I felt that it was of general orientation value for me and might divulge secrets.

At first, the general pathologists would not let me have the brains of the routine autopsies. They would just cut them up at the autopsy table—on the next day—and throw them out.

In order to obtain access to the pathological material, I asked them to train me in general pathology, which they agreed to do. So the first year I was there, in 1941–1942, I was doing general pathology, working at the surgical desk, doing autopsies, and showing them the advantages of studying the formalin fixed brain, the method used at the Mass. General Hospital. . . and they became impressed.

My main teacher there was Frederic Parker,[2,3] who was one of the most brilliant histopathologists of his day. He was head of the Mallory Institute of Pathology. Frank Burr Mallory, its founder, was retired and had an office nearby where I worked. And Kenneth Mallory, the son, was associate director. Parker took an interest in me. And he went through all of his teaching material with me, checking me on tumors and various diseases of all organs for the next year or two.

Parker had learned from Mallory, but Mallory said that Parker was at another level beyond him as a histopathologist. He was extremely clever in spite of his neurosis and phobia of most people. He wouldn't let them in his office, while he was sitting at his microscope. And he wouldn't look at any organ with blood in it. He really described, himself, the kidney pathology of diabetes. He wrote with Soma Weiss on chronic pyelonephritis, defining that as an entity. Everything he touched he carried beyond what was known. He liked me; I seemed to make him comfortable. I was always very obsequious in his presence. Of course, I tremendously admired him. Full of self-doubts, he'd go away for a few weeks and come back and lock himself up and test himself on slides to make sure he was all right.

So it was a marvelous opportunity for me to be indoctrinated in general pathology. (I had had only the usual second year course in medical school in pathology). I attended every week all their histopathologic conferences in general pathology for several years after that. [see Figure 20]

RL: *You were carrying on your neuropathology responsibilities during this period of training in general pathology?*

RA: That's right and then by the end of that time I was so completely accepted that I had access to everything in Mallory, as well as the animal laboratories and experimental units.

RL: *As far as you know, at this time or previously, had anyone taken this tack: to carefully examine every brain? There were so many autopsies being done in those days, that there was a lot of material to study.*

RA: I don't think I knew of any one at the time.

RL: *Were they not doing this in Los Angeles?*

RA: Courville was getting a lot of specimens but they were mainly neurological specimens that had seen and followed by the neurologists there.

The other decision, that I made, was to initiate, with the approval of Denny, a clinicopathologic conference as a teaching method. I set up a weekly demonstration of a case that had been seen by the clinicians. All the clinical data were presented before the brain was examined. And the clinicians were asked to predict what the pathology would be. This was a way to test the validity of some of their clinical concepts. So, the idea of presenting the clinical data and letting competent clinicians argue the case and then showing the pathology I thought was a worthwhile enterprise. They were well attended. People from MGH, Brigham, and Beth Israel came over to Boston City to these conferences on Tuesday afternoon; I'd always have one or two exemplary cases. This went on the whole time I was there. This allowed an ample opportunity to stress the anatomical aspect of the lesion in relation to the declared symptomatology. I came over the ten-year period to attach significance to those relationships. In these conferences there was no cellular pathology; it was all anatomical pathology. [see Figure 21]

RL: *Did you cut the brain into slices prior to the session?*

RA: Usually not, unless there was a likelihood of a microscopic lesion being the only one. Part of the exercise was the surprise of what would be seen. Sometimes the lesion would not be visible. And that was important too, when all the clinical change that had been discussed was not showing up on careful sectioning of the brain.

RL: *That is a sobering experience.*

RA: Yes, and instructive. Sometimes we would get into extreme arguments. I remember one case that we had at City Hospital that I thought was straightforward Parkinson disease in an elderly woman. And Denny-Brown came by on the weekly round and asked the residents what Dr Adams had thought. "He said it was Parkinson disease." And Denny said, "Well, any fool would know that's wrong. This is arteriosclerotic Parkinson disease." (I had been taught that there was no such thing.) The person died of a pulmonary embolus. We sectioned the brain at brain cutting conference and found a pale substantia nigra. I pointed out that sometimes clinical impressions were incorrect (*chuckle*).

After a few years Ray Adams' reputation as a neuropathologist grew. Brains, usually formalin fixed and uncut, were sent to him from around the world. C. Miller Fisher recalls that about 100 brains a year came from outside the Boston City Hospital. The brain cutting sessions became popular; internists and surgeons attended. "It was quite a show," Joseph Foley recalls.

RL: *Was there any neuropathology book that guided you when you took charge of neuropathology at Boston City Hospital?*

RA: I don't recall any at that time, no. Greenfield had written a small book, not the major work that he did later. But I don't think that had enough in it to make a difference. Spielmeyer's book on the nervous system was available, and I went through that.

RL: *Was the Spielmeyer book in English?*

RA: No, Spielmeyer was in German, but it was a small book and easy to comprehend. It's very elementary and essentially about cellular neuropathology and reactions of cells and glia.

RL: *Had you learned German in high school?*

RA: No. German was not offered. I was in high school right after World War I, and Germany was in bad odor. They gave only Spanish and French. I took a night course in German, when I was at Boston City Hospital, because some of the best articles on neuropathology were in German.

RL: *It sounds like you carried a huge workload at Boston City Hospital.*

RA: Well we were there long days and many evenings, working on material. In fact I was the only one to take the brains out, five or six a day. Fortunately I didn't get tuberculosis; about a third or a fourth of the younger pathologists came down with TB. Later I had fellows working with me—Jan Cammermeyer, Jan Stevens, Subramony Iyer, Henri Vander Eecken, C. Miller Fisher . . . Each one would be assigned a subject to study, and we would work it out together. I had lots of time to devote to investigative work. I tried to work in areas of neurology that were not well cultivated, cerebrovascular disease and nutritional disease. Muscle was a relatively neglected field.

RL: *Did you do any clinical work?*

RA: I visited on the neurology ward, one to two months a year, and I saw consultations with the residents in the afternoon or evening. At the same time I was attending neurology conferences every Saturday with Derek Denny-Brown and Houston

Merritt. So I saw a lot of clinical neurology. Then Denny-Brown went to India for a year, back in the British Army, and I looked after the neurology service myself, as well as continued in neuropathology. So I had a chance to gain experience, to mature as a consultant and as a clinician, which was an extremely valuable period. Houston Merritt had been serving as a consultant to the Pratt Diagnostic Hospital. When he left Boston in 1944–1945, I was invited over there to give a few lectures on neuropathology. And I formed quite good friendships with people at that clinic, which later became New England Center Hospital. For about five years I would see consultations. I'd see them once and try to make up my mind what to do.

RL: *Tell me more about this moonlighting job at New England Center.*

RA: I established a delightful relationship to the Tufts University staff. There were outstanding people there that were mainly Jewish refugees from Germany; it was during that period, when Hitler already was forcing people out. Tannhauser, a brilliant investigator, was one of them. Another was Iggersheimer—a neuro-ophthalmologist who was the first to demonstrate the spirochete in the spinal fluid in neurosyphilis. They got so that they depended on me for all of their neurology. It was a very good period for me.

It gave me a broad contact with some fine physicians. And through them I became acquainted with a rather considerable Jewish community here in Boston. Amongst the Boston symphony players were quite a number of displaced Jews. And so they would always call on me because I knew these Jewish immigrant physicians. Patients with finger trouble of the fourth finger of the right hand and viola players with elbow trouble and trumpet players who lost their lip. A fascinating period of my life. So I became a kind of neurologist for the symphony orchestra.

RL: *Were there no other neurologists at New England Center?*

RA: They had two other neurologists of great renown at Tufts. One of them was Hauptmann[4] who discovered phenobarbital; he was quite well known in Germany. I only saw him once or twice. The other was Kurt Goldstein,[5] a German, who was world renowned for his theories of cerebral function. Goldstein was on a grant from Rockefeller Foundation, which was trying to repatriate displaced German Jews.

RL: *Why did they consult you, if they had these prominent neurologists there?*

RA: These two people were not very helpful in diagnostic neurology. They took no interest or any real part in teaching or seeing patients. They had their own little research projects. They never quite adapted to American medicine. They went their own way, did their studies. Hauptmann did some consultative work, but rather felt that he didn't belong. A pleasant person, I thought. Goldstein was a very autocratic person, who tended to dominate every group that he joined. And the residents didn't like him. He visited a month or two on the wards of the city hospital neurology service. He didn't seem to be able to adapt to medical problems that led to nervous system disorders, and he took rather strong stands. One hilarious moment occurred, according to the residents. (I wasn't there.) He had been shown a patient that was quite rigid, and he decided that this man was hysterical.

The residents protested; they thought he had an extrapyramidal difficulty. In order to prove his point Goldstein took out his pocket watch and threw it to the man, expecting him to immediately catch it. The watch fell on the ground and broke apart, wheels flying around. He was mortified. He didn't say a thing—just walked on. But he was doing quite interesting work. He was highly respected in world neurology.

RL: *Had you had contact with Jewish people at Massachusetts General when you were a trainee?*

RA: No one, who was head of service or in a prominent position at Massachusetts General, was Jewish at the time. There were a lot at Pratt because Joe Pratt made a special effort to help displaced Jewish people.

RL: *Do you consider Merritt one of your teachers?*

RA: Oh yes. Denny-Brown too. I learned a lot from both. I was constantly exposed. I was fortunate. Merritt and Denny-Brown helped me tremendously. You probably have never been in a completely research institute; we were living off that gift of Alan Gregg of the Rockefeller Foundation, and we were full time—not many full time places in neurology in that era. So we lived day and night with the clinical material.

RL: *Tell me about Merritt.*[6]

RA: Well he was a superb clinician and a good poker player, and he was unpretentious, an open person, very bright. He had no great use for detailed pedagogy. He didn't style himself as a great teacher. One of the faults of his teaching was that he never would go through the steps of his thinking whereby he would reach the diagnosis. So it would be a matter of a resident presenting some data, and he would tap a reflex or do one or two things and make a diagnosis and walk off. Well, that was spectacular because he frequently was right, but no one could figure out how he reached his conclusions. He played on that in a way, enjoyed perplexing the student. He had a number of characteristic tricks. If he had a patient with any kind of spinal cord disease, he would quickly recognize it as such. If he didn't know what the cause was, he would assert, in a very dogmatic fashion, that it was syringomyelia. When you asked him how he knew that, he would casually say, "Well, you try to disprove it." He was so bright...I suppose there was no one of his day who was a better clinician than Merritt. I enjoyed him tremendously.

The relationship between Houston Merritt and Derek Denny-Brown,[7] was always a very complex one. There was endless conflict. Part of it was understandable in terms of personality. Part of it was understandable in terms of their own clinical experience. Merritt had been brought up in neurology with Cobb, Putnam and the group at the city hospital and was experienced with the rough and tumble type of neurological case that you find at a municipal hospital, lots of alcoholism, great numbers of traumatic cases and strokes. As a clinician he was much superior to Denny-Brown, though Denny-Brown was, of course, an outstanding neurophysiologist, trained in Sherrington's lab as a Bate fellow. He went to London later because he wanted to go into clinical work. He was at Queen Square, for several years, where he attached himself to Charles Symonds, and he worked with Greenfield in neuropathology for a time. He was more experienced with classic neurology, which was fine; it was a rather different type of case, which would be sent to a neurological center—not the general hospital type. So they had different clinical experiences.

The other point was that Merritt was a rather easygoing, jolly fellow. Derek Denny-Brown was rather tense, excitable and temperamental. Somewhat arrogant, he would try to assert his dominance as a clinician and often would fail because of lack of experience with city hospital-type neurology. That set up a kind of a rivalry between them—not really intended, I don't think. Denny was very assertive and didn't get along with people very easily. He was intolerant of opinion, mediocrity. In fits of irritation he would castigate senior people. Two or three of them resigned because of it... Swank and others.

RL: *Tell me more about Denny-Brown.*

RA: Denny-Brown would get quite mad at me at times. Whenever he would lose temper with me, he would quickly make it up. I was, I suppose, the only person who stayed there for ten years. He used to criticize me openly and harshly in public to a point where it was embarrassing. Yet, when I was considered for the appointment at Mass. General, he strongly supported me.

RL: *Didn't it bother you that he would lose his temper?*

RA: No, I just looked upon it as a character trait. I admired his extreme intelligence and wide experience. He was an excellent physiologist. His training with Sherrington had been superb, and his doctorate thesis with him was highly admired by neurophysiologists. He could have stayed in neurophysiology and would probably have been world renowned. I learned a tremendous amount from him.

RL: *What was his clinical strength?*

RA: He had a good eye for clinical problems. He was an excellent histologist and had considerable background in neuropathology, wrote up that paper on the paraneoplastic neuropathies. He had developed the technique of using celloidin embedded material and axis cylinder staining. I was privileged to look at the material.

He wrote a classic paper on basal ganglia disease and a monograph, which was widely appreciated, reviewing the world's literature on frontal lobes. Denny was very skilled in classical neurology and talked very well. His lectures were excellent. He was certainly a scholar, and he instilled respect for scholarship in the residents, who trained with him. I think he was aware of his temperament and was himself upset with it.

RL: *He sounds difficult.*

RA: Yes, he would make things difficult, but often he would have very good suggestions. Some of his speculations would be a bit off base. It was typical of Denny to go off on a wild tangent on the basis of one incomplete case. Yet, when it came to analyzing the physiology or the literature on physiology, he was superb. He was very tense and wanted to be involved in everything. He didn't want anyone to get ahead of him. I managed to get around this pretty much by placating him.

He had a peculiar way. I had collected fifty cases of torticollis. I had a careful description of cases. I gave them a battery of psychological tests, and I thought they were no more abnormal psychologically than another group that didn't have torticollis. I started collecting these cases as a resident because Jost Mikelsen, who was a neurosurgeon at Mass. General, used to have me look at them before he operated on their necks. At that time the standard procedure was to denervate the neck muscles. It was a pretty radical procedure, but a fair number of them straightened their heads out. And I was quite convinced it was some kind of movement disorder; I proposed to write it up. I told Denny about the data, and he said, "Well, that's nonsense! Don't dare publish such rot as that; this is a psychogenic difficulty." I never did publish it. I was upset about that.

RL: *For what else was Denny-Brown known?*

RA: He had very good EMG studies of denervation. Another very fine study was his work on the effect of a concussive head injury on animals. He showed very clearly, with someone at Oxford, that, if you deliver a blow to the head of an animal, with the skull, fixed in one position so it can't move, all you did was smash the skull—you did not produce concussion. But if the head was not fixed and there was mobility of the brain and skull, at once you obtained a concussive effect. This mobility of the brain in relation to the skull is also the basis of frontal lobe contusion. That brilliant observation has held up. And also he studied bladder function with Robertson of Australia, one of the first good studies of physiology of bladder. So he had a tremendous influence in neurology. I was full of admiration of him.

RL: *What happened to Merritt?*

RA: Merritt and Denny-Brown never hit it off very well. There was always a struggle. It was awkward and caused the residents to take sides about that time. Merritt appreciated that and, when Montefiore offered him a job, he left Boston. He later became head of the Columbia Neurological Institute and then dean of Columbia, very effective.

RL: *What type of hours did you keep, in the nineteen forties, while you were at Boston City?*

RA: Well, they were long hours. At one time, when Denny-Brown was called back into the British army, I had the full neurology research unit on my shoulders; I was alone there, teaching half of the Harvard class in neurology. And at the same time I was spending three afternoons a week at the New England Center Hospital. I'd go there at lunchtime and come home at eight or nine, having seen as many as eight or ten neurological consultations and having done a myelogram with Alice Ettinger. So it was a busy period for me.

RL: *Would you get to work at 8 o'clock?*

RA: Oh, yes. I would work in the garden for an hour or two in the morning and then go into the hospital. I remember spading about an acre of ground for the first planting of crops.

Notes

1. Beatty J. *The Rascal King*, De Capo Press, New York, 1992, 571 pp.

2. Rosai J., ed. *Guiding the Surgeon's Hand: The History of American Surgical Pathology.* American Registry of Pathology, Washington, 1997 (see Chapter 6, Surgical pathology at the hospitals of Harvard Medical School by Robert E. Scully and Austin L. Vickery.)

3. Robbins SL, Tenney Jr. B., Frederic Parker Jr. MD. *Lab Invest* V9, pp 3–6, 1960.

4. Krasnianski M, Ehrt V, et al. Alfred Hauptmann, Siegfried Thannhauser and an Endangered Muscular Disorder. *Arch Neurol* V61, pp 1139–1141, 2004.

5. Quadfasel FA. Aspects of the Life and Work of Kurt Goldstein. *Cortex* V4, 113–124, 1968.

6. Adams RD. Obituary H. Houston Merritt. *J. Neurol Sci* V45, pp 391–392, 1980.

7. Foley JM. Derek Ernest Denny-Brown 1901–1981. *Ann Neurol* V11, pp 413–419, 1982.

Return to Massachusetts General Hospital: The Early Years, 1951–1954

After ten years at Boston City Hospital Ray Adams was being courted by Tufts, by some southern medical schools, and by Massachusetts General Hospital. After Ayer had stepped down as neurology chairman at Massachusetts General Hospital, Charles Kubik had become acting chair. Naturally, Ray Adams was interested by the opportunity to replace Ayer. Although the hospital and medical school did not make an attractive offer, he finally agreed to return to Massachusetts General. Soon thereafter the Montreal Neurological Institute tried to hire him away.

RL: *At some point you received a call about the possibility of your moving over to Massachusetts General Hospital.*

RA: Yes. That was a long negotiation. Ayer had retired. The problem was that I was an associate professor, full time, at the Boston City and they said they didn't have money for a full time director at Mass. General. (Ayer had been part time.) So I was reluctant to take the job. And we went through about a year of back and forth negotiations. Finally George P. Berry, who was then dean of the medical school, brought me in and asked if I trusted him. I said I had no reason (*chuckle*) not to. (He was a very powerful figure.) And he said, "Well if you trust me, take the job. . . we'll work it out later." I wasn't very enthusiastic about that, but nonetheless did finally take it. They had a salary of $12,000 based on a fellowship which was being paid by the National Multiple Sclerosis Society. The hospital was not putting anything into it. Nor was the medical school. [see Figure 22]

RL: *How did this salary arrangement work out?*

RA: It was less than I had been making before. I was living on that salary plus seeing a few patients. Then, about October, the Multiple Sclerosis Society went broke. So my fellowship was terminated. Berry was mad as anything about their failure to carry through on the promise of the fellowship. Konrad Trager, who was president of the society, was forced to sell a house in Washington, DC, that the society had acquired. They finished out my first year's salary on part of the proceeds of that house. That gives you some inkling of Harvard medicine at that time; very stingy, they wouldn't free up any money.

In the second year, David Crockett, who was a fundraiser at Mass. General, obtained a King Trust Fellowship for me for several years and additional funds from the medical school and hospital.

RL: *Please tell me more about your move to the Massachusetts General Hospital.*

RA: Firstly, an orienting idea, obtained from my work at the Boston City Hospital, is that the neurology that's done in a brain institute, like Queen Square, is very different from the kind of neurology that's done in a general hospital. There were proposals by neurosurgeons that neurology and neurosurgery together raise funds and build a separate institute apart from Mass. General, Beth Israel, Peter Bent Bingham and Boston City Hospitals. I disapproved. I disagreed with that point of view. I realized, at that time, the difference between an institute of neurology and neurosurgery, such as Penfield had established in Montreal, and the more conventional type of neurological service at a general hospital. The latter type, I thought, we would have at the Mass. General Hospital.

The second point: Merritt felt very strongly that neurology was a dying specialty, that it was being dissected away by infectious diseases experts, neurosurgeons, psychiatrists and that there'd be very little left. I was critical of this thinking. I thought the fault of neurology was the neurologists themselves. They had too limited a view of neurology, a perfunctory approach to cerebrovascular disease, and little interest in peripheral neurology. It was with these ideas that I went to the Mass. General Hospital. I discovered on arrival that there was a small ward, obtained by James Ayer. This had three wings, one for neurosurgery, one for psychiatry and one for neurology. Also the neurologists were seeing only a small proportion of the hospital cases that had neurological diseases. The majority of the patients with neurological diseases were being seen only by internists and pediatricians. The stroke cases were divided up. We saw one out of every four. Or, if they had something very unique, as a syndrome, we might see them. And the pediatric cases were out of our sphere entirely. Higgins, the professor of pediatrics, would not allow a neurologist on the premises. (This was also true of the chief of pediatrics at Boston City Hospital, Martin English.) We had afternoons to do what we wished. We had to work in the outpatient clinic in the mornings. We would see an occasional consultation in the afternoon and an occasional case in the emergency ward.

So the neurology service was extremely small and limited in its scope. I felt, in moving back to the Mass. General, that the first thing to do would be to see if the neurology service could be extended to include all of the neurology cases in the hospital and to see if we could extend the sphere of neurology into the then borderline areas, pediatrics, psychiatry, mental retardation and stroke. Obviously, with two residents alternating nights and weekends, one could not do that. So that required that the service be enlarged despite the limited funds. (I told you earlier how little financial support the medical school and the hospital provided at the time.)

RL: *What did you accomplish during your first few years?*

RA: I tried to integrate my affairs with the people that were at the Mass. General. There were several able people: Robert Schwab, Peirson Richardson, Ed Cole, Henry Viets and several other visiting neurologists. I wanted to make sure I didn't interfere and, if anything, I wanted to help them with their work.

Secondly, I wanted to develop a program of research there that didn't exist before. In acute metabolic disease I selected Maurice Victor, who came with me from Boston City, as the first new staff person. In experimental disease I installed Byron Waksman as an investigator in our unit. He had been working with Morrison in neuropathology. I knew Waxman from my days at Boston City Hospital. (After Morrison fell ill, Waksman had brought his experimental material to me, asking for help on the interpretation of neuropathology of neuro-immune disease.) We also wrote a whole series of papers together on diphtheritic and demyelinative polyneuropathy. I was spending about half of each day in neuro-immunology during that period of time.

Thirdly, I was trying to orient myself to the medical service, in general, of which I was still a part, like cardiology or gastroenterology. Walter Bauer, an outstanding chief of medicine, made it clear that I could act independently. I went to their conferences as often as I could. They rotated their residents through neurology, as they had before.

RL: *What else happened during those first years at MGH?*

RA: I had a very fortunate break. George Thorn, Hersey Professor of Physik at Peter Bent Brigham, invited me to become an editor of the second edition of the Harrison textbook of general medicine.

In the first edition of the book, the five editors, Bill Resnik, Harrison himself, Max Wintrobe, Paul Beeson at Yale and George Thorn—decided not to have any neurology. Then they got cold feet about the whole thing. They decided, at the last moment, to solicit Houston Merritt, who was, by then, at Columbia at New York Neurological Institute. He was extremely occupied—he'd become dean of the medical school, and he turned the assignment over to Sciarra. Merritt had no time and didn't put much effort into it, and it was very unsatisfactory.

So, when they were preparing the second edition, the other editors asked George Thorn to approach me to see if I would do it. I agreed. They just wanted some chapters, but I sat to, and wrote fifteen or more chapters one spring. That must have been about 1952 or 1953; I don't remember exactly. I wrote chapters on those aspects of nervous system disease that every internist and general physician was bound to see, things like disturbances of consciousness, disturbances of sleep, convulsions, all forms of motor disorder, sensory disturbances and neuritis. They wanted me to just be a consultant on the textbook, but Harrison was sufficiently impressed with the writing that he convinced the others that I should be a full editor. This was very fortunate because it provided a greater income than I ever received at Harvard.

RL: *How was Harrison connected with all of these northern people?*

RA: He had been at Peter Bent Brigham, Vanderbilt, and was widely known as a teacher and a cardiologist, chairman of Birmingham, Alabama. He was a marvelous character.

RL: *When the Harrison textbook came out—I realize that you were not part of the first edition—was the Cecil Loeb textbook already established?*

RA: Cecil had been going for several editions, but it was in the format of the old fashioned text books of medicine with chapters on each of the common diseases. But the Harrison (and I think that I had some influence on this right from the early days) had a section on the principal manifestations of disease and their anatomy and physiology and then a discussion of categories of disease, and then a discussion of individual diseases. This format was important to orient a reader to a category of disease like stroke before discussing the individual diagnosis.

RL: *Did the first edition of Harrison's textbook have that format?*

RA: Well, to a slight extent but not nearly as much as the second and third editions, where almost a third of the book was given over to a discussion of fever and other aspects of general medicine. And that format was, I think, the basis of the success. One of the representatives of McGraw Hill recently told me they had sold 2.3 million copies.

RL: *Did you speak at the meetings of the editors on behalf of this approach?*

RA: Yes, I urged that it be increased; that would be the place where the second and third year medical students would get oriented in general medicine. That's where they would turn to in order to have a full discussion of fever or fainting or consciousness in general or some aspects of infection. Very soon the Harrison was selling better than Cecil, which continued, for a time, its old fashioned plan.

RL: *Cecil came to copy Harrison eventually.*

RA: Yes, it changed gradually—increasingly had a section on the general aspects of disease. But I think that Harrison continued to do it better than Cecil.

RL: *Tell me about your negotiations with the Montreal Neurological Institute.*

RA: About 1954 Wilder Penfield decided to retire. He had been a tremendous force in American neurosurgery. The trustees of the Montreal Neurological Institute thought that in the next generation there should be someone that could promote and expand the neurological side of the institute. Montreal had been mainly neurosurgical.

RL: *Do you know how your name came to the fore?*

RA: No, I was about the right age. I had been considered as a candidate for the directorship of the new neurological institute in Bethesda. And my writings.

RL: *Only ten years after completing a psychiatry fellowship, you were being recruited to become the director of the Montreal Neurological Institute.*

RA: I had spent that ten-year period in neuropathology and neurology, and I had made my reputation, such as it was, in that field. It was enough to attract the ad hoc committee that would make the selection.

RL: *Tell me about the committee.*

RA: I think it was Carmichael of London and Symonds of London and Allen Gregg of the Rockefeller Foundation and Stanley Cobb. McGill asked them to select someone for directorship of the Montreal Neurological Institute, and for the professorship of neurology and neurosurgery. And I was chosen for the post. Penfield came to see me, and I went to Montreal a couple of time and talked to the principal people. I couldn't decide what to do. Penfield said that he would stay out of the way. He knew that he was so highly respected that it would interfere with anyone, especially a non-neurosurgeon, coming and taking the post. He would go to Greece or to the Rockefeller Foundation and their institute, and stay there for two years. But I was still reluctant to go because I had just finished bringing several people into the department at Mass. General. I thought I would let them down, in a way, so I refused. Also, the fact that Montreal was interested in me caused Dean Berry to consider offering me the Bullard Professorship; at the moment Stanley Cobb was retiring from the Bullard Professorship at Harvard. I remember giving a neuropathology conference at the Veteran's Hospital. Berry came out during that conference, called me out and said that he would assure me of the Bullard Professorship and full support, if I would not take the Montreal offer.

RL: *What was the meaning of the Bullard professorship to you?*

RA: Well it was a key appointment at Harvard, and it had been in existence about thirty years. Southard had been the first Bullard professor, Cobb the second. It was a highly respected post. It was part of the old bargaining game in scholastic affairs. Another condition was that, if I would stay, David Crockett promised an entire floor of laboratories in the new building that was going up at Mass. General. And also later they found other support for me. So they made it very much more attractive at Mass. General.

RL: *The formal letter from Dean Berry, dated December 19, 1953, implied that you would get the Bullard professorship.*

RA: It was written very urgently because Penfield[1] had been down a number of times to get me to go to Montreal.

RL: *It says, "Were you to be appointed the next Bullard professor, you would get $25,000.*

RA: I was supposed to pay Maurice Victor and Miller Fisher and Ruth Symonds out of that twenty-five.

RL: *Is that what it says?*

RA: No, that's the way that it turned out. He was trying to block the appointment at Montreal.

RL: *You received a letter of January 7 from Wilder Penfield. You obviously had told Penfield that you were not coming to Montreal. Did you have a high opinion of Penfield?*

RA: Oh, yes. He was, I suppose, the leading figure in North American neurosurgery after Cushing.

RL: *Were they the two major neurosurgeons of the twentieth century?*

RA: That's right, but Penfield did something more; he established an institute. Cushing could never get anyone to work with him; he was a rather disagreeable personality. So was Dandy. They were from that school of neurosurgery that started cursing from the time they entered the operating room and blasted everyone off.

RL: *Did Penfield have more of a neurological bent?*

RA: Yes and neuropathologic. Those three volumes on cellular neuropathology—he started that work with Ramón y Cajal, when he was in his laboratory, as I recall. They were written by world authorities. He had a lot to do with it. He was a man of parts. He built an enormous institute, superb, and he brought people together. He was a delightful personality, kind and generous, supportive of young people: I was much impressed with him.

Note

1. Penfield W. *No Man Alone: A Neurosurgeon's Life*. Little Brown & Co., Boston, 1977.

Sabbatical Year in Europe 1954–1955

Within months of his appointment as Bullard Professor of Neuropathology, Ray Adams left for a sabbatical year in Europe. The highlights of his trip were his interaction with van Bogaert, the neuropathologist in Ghent, and his sojourn in Paris with Alajouanine, the Charcot Professor.

RL: *I was hoping we could talk about your sabbatical year in Europe.*

RA: Yes. I had been at Harvard for thirteen years by the time I was elected Bullard Professor of Neuropathology, and I felt, therefore, entitled to a sabbatical. I applied also for a fourth year of my Rockefeller fellowship; it was granted.

    I left my house in Milton in the hands of John Walton. I bundled the family into a station wagon and drove to Montreal. There I saw Miller Fisher and persuaded him to leave his post at Montreal General Hospital and come to Boston as a staff member at Mass. General and as an assistant professor at Harvard.

    The car was put on a steamship and we all went to England. I had the entire family, my wife Elinor and the four children, the youngest about eight or nine years old. We landed in western England and drove in Wales, England and Scotland. We put the car on a boat and went to western Norway, from which we made the trek to Oslo.

    I began visiting neurology departments at that point. I didn't visit any in England except in New Castle on Tyne, where Henry Miller[1-3] was professor of neurology. That was a very strong department. Miller was a brilliant clinician and a very colorful and influential speaker. He advanced provincial neurology in England more than any other person, I would say.

RL: *So you went on to Oslo . . .*

RA: Yes. Monrad Krohn[4] had written a little book on neurological diagnosis that went through many, many editions. It was well written and quite appropriate. He was a very colorful gentleman, of the old school, well educated, fine speaker—ruled neurology completely in Norway. His only contribution really was the little book.

I didn't think he had taken full advantage of the University of Oslo. There were some very fine people: Alf Brodal, who was perhaps the best known neuroanatomist in western Europe at the time, Jan Cammermeyer, who was well trained in neuropathology and had come to work with us in Boston for about a year and a half, and Refsum, a young man who was interested in epilepsy and came to Boston to work with William Lenox.

Refsum later succeeded Monrad Krohn. He wrote up a series of cases of familial polyneuropathy. Later a German worked out the biochemistry of what became known as Refsum's disease. I suppose it was his major accomplishment to promote the study of familial disease. I had a good opinion of him.

RL: *Where did you go next?*

RA: After spending about a week with the Oslo group, I moved on to Sweden. This was a rather curious situation. Kugelberg[5] and Wohlfart[6] were the two leading neurologists in Sweden at the time. By the time we were there, Kugelberg had just been selected as Antoni's successor and head of the department in Stockholm. Kugelberg was a brilliant neurophysiologist, a charming person. There wasn't interest in all sides of neurology, as far as I could tell.

Gunnar Wohlfart had already moved down to Lund in southern Sweden. Wohlfart was very upset about not being selected as professor of neurology in Stockholm. One of the reasons Wohlfart failed was that Derek Denny-Brown in Boston had been one of the referees about the chairmanship of neurology, and he had pointed out that Wohlfart was not as talented as Kugelberg. This opinion was printed in the Swedish newspapers. When I explained to Wohlfart that I had nothing to do with this, he actually arranged for me to stay with him in Lund. Wohlfart had written extensively on muscle dystrophy and other muscle diseases. So we had common interests. I spent a good bit of time with him. He was building up a department and was obviously an experienced neurologist with interests that extended throughout the realm of neurology.

After a week we went over to Copenhagen and met Buchthal[7,8] and his wife. He was very interested in muscle pathology at the time. We were discussing the meaning of large fibers in dystrophy and also the basis of the fibrillations in polymyositis. A contribution he made (and I was very impressed with it): he showed for the first time that many of the motor units in dystrophic and myositic disease were smaller than normal due to the fact that they were depleted of the full complement of muscle fibers. He didn't account, as I recall, for the enlargement of motor units, when a motor unit had been denervated. That was done by a Swedish worker. I also talked to Buchthal about fasciculating muscle fibers. I asked where the excitation of fasciculation occurred. I remember challenging him to show whether the fasciculation potentials were those of normal motor units. He said that he did not know but that he would find out. He later wrote to me about his subsequent research on this question. He showed that these were normal units. His careful analysis of motor units supplemented the work of Derek Denny-Brown and his associates in EMG. He was a very able physiologist, and he knew a lot about neurological medicine in general.

From there we traveled south to Amsterdam and Utrecht and spent some time with the neurologists in both places but did not stay long. Went on then to Belgium, where we spent time with Henri Vander Eecken a former fellow of mine. (He was finally chosen as chief of neurology for Ghent. He was able to build a new institute and put neurology on its feet in Ghent.)

Then I went back to Paris by train and I sent my family and our car by boat to New York. From Paris, I returned to Ghent. Almost immediately I went to van Bogaert's laboratory where I spent weeks. Van Bogaert[9] welcomed me, very generous with his time and material. I admired him very much. He was the most eminent neuropathologist in Europe at the time and had a neuropathological collection. I saw him each morning, and we would discuss cases from his files.

I thought it would be worthwhile to talk to van Bogaert about my observations on striatonigral degeneration. Henri Vander Eecken and I had worked up a case that I had seen one evening for Dr Max Finland in the Boston City Hospital. There had been a striking and gross atrophy of the putamen, in a patient that we had seen as a rigid Parkinson. I went out to see the wife of the patient, who told me he had frequent syncope. The nigra was involved too. The patient came in one night and died of some intercurrent disease a day or two later. Henri Vander Eecken and I had collected three or four cases at MGH. (I did not have access to the spinal cord in these cases.) Van Bogaert looked at my material, had never seen a case like it. We finally wrote this material up with him as a case of primary nigrostriatal degeneration, sometimes associated with cerebellar atrophy and with frequent fainting. [see Figure 24]

RL: *The terminology has evolved. You used the term, striatonigral degeneration. Currently the term, multiple system atrophy, is popular. Do you have any thoughts about the change in terminology?*

RA: Well, I have no objection to the term multiple system atrophy but, of course, there are other multiple system atrophies too. So the fact that multiple systems were involved in a degenerative disease is not a distinguishing mark.

RL: *What do you consider van Bogaert's major contributions to the literature?*

RA: Enormously productive, he had written so many articles that were fairly original or enlargements of things that had been written before. Van Bogaert got all the good brains at Institut Bunge because he would include the referring neurologist as coauthor. Van Bogaert and Bertrand wrote a paper on Canavan's disease. Van Bogaert was very important in describing myoclonus and cerebellar ataxia in a subacute disease related to previous measles infection, SSPE. He wrote the best description of that condition and its pathology. I remember sitting with him in the balcony at the microscope. A patient was being led across the lower floor by his parents. An adolescent boy, he was staggering and twitching, and Van Bogaert looked over and said, "There's a case of it." He could recognize the clinical part very well. SSPE is almost nonexistent now, since we have measles vaccine.

RL: *Where did you go after your time with van Bogaert?*

RA: Henri Vander Eecken and I traveled to all the German Universities.

Hallervorden[10] was in the laboratory of Spatz[11,12] in Giessen, but Spatz deferred to him for careful clinicopathological studies. Spatz was vivacious; Hallervorden was gruff. Hallervorden had long experience and was much admired by van Bogaert. I was quite impressed with both Hallervorden and Spatz. Hallervorden, however, was under intense criticism because he had accepted and examined the brains of hundreds of retarded individuals and Jews, who had been killed by the Nazi party.[13-15]

It was in Würtzburg where we met Schaltenbrand.[16] He was a very erudite and skillful clinician. He was under considerable criticism. He had injected human extracts from multiple sclerosis patients under circumstances that were criticized— not a Nazi era experiment, after that time. He wrote a stereotactic anatomical atlas with Alajouanine and Percival Bailey.

In Freiburg am Breslau, there was an institute run by Oskar and Cecile Vogt.[17,18] We went to see the Vogts on a Sunday afternoon; we found them walking in the garden. In many ways Cecile was more objective and dependable than her husband, Oskar. [see Figure 23]

The Vogts had spent two years setting up an anatomical institute in Moscow, much of the work of which related to studying Lenin's brain. They took part of the sections back with them to Germany.

RL: *What did Lenin's brain show?*

RA: Old ischemic infarcts.

RL: *Lacunar infarcts?*

RA: No, no.

Oskar was a little bit confused and got the idea that Paulette Vander Eecken was a neurologist. So he had her sit beside him and showed her in the microscope different things. She had no idea about what he was demonstrating.

Henri van Der Eeken and I stood in the back. Occasionally Cecile was trotting around finding things that Oskar wanted. It lasted a couple of hours. Toward the end he was getting mixed up, and she persuaded him to rest for a while. He was in his dotage.

The next day he wanted us to come and review the work of many young assistants. He had a two-floor institute. The lower floor was a whole floor of laboratories. Each assistant had a room. He would knock on each door, and a very well-disciplined student would open the door, bow respectfully and give a brief recitation of what he was doing. So, all in all, it was very agreeable visit.

In Munich we did visit Spielmeyer's laboratory; Spielmeyer was no longer alive, as I recall. He was the most prominent German neuropathologist of his day. Between the wars a good many Americans went to study in his laboratory—Stanley Cobb and Houston Merritt are examples. His books and articles were highly regarded. He probably made too much of very subtle Nissl changes in fixed tissue. Spielmeyer was correct when he completely refuted Vogt's ideas about abnormalities in cerebral cortical cells in schizophrenia. There was not a very good understanding between them.

RL: *What was your overall impression of German neurology?*

RA: Well, the only outstanding clinical neurology that I observed after the Second World War was in Paris and London and some in New Castle. Germany was producing almost nothing at the time. It's only in the last few years that they're coming back very strongly.

RL: *That related somehow to the war and emigration of talented people?*

RA: Both, yes. They were very badly hit. And Japanese neurology, also, which was quite strong before the Second World War, mainly much influenced by Germany, also went down to a very low level. It came back much faster than it did in Eastern Europe.

RL: *To what do you attribute the affinity of the Japanese and Germans in medicine?*

RA: Well, it was a common practice for young Japanese neurologists or aspiring neurologists to go to Germany for graduate study. That stopped, of course, during the Second World War, and it probably stopped during the First World War too. So the German influence on Japanese medicine was very much reduced. Chinese medicine, in general, was also influenced much by Germany. American influence was also evident after the First World War, when Rockefeller Foundation fellows were being sent to Peking.[19] I was supposed to go for two years to Peking Union Medical College after the completion of my three-year Rockefeller fellowship. It was only because of the beginning of the Second World War that I didn't go.

RL: *Why would you have gone to China?*

RA: Well, it was sort of understood that as part of your commitment, upon the granting of a Rockefeller fellowship, that you would go and help and participate in this particular Chinese medical center, and a good many people of my age and development did that. It was mainly the Rockefeller Foundation's interest, I think, in helping medicine develop in China.

RL: *After Germany you returned to Paris.*

RA: I spent the last four months or so with Alajouanine[20] and his assistants, Lhermitte and Castagne. Alajouanine was very gracious. I stayed at Maison Belgique, a dormitory outside Paris built by the Rockefeller Foundation. I went each day by subway to Salpetriere. I made rounds with them. I attended all of Alajouanine's conferences, which were brilliant. They would present two or three cases. He would invite discussion and then he would express his opinion. Alajouanine was Charcot Professor, one of the most brilliant clinicians in France, an acknowledged scholar. He had a broad view of cerebral disease, wrote extensively on vascular disease,

disease of the basal ganglia and thalamus and cerebellar disease. He wrote brilliantly, coming out with one or two monographs a year. His monographs on frontal lobe and temporal lobe were very informative. The kindness of the man—he put everyone at ease, assistants, patients and others. He was not an arrogant man, very humble yet very impressive with his extensive knowledge.

In the afternoons I was able to see some neuropathology in a way, but Bertrand, the neuropathologist, was never there. I would look over some of the cases he had published.

RL: *Why did you choose to spend so much time at Salpetriere?*

RA: Well, Salpetriere is the great center of French neurology, and, since I read and spoke French, that seemed to be a very good place for me to go. Of course, through Derek Denny-Brown and his various visitors from the National Hospital, Queen Square, I was pretty well steeped in British neurology at Boston City Hospital. So this was an alternative. Paris seemed to be the ideal for me.

Furthermore, it enabled me to see the French style of interviewing patients, conducting lectures and seminars in that institute, which went back to the time of Charcot and Raymond, Pierre Marie, Guillain; it's a long chain of brilliant neurologists. Many very famous practitioners, who were not strictly academicians, were there too.

RL: *Could you comment on the French style?*

RA: You can't help but admire the thoroughness of their scholarship in the field. If you look over the publications in the last 100 years in Revue Neurologique, you find that everything that's important in neurology has been touched upon. The scholarship in every phase of neurology is admirable. And it rivals that of Queen Square. The French are very proud of that.

RL: *You mentioned their method of interviewing patients.*

RA: Well, they were very systematic and they put on excellent clinical demonstrations of phenomena. And if you look through many of the publications of Charcot[21] himself, the way he brought out some of the details of the clinical side of neurology, you could not help have considerable admiration for the level of clinical neurology.

RL: *To what do you attribute the celebrity status of Charcot? People always refer to him as a special person in neurology. Was he that much more important than some of his Anglo Saxon or German contemporaries?*

RA: No, but he was one of the first to combine, in a very scholarly fashion, the clinical expression of diseases of the nervous system and their anatomical bases. I think that he contributed something to everything that he looked at. He was wrong about certain interpretations but, on the other hand, his general clinical–pathological approach sort of set the French standard. And, of course, he held one of the first chairs of neurology in the world.

RL: *Was his influence magnified by his books?*

RA: It became extended, of course, because many scholarly Americans read French, and the source of much of their knowledge, during the nineteenth century, was from his writings and those of Hughlings Jackson and Gowers. And the successors of the

Charcot chair of neurology have always been quite famous people, who made major contributions. Alajouanine was the one I became well acquainted with. I thought he was superb.

RL: *Did you feel any affinity toward Duchenne when you reviewed his works?*[22]

RA: Well, I could not but admire his scholarship. He not only was a very astute clinician, but he was able to isolate disease. I think he was the one who clearly was able to separate tabes dorsalis from the other forms of ataxia, and I believe Charcot himself had a great respect for him. He would, I was told, often ask him to see a puzzling case to help out in the diagnosis.

RL: *Did you know the older Lhermitte, Jean Pierre, the one for whom Lhermitte symptom is named?*

RA: I had dinner with him. He was a very, very original fellow. He made a lot of excellent observations. He was a Catholic, and he was the neurologist for the Shrine at Lourdes. He went every year with a train load of patients and made careful notes on their ailments and what happened. He never saw anyone, who wasn't hysteric, improve. He thought it all was a matter of spoofing. He was a very provocative man. He'd make statements just to excite you. He wanted me to explain why Parkinson disease always affected the left side first. (*Laughter*) He'd do that all through the dinner hour; he was eighty-some at the time.

Notes

1. Walton J. Obituary Henry Miller (1913–1976). *J Neurol Sci* V30, pp 423–425, 1976.

2. Henry M. *Med J Aust* V2, p 844, 1976.

3. Obituary, Henry Miller. *J Neurol Sci* V30, pp 423–425, 1976.

4. Cohen, M., Vidamer D. Two Norwegian Neurological Giants. *J Med Biogr* V6, pp 194–199, 1998.

5. Edstrom L, Lennart G. Obituary, Eric Kugelberg 1913–1983. *Muscle Nerve* V8, p 258, 1985.

6. Aird R. Karl Gunnar Wohlfart March 9, 1910–March 23, 1961. *Neurology* V7, pp 839–840, 1961.

7. Trojoborg W. Fritz Buchthal, MD (1907–2003). *Neurology* V62, pp 1482–1483, 2004.

8. Horowitz S, Krarup C, Frirz Buchthal MD. *Muscle Nerve* V30, pp 1–2, 2004.

9. Baeck E. Ludo van Bogaert and the Bunge Institute. *Eur J Neurol* V12, pp 181–88, 2005.

10. Richardson EP, Julius Hallervorden. In Auschwitz, *Founders of Child Neurology*. Norman Publishing, San Francisco, 1990.

11. Kahle W. Hugo Spatz (1888–1969). *Z Mikrosk Anat Forsch* V82, pp 1–6, 1970.

12. Krucke W. Hugo Spatz (2 September 1988–27 January 1969). *Verh Dtsch Ges Pathol* V54, pp 598–605, 1970.

13. Shevell M. Racial Hygiene: Active Euthanasia and Julius Hallervorden. *Neurology* V42, pp 2214–2219, 1992.

14. Aly G, Chroust P, Pross C. *Cleansing the Fatherland Nazi Medicine and Racial Hygiene* (Belinda Cooper trans.). Johns Hopkins University Press, Baltimore, 1994.

15. Strous RD, Edelman MC. Eponyms and the Nazi Era: Time to Remember and Time for Change. *Isr Med Assoc J* V9, pp 207–214, 2007.

16. Georges Schaltenbrand (1897–1979). *J Neurol* V223, pp 153–158, 1980.

17. Jones, EG. Two minds. *Nature* V421, pp 19–20, 2003.

18. Klatzo I, (with Gabriele ZuRhein), Cecile, Oskar Vogt. *The Visionaries of Modern Neuroscience.* Springer Verlag, 2002, 130 pp (*Acta Neurochirurgica* Supplement 80).

19. Jonas G. *The Circuit Riders: Rockefeller Money and the Rise of Modern Science.* WW Norton & Co., New York, 1989.

20. Lhermitte F, Lecours, AR, Signoret JL. Obituary Théophile Alajouanine (1890–1980). *Brain Lang* V13, pp 191–196, 1981.

21. Adams RD. Influence de Jean Martin Charcot sue la neurologie l'enseignement—médical et la psychologie aux Etats—Unis. *Bull Acade Natle Med* V177, pp 877–881, 1993.

22. Adams RD. Armand Duchene (1806–1875). In Haymaker W, Schiller F. (ed.), *The Founders of Neurology* (2nd ed.). Charles C Thomas Publisher, Springfield, IL, pp 430–435.

The Bullard Professor: Massachusetts General Hospital 1954–1977

After his sabbatical year in Europe Ray Adams returned to Boston and created the first modern department of neurology with many subspecialty divisions. In a division of neuroimmunology Adams and Byron Waksman continued the study of demyelinative disease of the central and peripheral nervous system. With Maurice Victor[1] he continued to study acquired metabolic diseases of the nervous system. C. Miller Fisher,[2,3] who had arrived from Montreal, headed a division for study of cerebrovascular disease. Philip Dodge[4] was recruited to head up pediatric neurology. A few years later Richard Sidman was recruited to head a division of experimental neuropathology, where Paul Yakolev[5] continued his study and teaching of neuroanatomy. During the decades of further expansion, the resident staff grew from a handful to twenty-four, and Ray Adams created an original program of resident education. Research space grew from a few rooms to eight floors of laboratories by his retirement. These productive years were punctuated by conflict with the departments of pediatrics, psychiatry, and neurosurgery and with the medical students and the medical school dean. [see Figures 25–28]

RL: *Tell me about your return to Massachusetts General Hospital from the sabbatical year in Europe.*

RA: Miller Fisher continued our studies of cerebrovascular disease. He took that over when he came in 1954.

RL: *Maurice Victor already had been there.*

RA: Yes, Maurice was working with me on metabolic diseases of the nervous system, anemia, hyperammonemia, and vitamin deficiency states. So we were fairly active in investigative work, I think, for the first time at the Mass. General. And I was extremely pleased at how the service was shaping up.

RL: *How were you supporting these doctors?*

RA: By here and there and fellowships and things like that. Hit or miss. . .never on a very secure basis. The people that we had working were not at all demanding. They were just pleased to be part of a developing service.

RL: *You were on the search committee that chose Stanley Cobb's successor as psychiatry chairman.*

RA: Yes. The committee chairman was Alan Butler who was the chief of pediatrics. Dean Clark, who was director of the hospital, and myself were strongly opposed to Lindemann and anyone in psychoanalysis. And that committee went in circles, trying to select someone for a period of about two years. And finally, Clark came to me and said that "it was useless; you'd better just give up," and Lindemann was appointed. Lindemann[6] got involved in social psychiatry, studying the effect of moving the Italian population, living behind the hospital, to other places. I think that was a weak appointment. Dean Clark and I were the only two on the committee opposed to Lindemann's appointment.

RL: *How did you organize the neurology residency program?*

RA: I favored the notion that it is better to have the first-year resident exposed not only to inpatient neurology but also to the outpatient clinic neurology, emergency ward neurology, neurosurgical neurology, and to neurophysiologic techniques. That's such a variety of things. He can't spend enough time to be expert in all of these fields, but he will know what is within their compass, whether he is attracted to any of them, as a possibility for his own further development. After a year spent that way, we moved them to neuropathology for the study of disease process during the second year. Then, for the third year, they were senior residents, with the background of the first two years.

One of the most successful steps was to rotate our residents through neurosurgery. Before that, neurosurgical residents and neurology residents were in constant conflict, fighting over whether a lumbar puncture should be done on a patient. The neurology residents would say "no" and the surgical ones "yes," and they would go to the chiefs, and we would get together and argue. Very bad feelings in general. I was sending some cases to the Leahey Clinic, where the surgical results were good.

RL: *This is a 1961 letter from Walter Bauer that implies that there is a breach between neurology and neurosurgery.*

RA: He was chairman of medicine. Our residents were clashing. And I decided to rotate every resident three months in neurosurgery because they had to learn to live with neurosurgeons. They could be helpful both before and after operations, and that put the quietus on the whole matter of disagreement between the two services. Also we accepted the neurosurgical residents for three months and then for three months in neuropathology. Then Bob Ojemann came along and was a superb neurosurgeon, very gentle. So we were all working as a team together, and everyone had friends on the other service.

We also arranged for each adult neurologist, in his third year, to have a three-month exposure to newborns in the critical care unit and to children's neurology. It was during this period that they went to the Shriver Center and were exposed to patients in our evaluation clinic and to those being studied for various diseases. I gave conferences every week on such cases.

RL: *What other changes did you make?*

RA: I felt strongly that every neurologist should be exposed to some psychiatry. And I tried to arrange for a rotation through Eric Lindemann, who succeeded Cobb as chairman. He was strongly against it and was very upset with me because he was aware of my unwillingness to accept psychoanalysis as a valid approach to psychiatry. He was not at all sympathetic to neurology or to me. (He knew of my opposition to his appointment.) Eventually, he agreed that we could send our resident for two or three months under the direction of one of his assistants. All of the residents, psychiatry and neurology, would not wear uniforms. They would sit with nurses and patients and talk about their sex lives and their personal problems. Our residents rebelled and went on strike after about six months.

So then I decided to go out to McLean Hospital. This was still in the 50s. I found the director a rather inept man, quite willing to let our residents come out there. In fact, he even agreed to pay for one resident a year, if we could rotate one every three months. And at that time I started going out. And I placed there one of our staff in neurology, to be the neurologist for McLean, to see neurological consultations or psychiatric cases with some neurological aspects. Our residents were working up cases like regular residents in psychiatry. So we were one of the few services in the country that included psychiatry and neurosurgery as part of our rotation.

Between these rotations and seeing neurological consultations in the general hospital and seeing an increasing proportion of the stroke cases and having a commitment to spend some time in the emergency ward, which had suddenly enlarged to about nearly 90,000 cases a year, our residency was probably as varied as any in the country. That and the rotation in neuropathology made it quite distinctive. Our general idea was that you didn't have to spend a lot of time in any of these fields. You had to know what is included in each field and to get some exposure to it, rather than spending the first year just seeing cases of stroke and multiple sclerosis and things like that. So I was pleased with how the service developed.

RL: *Tell me more about the neuropathology rotation in your residency program.*

RA: I had decided that the residents should spend their second year working full time in the neuropathology lab. This included removing brains, spinal cords, nerves, and muscles and preparing representative blocks of tissue for microscopic study. I would supervise them to some extent on Tuesdays, when the most interesting cases were the subject of our weekly brain cutting in the afternoon. We had a microscopic conference in the evening. In the spring, the residents attended a six-week course in neuropathology and served as instructors of Harvard Medical students. Without a single exception the residents considered that period, when they studied neuroanatomy and pathogenesis of disease and neuropathology, their most valuable year of education after medical school. I think that our service was the only one in the country that offered that kind of training.

RL: *Tell me about the gross brain cutting.*

RA: I think I had a fairly active role in developing the clinicopathological gross conferences over at city hospital, and I transferred them immediately to the Mass.
General. In traveling in Europe, I had never seen a place where clinicians were
brought together and were asked to analyze the clinical data of a case in hand
and where the gross pathology would then be exposed. The clinicians in general
tended to be arrogant and considered any challenge to their ideas below their dignity. I found that it was very helpful to everyone to ask good clinicians to analyze
the data and then to show the nervous system lesion and to be able to validate
certain concepts of neurophysiology, psychology, anatomy and so on.

I believe at the Boston City we had the first such conference weekly, certainly
in the Boston area. I never saw that at Salpetriere or Queen Square. I remember seeing Greenfield[7] cut brains. He would try to put together the anatomy and
the histopathology, but he almost never had a clinician there, unless the clinician
just wanted to see what his patient had at autopsy. Charles Kubik never had such
conferences. I learned about the anatomy of lesions from him—the neurologists
and psychiatrists never came—I was a privileged audience. So I think this macro-
scopic conference proved to be a valuable method, at Mass. General, where it still
is carried on regularly and is well attended.

RL: *Tell me about the microscopic conferences.*

RA: We started something else that was extremely interesting and valuable. On the day
of our neuropathology gross conference we would stay over in the evening and
have a microscopic conference, where we would start with an array of sections
of a case. Everyone would study them without knowledge of the case and try to
reconstruct the gross pathology and to predict the underlying disease and what the
clinical picture must have been.

Our residents and fellows all attended; each one would study the sections
and express his opinion. I would summarize the findings and diagnosis. Peirson Richardson,[8-10] who selected the cases, would finally reveal what the disease
was. This type of study showed the weakness of present-day histological methods...served as a way of reevaluating them. In other words it challenged the
microscopic pathology of disease and challenged the neuropathologist. The blunders that we made were instructive. We had a neuropathologist from England that
was most well known for his work in children's neuropathology. We showed three
cases: one was Down's syndrome, one was cretinism, and one was autism. He could
not make a diagnosis from a large array of microscopic slides in any of these three
cases. So I think that conference was a development, of which I was very proud.

RL: *What was the impact of requiring the year of neuropathology training in the second year
of neurology residency?*

RA: The residents, after this year, leapt ahead two or three years in their grasp of clinical
neurology and usually authored one or two papers in some related subject.

RL: *Did you have a particular approach to selecting residents?*

RA: No, you really can't. I think you pick the ones that sort of impress you as being
bright, able, and personable. Whether an applicant is well mannered has to be

taken into account. Many of the first residents, that we had, were mediocre. But, increasingly, we obtained applicants that were highly talented. And it turned out that probably 75% or 80% of them went into academic medicine.

RL: *It is said that you would occasionally take a resident who was atypical.*

RA: Yes, if they were brilliant and able in some way or other—not conventional. I always thought that if you had seven sound residents, we could handle one like that.

RL: *Did any of those work out well?*

RA: You never could tell. John Barlow lasted about six months as a resident. (Weiner at MIT thought that, of all the physicians he knew, Barlow was the brightest mathematician.) He stayed on, working in neurophysiology with Molly Brazier in my department. He stayed a neurophysiologist. Dick Sidman stayed a year as a resident and did some neuropathology. Ken Wolf[11] was a brilliant pianist, a prodigy who graduated from Yale at the age of fourteen or so and was interested in the nervous system. So I took him on. After three months, he went over to our experimental neuropath lab at Harvard with Dick Sidman. And then he went to University of Massachusetts as professor of neuroanatomy.

RL: *Did any of the brilliant, unconventional people end up as clinical neurologists or professors of neurology?*

RA: Not really.

RL: *Tell me more about your approach to resident education.*

RA: I encouraged scholarship and always to be searching out something new in every patient and to read extensively so they would know, to some extent, what was already known and what wasn't known. Throughout their exposure they were encouraged to make careful clinical observations, to write up their observations, and report them in journals. I used to chide them with the remark that an observant person could not work on the adult service for a month without finding some phenomena that had never been described and was in need of careful study.

RL: *You told me that you supported the development of residents and fellows by putting them on to a subject and then letting them study the topic. You had to have the right kind of person, didn't you?*

RA: Well, yes; I never figured a way of determining whether someone, who wanted to do research, really would turn out to be any good at it.

RL: *There was no predictor?*

RA: I didn't think there was. Someone would come along and be sort of flubbing around and turn out very well. Another fellow would come in, spouting ideas a mile a minute, big talker, and would never do a thing. I don't think that you can look at a man and tell whether he's going to be an original thinker and highly productive investigator. So my tendency was, if they wanted to try themselves out for a year in research and continue teaching and making rounds, to give them all a chance. At the end of a year it would usually turn out that those, who were inept, would decide that they didn't really want to do research.

RL: *You played tennis with residents. Would you just hit the ball around or would you try to win the game?*

RA: No, I would always try to win. And I always took pleasure in taking a resident, who was a little bit cocky, and beating him on the tennis court.

RL: *I see that you were seldom the sole author of a paper.*

RA: I must remark that very often, when someone else was involved with me, they were junior members of the staff, and I had put them on the problem. Then I had written the article, mostly by myself, putting their name on it.

RL: *That seems very generous.*

RA: I thought that was a good policy because it helped young people get started. For example, most of the chapters in Harrison's *Principles of Internal Medicine* were coauthored with residents and research fellows, but I had written them pretty much myself.

RL: *Did you ask them to help in any way?*

RA: They went over the chapters, and we talked about it and I put their name on the article. I always thought that, in writing with some younger person, their name should come first to help them enter the field of neurology or neuroscience. And, if I didn't contribute most of the ideas or a good part of them and didn't take an active part in writing, I would leave my name off altogether. I abhorred the practice, common in Europe, of a chief of service putting his name on everything that came out of his department.

RL: *That happens in this country also.*

RA: It happens in places but not to the same extent as I saw it happening in Germany and Switzerland.

RL: *Did you ever use your residents as a way of educating yourself?*

RA: I did that continuously.

RL: *Can you tell me about that?*

RA: I had always had the great advantage of having access to the minds of very bright young doctors. Many of them had come with advanced degrees in science, and others were extremely observant, excellent physicians in internal medicine or pediatrics. So, there were continual discussions and exchanges of ideas and questions on both sides, mine and theirs. That also pertains to the junior members of our staff. Frequently, in discussing some phenomena, it's rather difficult, in retrospect, to know whether your ideas come from yourself or from exchanges with them. We would regularly have meetings, luncheons together, and we'd be discussing every kind of problem. You know very well that their questions and your questions are eliciting answers, the origin of which you forget. So that type of exchange is very important.

RL: *There was a polio epidemic.*

RA: When we had a poliomyelitis epidemic, about 1955 I think, we had many hundreds of cases in a month at the Mass. General Hospital. I remember that we had forty-four of them on respirators at one time, and that was a huge problem. The mortality was quite significant. The residents did their best to try to manage the cases without much tutelage—there was about 25% mortality.

RL: *Were those "iron lung" respirators?*

RA: Yes, the old Drinker type. Cecil Drinker was a professor in the Harvard School of Public Health. He invented the "iron lung."

RL: *Were they electrically powered?*

RA: Yes, if the electricity went off, you were frantic. You had to have someone with the patient 24 hours a day, lest he choke or something like that happen. I remember having to get some recruits from the nearby naval station to help look after our respirator cases. We never stopped admitting patients at the Mass. General, and the hospital was virtually taken over. All of the wards were full with polio during that epidemic, and we had a high mortality. I'm sure we saved a good many, but we had no treatment at all. We were getting two, three, four patients an hour at times.

RL: *Let's turn to your international activity. Please tell me about your relationship with Switzerland.*

RA: The real contact with Lausanne[12] came around 1959. I had gone to England to attend the 100th anniversary for the National Hospital of Neurological Disease, and I remember commenting on some papers that were presented there. At the time Michelle Jequier happened to be in attendance, and we met. He asked if I would come to Lausanne and spend some time and give some lectures to the residents or assistants in his division of neurology. I agreed.

So we went there. Each day I would go in the morning to his service and sometimes in the afternoon I would give a talk to the assistants. I discovered very soon, when I attempted to lecture in English, that despite their versatility with language, most of the assistants could not speak English. So I quickly turned to French and began trying to perfect myself in the language well enough to give my talks and clinics in French. And, of course, in interrogating patients, it was necessary to speak their language. (Lausanne is a French-speaking part of Switzerland.) I was able to get along fairly well, and toward the end of the summer I gave a final address to them in French.

It was sufficiently successful that he asked if I would make arrangements to come back another time and perform the same service. I think a couple of years lapsed before I went back, but that was the start of an activity which eventually resulted in my being in Switzerland from July 1 to Labor Day each summer for almost nineteen years.

RL: *Did anybody complain about these long absences from Mass. General?*

RA: They came to accept it.

RL: *Was there any resentment?*

RA: I don't know. I received appointment as an adjunct physician, University of Lausanne. I still retain that position. The second time I went, Jequier very kindly had arranged for me to rent a villa about 15 kilometers from the center of Lausanne. That was very agreeable. And then in the afternoons, I resumed playing golf, which I had not done since my college days.

Neurology was in a curious state there. Jequier was not given anything more than a very nominal title in the University; it was all under internal medicine. He had no standing in the university affairs; all that was taken care of by the rather autocratic professor of internal medicine. He was strongly averse to giving any degree of autonomy to neurology. He thought it was just part of medicine, and that was that. We had many discussions about it, and I found him extremely rigid and resistant to any ideas. We had several rather heated exchanges over lunch tables in restaurants. So it was impossible to work through him.

Finally a strategy, that occurred to me, was to elevate Jequier, who was a very polished clinical neurologist and knew neuropathology fairly well. I invited him to Massachusetts General Hospital for a month as an exchange professor. So that was a credit to him and an indication to the university that, although they didn't recognize him as a professor, Harvard University would. And that was the beginning of a series of changes that gradually came about. About three or four years later, they moved neurology to two floors in a new building, an excellent physical plant. And Jequier was then elevated to what they call a, "professor extra-ordinare"—sort of a part-time professor.

And I, in the years that followed, would go there and see patients twice a week, I think. I would have an early afternoon outpatient clinic, in which the assistants would present to me a case. Sometimes, I would tell them about something, they had never heard of. I remember an amusing incident. I had been at the American Neurological Association meeting in Atlantic City, when Steele and Richardson had presented their material on supranuclear ophthalmoplegia. One of the first cases they presented to me, when I went to Lausanne, was a case of that. They had never seen it. I remarked that, "This is a very well known phenomenon in the States; we're quite familiar with this rare disease." Of course, I had never seen a case myself!

The clinics were often very interesting and quite stimulating to me. On the other mornings I would go to neuropathology. Ted Rabinowicz[13] was in charge of neuropathology. He had been brought there after having been educated in Munich in the old clinic of Spielmeyer. He was one of my closest friends in the years that followed. He was a charming, bright, wonderfully sympathetic fellow.

Through the support of Jequier, and the chief of pathology, they gave him an entire floor of laboratories including an electron microscope. It was established as the autonomous Institute of Neuropathology. (This was a huge institute with about 2,000 or 3,000 autopsies a year.) He had access to that material, as well as extraordinary material on children's diseases. Through Rabinowicz, I had a laboratory there and my own microscope. Each morning I would have laid out before me the most interesting of the past year's children's neuropathology, and I had access to the various books on neurology and neuropathology in his library. And I would talk to the residents and fellows; it was a delightful experience.

Later Rabinowicz spent six months in our department in Mass. General, and Richardson spent six months in the Institute of Neuropathology in Lausanne. So there was a good exchange there. In the meantime, as Jequier's status improved, we began to exchange residents and fellows.

And they had no children's neurology in Lausanne. There was a professor of pediatrics by the name of Gautier, who was very sympathetic to the idea of having children's neurology. He arranged for me to have clinic presentations in the afternoons. I did that five or six times on topics that were relevant to children's neurology and he was very supportive. Later, he sent a man named Deonna to us in Mass. General; he spent three years as resident, then two years in pediatrics and since then he's been the children's neurologist for the University of Lausanne. I visited him five years or so ago; he had an excellent service with one or two extremely well-informed assistants with large clinical experience. There were others that came over on our service.

RL: *Could you summarize your effect on neurology in Lausanne?*

RA: I introduced them to clinical demonstrations with live patients; they hadn't done that before. I was helpful in getting neurology independent from internal medicine and encouraging the development of a division of children's neurology. Under Jequier and his successor, Lausanne became the strongest neurology department in Switzerland.

RL: *Tell me about your contribution to Lebanese neurology.*

RA: The main thing, that I helped with, was the arrangement for their residents to come work on our service at MGH. Many returned to Lebanon and occupied important places in medicine there.

Fuad Sabra was a fellow with us and became the chief of neurology at American University. Atwah, his successor, spent three years as a neurology resident with me. Rosemary Boustamy spent four years with us and is about to hold the first endowed chair of neuroscience at American University. Jean Rebeiz worked four years in neuropathology with Peirson Richardson and me and went to American University as chairman of Pathology and of Neuropathology. The chairman of pediatrics at American University was with us for three years. I went there quite a number of times to give lectures. I gave the second Penfield lecture there.

RL: *Please comment on your experience with medical student education.*

RA: It has distressed me that there's a tendency to curtail the amount of science in the first two years of medical school, assuming that such matters as cell chemistry genetics, statistics, etc., taken in the university before they come to medical school, are adequate. The tendency now, to an increasing extent, is to accede to the student's desire to immediately become a doctor and start wandering around the community with a stethoscope around his neck, taking on the care of poor patients. It would seem to me that the advances in science are so rapid and extensive that, if anything, we should extend the amount of education in the sciences so that a student will be able to understand and apply them to the medicine of the future.

I gave a course in neuropathology, as the basis of clinical neurology and psychiatry. That course was accompanied by twelve lectures and patient demonstrations in clinical neurology, six with Denny-Brown and six with me at the Mass. General. The neuropathology course lasted a month. Each session included an hour lecture followed by two hours of study of slides of representative diseases in the laboratory. The first three lectures were on histopathologic reactions, the next six on categories of disease (vascular, neoplastic etc.) and the last three on correlative neuropathology (organ pathology). I thought it was the best course in neuropathology of any medical school in the country.

Introduction to Neuropathology was really an exposition of the material of the course. The year that it was published the students protested and decided that they would not go to the laboratory and look at representative slides of diseases. It was during that period, when there was an uprising all through the universities. They were tired after the fall, winter, and spring sessions of the second year. They went to the dean and protested, and they said that they wouldn't continue the course, unless I gave each of them a free copy of the textbook. I refused to do that. They told the dean that I was unreasonable. The dean reported this to the curriculum committee, and they thought there was too much neuropathology. I refused to shorten the course, and Dean Robert Ebert said that I didn't need to teach at Harvard anymore. So I never taught neuropathology again after that textbook came out. That was 1968. I had inherited the general format of my course from Stanley Cobb. It had lasted twenty-five years. Dick Sidman took over and abbreviated the course, merged it with a course in neuroanatomy, as I recall. At any rate, I was relieved because it tied up my whole spring, preparing slides and getting instructors.

RL: *As an educational method, you tended to emphasize the exposition of individual cases as opposed to the lecture method. Can you comment on the history of this approach at Massachusetts General Hospital?*

RA: Yes. Going back to the time of James Jackson Putnam in the 1870s, 80s, 90s, the Ether Dome presentations had always been a demonstration of a patient and a solicitation of the opinions of members of the staff about diagnosis and therapy. I felt that was a good program and should be continued in neurology. My predecessor, Ayer, did that regularly, always with a patient. And his secretary Miss Gryzebienowska (known as Miss G. because Ayer could not pronounce her name) always made a shorthand recording of the main features of these cases and the response of the staff. They were published each year in a volume of Ether Dome cases in neurology. I continued that.

RL: *How long had the clinicopathologic conference tradition been going on at Massachusetts General?*

RA: CPC was actually initiated around the turn of the century. There was always a detailed presentation of all the clinical details of a case that an invitee would analyze and diagnose. There followed a presentation of the gross and microscopic pathology and the final diagnosis. That was actually set up by Hugh Cabot,[14] who was professor of medicine. I think the idea was suggested by Walter B. Cannon. Talking to a famous scholar in the law school, Cannon got the idea about 1900, that case study was a method that could be transferred to medicine. The plan was adapted in medicine, in the first decade of the twentieth century, and there are a whole series of books that contain these cases.

RL: *Who was Cannon?*

RA: He was one of the most famous professors at Harvard Medical School. He worked out the physiology of the autonomic nervous system, the use of barium for gastrointestinal display, and the subject of denervation hypersensitivity. He was a brilliant researcher, who should have gotten a Nobel Prize but never did.

RL: *Miller Fisher told me that many from your earliest groups of residents became national figures.*

RA: I made a list of people who had been trained there . . . I gave it to Anne Young. The majority held professorships. That has been one of the outstanding features of the neurology service at Mass. General, the number who have pursued an academic career.

RL: *Do you have any summary comments on your training programs?*

RA: We were getting some of the better residents in the country, and it turned out that about 75% or 80% of the residents wanted to do research, to add to knowledge, and it was common practice for them to obtain, for two, three, four years, a research fellowship from NIH. One could obtain such fellowships almost for the asking. And, as a result of this type of residency and of exposure of some field of neuroscience for two or more years, the majority of them then went into academic medicine.

We began to receive young neurologists, who had been through a residency or assistantship, and wanted to come and work in neuropathology or neurophysiology in our department. Thus we had an interesting group of fellows as well as our own past residents. I calculated there must have been 200–250 residents and fellows during that period, when I was chief of service, who later became professor of neurology at some university in the world. There were eight of them, I think, in Australia, two or three in South Africa, a good many in Western Europe and England. So, from the point of view of academic neurology, I would say that our program proved to be quite a good one. That was the state it was in, when Joe Martin took over in 1977.

RL: *What did Joe Martin do?*

RA: He expanded the department to the fields of neuroendocrinology and genetics. He was more popular at the hospital than I was.

RL: *What do you mean?*

RA: I was not highly regarded by the other services at the Mass. General; they thought I was neglectful because I didn't attend committee meetings or faculty meetings. I did go once a week to the Chiefs of Staff meeting, but I usually went late. It was probably a defect in my personality.

Notes

1. Johnson RT. Maurice Victor: 1920–2001. *Ann Neurol* V50, p 831, 2001.

2. Trobe JD. C. Miller Fisher: The Master of Clinicopathologic Correlation.

3. Adams RD, Richardson EP. Salute to C. Miller Fisher. *Arch Neurol* V38, pp 137–139, 1981.

4. Cole H. Health-Care Heroes: Dr. Phil Dodge. *St. Louis Business Journal.* November 11, 2005.

5. Kemper T. Paul Ivan Yakovlev. *Arch Neurol* V41, pp 536–540, 1984.

6. Satin DG. Erich Lindemann: The Humanist and the Era of Community Mental Health. *Proc Am Philos Soc* V126, pp 327–346, 1982.

7. Obituary, Joseph Godwin Greenfield. *Lancet* V1(7019), pp 540–541, 1958.

8. Richardson Jr. EP, Astrom KE, Kleihus P. The Development of Neuropathology at the Massachusetts General Hospital and Harvard Medical School. *Brain Pathol* V4, pp 181–195, 1994.

9. White TH, Pope A, Adams R. Dr. Edward Peirson Richardson, Jr., Harvard University Gazette, December 16, 2004.

10. Hedley-White T. In Memory of Dr. Edward Peirson Richardson. *Brain Pathol* V9, pp 415–417, 1999.

11. The Shoes of a Man, *Time*, Monday, November 21, 1949.

12. Jequier M. Neurologie lausannoise. *Rev Med Suisse Roman cle* V94, pp 873–885, 1974.

13. de Courlen-Myers GM. In Memory of Theodore Rabinowicz (1919–1995). *Brain Pathol* V5, pp 195–196, 1995.

14. Crenner C. Diagnosis and Authority in the Early Twentieth-Century Medical Practice of Richard C. Cabot. *Bull Hist Med* V76, pp 30–55, 2002.

Building Pediatric Neurology

Development of child neurology at Massachusetts General Hospital was delayed by the resistance of the department of pediatrics. Eventually, with the help of the National Institutes of Health, Ray Adams established a formal program for educating residents in pediatric neurology. With a Kennedy Foundation grant and the support of the hospital trustees, the Kennedy Laboratories for research were built on top of the Burnham Pediatrics Building. Additionally, Ray Adams was the central figure in the founding of the Shriver Center for mental retardation on the campus of Fernald School. At this institute, laboratory research, clinical observation, patient care, and resident education flourished. By building these programs and through his own writings, Ray Adams assumed a prominent role in advancing pediatric neurology as a formal field of study. [see Figures 29 and 30]

RL: *Tell me about the pediatric aspect of your own neurology training.*

RA: As a resident at Massachusetts General I had no exposure to pediatric neurology. Higgins, chairman of pediatrics, forbade neurologists from coming to the pediatric service.

RL: *Had you exposure to child neurology at Boston City Hospital?*

RA: The chairman of pediatrics, Martin English, had no respect at all for neurology, and he refused to allow anyone from the neurological research unit on the wards of the children's building. He was very arbitrary and argumentative and influential, since he was a trustee of the Boston City Hospital. Occasionally a neurologist would sneak into the pediatric building at night. I remember going over to see an adolescent girl, paralyzed by a spinal epidural abscess; the pediatricians had called it polio. So, all of the pediatric neurology was beyond the preserve of the neurological service. That bothered me considerably.

I realized that I knew very little about children's neurology. To acquire experience in the field I made an arrangement to consult each week on neurologic cases at the Boston Floating Hospital. I agreed to examine children that they'd be puzzled about, as part of my work at Pratt Diagnostic Hospital (later New England Center). In two to three years I acquired a fairly large experience in children's neurology. I decided, by virtue of my experience at the Boston Floating Hospital and New England Center, that pediatric neurology would benefit if joined to an accredited neurology service and that an adult neurology service would also benefit. Of course, pediatricians were, for the most part, opposed.

RL: *What happened when you left Boston City Hospital and returned to Massachusetts General Hospital?*

RA: When I went to the Mass. General I encountered the same problem as at Boston City Hospital. Higgins was still chief of pediatrics. He resisted any formal relations with adult neurology, insisting that the neurologists were ignorant of children's problems. He would not let any of the neurologists see his cases on the pediatric service.

RL: *Why did you have this difficulty with the pediatricians at both Boston City and Massachusetts General Hospital?*

RA: National problem. The pediatricians were autonomous.

RL: *Did they feel that they knew everything about children's neurologic problems?*

RA: Yes, and that the neurologists did not. Certainly none of the neurologists at Mass. General were experienced with children. They (the pediatricians) were probably correct. On the other hand, the pediatricians had no formal training in neurology or neuropathology, and their attitude stultified the emergence of pediatric neurology.

At that time there were only three neurologists specializing in children's diseases. One was Frank Ford in John's Hopkins. The second one was Buchanan at University of Chicago and the third, Bronson Crothers at Children's Hospital in Boston. Bronson Crothers was the one we knew best, and he had never really been trained in neurology. He had very little concept of anything except birth injuries, about which he wrote very well.

During the 1930s and 1940s and before there was no place where a separate division of children's neurology existed, as far as I know. There had been some excellent studies of development of the nervous system by psychologists and neurologists, but they were working by themselves for the most part. Yakovlev began collecting anatomical material from mental hospitals in the 1930s and 1940s, but the cases had not been studied clinically. He assembled only isolated pathologic specimens and lacked normal controls.

RL: *How did things get moving at Massachusetts General Hospital?*

RA: At about this time, through the influence of Houston Merritt, the National Institute of Neurology and Blindness, it was called, decided that children's neurology
should be supported, and the first grants were given to Columbia University and to
our service at MGH. I think ours was the second. It was with that money that we
were able to get some adult neurologists trained in children's neurology. The first
one was Philip Dodge, who was in the Army at the time. He spent one of his years
in the army in pediatrics in Hawaii. When he returned to Boston, having already
had a neurology residency at Boston City Hospital, he was appointed an assistant
professor of neurology with a specialty in children's affairs.

About that time, when Phil Dodge was ready to help with that work, Higgins
had resigned and Alan Butler had replaced him as professor of pediatrics at Mass.
General. Butler was a gracious, liberal descendant of an old New England family.
He and I took a liking to one another. He understood the problem of neurology in
pediatrics very well and was extremely helpful in arranging for me and our residents
and staff to see all of the children's cases.

RL: *Tell me about your teaching of child neurology to residents.*

RA: Phil Dodge was eminently successful in setting up a training program. We decided
to always have one or two of the resident appointments in neurology spend their
second or third year in pediatric neurology. Phil and I decided that they all had to
do a year of adult neurology first, since you can't obtain a complete idea of how the
nervous system works from children alone.

RL: *Was there no model for that system elsewhere?*

RA: Not as far as I knew. And that plan has been pretty widely adopted. When Phil left
for Washington University in St. Louis, I did the children's neurology for a short
time again, and then Peter Huttenlocher took over. Peter was a fine neurologist,
had been through our program. And then, when he left for University of Chicago,
Bob DeLong came; he was highly successful.

RL: *Tell me about the origins of the mental retardation initiative.*

RA: With Butler's help we were able to approach the Kennedy Foundation, asking for a
grant to support child's neurology. The Shrivers had earlier contacted Dean Berry
at Harvard Medical School, but they were irritated by his response. When I heard
that the Kennedy Foundation was interested in giving money to Harvard, David
Crockett, our fundraiser, and I drew up a plan for research for mental retardation.
David Crockett contacted the Shrivers, who formed a committee.

Eunice Shriver bought their trustees to Boston. The committee was peopled
by two or three mental retardation supporters, who did not have any use for neurology. We had an all-day session. And I saw that it was going badly. We were asking
for three million; I thought we would get nothing. The committee included Camp-
bell who was a professor of medicine in Chicago. He had been a patient of mine.
So I took him apart during the lunch period and implored his help. He persuaded
some of them to change their minds, and by four o'clock that afternoon they made
an offer. David Crockett refused to accept it! He folded his arms, stating that such
a piddling sum was useless. Then they went to dinner instead of going back to the

airport. They came back and offered one million, two hundred thousand to support a unit to be called Kennedy Laboratories at Massachusetts General Hospital.

I received a phone call the following day from Joe Kennedy, saying that he had spoken to Cardinal Cushing who approved of it. (I suppose he felt better having the approval of the church for such a grant in Boston, and ours was the first grant they'd ever made for scientific study or medical investigation.)

RL: *I gather that Eunice Shriver was there for this meeting?*

RA: She was there as was Sargeant Shriver, her husband. A second research grant was made to Bob Cook at Hopkins. Then followed others at Chicago, Wisconsin, Stanford, and Peabody College in Nashville. Prior to our grant the Kennedy Foundation had supported homes for patients with mental retardation but not research.

Half of the money was saved, and the income was used for putting together the Kennedy laboratory staff. I used $500,000 to add 2 floors to the pediatric building at Mass. General for Kennedy labs. I brought in a number of people, experienced biochemists, Hugo Moser, who had been through our residency in adult neurology, Mary Efron,[1] a brilliant protein chemist, and Vivian Shih. Phil Dodge began working on metabolic diseases in animals and humans. Murray Sidman, the brother of Richard Sidman, put together a group of behavioristic psychologists. They used Skinnerian techniques that would be applicable to verbal and nonverbal mentally retarded individuals, and that would allow us to more completely assess their nervous system function.

That was the second or first pediatric neurology program in America. We had a very lively group then.

RL: *What do you mean by Skinnerian techniques?*

RA: Patients were put in testing situations, whereby they would be rewarded for a correct response but not for an incorrect one. The classic example, that we had, was a microcephalic idiot. Cosmo his name was. He was shown a circle, which would disappear if he punched a button but not if he saw an oval or some other figure. A correct response was rewarded. And they finally could, without using language at all, just giving him M and M chocolates for a correct response, but not for an incorrect one, show that he could distinguish an ellipse from a circle.

RL: *Was this study published?*

RA: Yes, it was published by Murray Sidman. It took a year to teach Cosmo the letters of the alphabet. He only had three partial words in his vocabulary. I gave a lecture on his performance in New Castle, England, showing a way of studying the function of the brain in nonverbal humans.

The point was to study his visual perception; you could not test it in any other way. Murray Sidman had perfected these techniques with three assistants. He not only used this method of rewards to get positive responses for vision. He later took over a ward at the Fernald School for those with the most severe behavioral abnormalities, all males, unable to keep on their clothes or eat from a dish or control their sphincters. He had them all under control within about six months, so that they could stay dressed, sit at a table, and perform quite satisfactorily.

RL: *I gather that this improvement came from rewarding their good behavior.*

RA: Yes. So within a year or two we had a research unit in the new laboratories in the children's building and a team of people, chemists, psychologists, neurologists, and neuropathologists, who were quite productive.

It went very well for a time, but when Alan Butler retired, we discovered that the new head of pediatrics, Nathan Talbott, was very much opposed to a separate neurology service. He would allow us to examine the neurological cases, which made up about 25% of pediatric admissions, but not to prescribe for them. He discouraged the admission of retardates. He opposed the promotion of Philip Dodge, who was a popular clinician and others, who had been trained by Dodge. Our relationship with Talbott was the main reason for moving part of the Kennedy labs to Fernald School.

I had already decided that a vast population of severe neurologic diseases was being consigned to mental retardation asylums and was out of the orbit of neuroscience. Fortunately, the superintendent of the Fernald School, Malcolm Farrell, was very receptive. Hugo Moser played a large part in getting the federal money to set up a separate institute at Fernald. It was to be a four-floor new building with an adjacent one-floor outpatient clinic building for evaluating patients with mental handicap.

It was built and opened in 1968. (We named it after Eunice Shriver, since she had been extremely helpful and supportive after the initial grant for the Kennedy Laboratories.) We were able to evaluate 2,000 patients a year on the grounds of Fernald School. Fortunately, the commissioner of mental health for the state of Massachusetts was a former teacher and colleague of mine, Harry Solomon. And he was very supportive, persuaded the state to contribute 1/3 of the money for the building of this institute. This was an excellent arrangement. It included a ward of about fifteen or sixteen beds; so we could take sick patients from Fernald School and give them good medical care. We would send them to the Mass. General, if their illness was severe. Most of the staff of Kennedy laboratory at MGH moved out to the Fernald School. The brilliant Mary Efron and her protégés, Vivian Shih and Harvey Levy, stayed at the Mass. General continuing their surveys of all the newborns. I moved my office over to the new part of the pediatric building and served as director of the Shriver Center. The Kennedy Foundation did not give money for the new building at Fernald School. That was all done by the federal government and state government.

RL: *Is the Fernald School the same institution where you had visited Paul Yakovlev for neuroanatomy lessons?*

RA: Yes, the same one.

RL: *So there was some scientific activity there already.*

RA: Only in so far as Yakovlev, who had moved into the state system, was able to collect some brains of individuals who had died there. He, I think, did very little in the way of study of disease per se.

Once we had that center paid for and open, we were in a position to pursue this interest of extending neurology to this whole field of mental retardation. The first thing that was undertaken was to obtain a general orientation in the entire field. Hugo Moser took the lead in this with the assistance of Lou Holmes, a pediatrician at Mass. General. They made a survey and a detailed analysis of all the main categories of neurologic disease that existed there. They found, in going through the Fernald material, there were 1,300 cases with central nervous system abnormalities. They divided them into those due to chromosomal disease, acquired injuries of various kinds, hereditary metabolic diseases, developmental abnormalities and so on. And they produced a superb atlas[2] that pictured each of the main diseases. They gave a summary of the clinical forms of the disease, the pathology with illustrations, the genetics, if there was such, the diagnostic methods, and treatment and means of prevention. That atlas was published in 1972.

RL: *Were you co-author?*

RA: No. I did not co-author that. I, as director of the Shriver Center, helped sponsor it. I encouraged Hugo Moser[3] and he engaged other authors. Some of the cases I had discussed at my weekly conferences. We talked over the whole format of the book and the format of case presentations.

It was interesting. About a third of the cases, more than a third, could not be categorized. They had some abnormality that we could not unravel. And about 20% had chromosomal abnormalities and about 20% had some acquired injury, and a very small percent had hereditary metabolic diseases that could be studied by biochemical methods. The latter group was expanded, and within a few years there were more than 200 hereditary metabolic diseases that could be identified by biochemical methods.

The next thing that was done was to organize the different divisions of the Shriver Center and recruit staff. We eventually had about fifty chemists, geneticists, neuropsychologists, and pathologists all working in this unit. We were able to get funds for animal laboratories. Hugo Moser became the director of the biochemical division, which was probably the largest part, and Vern Caviness and Roger Williams took over the study of developmental disorders of the human nervous system.

The next objective was to recruit a medical staff for the Fernald School itself. The physicians that they had been able to hire to provide medical care for the mentally retarded were often immigrants, who did not know our language very well, who were themselves trained in different ways and not familiar with medical practice here. So the staff of the Fernald School was really a motley group. I remember there was one Chinese woman who always prescribed tea for any sick patient that was in the Fernald School; she was never known to prescribe any other medicine. So, one of our objectives was to gradually replace these people with some of our neurology staff at Mass. General and to provide the kind of care that the patients deserved.

As part of the general education plan, we began to rotate our residents in their third year, while they were studying pediatric neurology, to the Shriver Center for a month. They would participate also in an outpatient evaluation center to see how the patients were studied, and, at the same time, they would make rounds on many of the inpatients in the Fernald School. So they were taught the importance of this part of neurology, which would certainly influence them in the years ahead. As a consequence, many of them became quite interested and pursued some problem within the field.

We also studied the older people who had resided in the Fernald School all their lives. And in going through that material, we found that there were a good many people who had been at Fernald School just because there was no other place for them to live. They were not very severely affected. They were discharged.

From that time I began lecturing here and there on the whole matter of mental retardation, pointing out that probably the largest group of cases of central nervous system disease in America resided in institutions for the mentally retarded. If you accept the figure that 0.5% of all the population are severely mentally retarded and 3% are mentally backward to the point, where often they cannot properly look out for themselves without assistance, you can see how large a category of potential disease must exist in this field. It had hitherto been neglected by medicine. These cases were cast into homes for the retarded, most of them taken over by the state and run very badly. Pediatricians had almost nothing to do with them except to see them before they were sent to the institutions for the mentally retarded, and there was virtually no research going on in the field.

So we felt that we should take the initiative and extend the periphery of neurology to include this large category of disease. Joe Volpe, who's now Professor of Neurology at Boston Children's Hospital, was a product of this environment as were Paul Rossman, professor at Tufts, and Daryl Devivo, professor at Columbia. Volpe and I wrote a paper on the pathology and the developmental derangements in Zellweger disease. My wife, Maria, and I published a paper on the new horizons in child neurology and brought together some of the outstanding works that had been put together by psychologists. I had an extensive paper on neurocutaneous diseases in Fitzpatrick's two-volume dermatology text. With Elizabeth Dooling I had written a paper on the brain of posthemiplegic athetosis, studied in serial section from the Yakovlev collection. My wife and I put together a paper on the effect of maturation on the form of seizures at different periods in life. Rebiez and I wrote a paper on the dystrophic changes in the cerebral cortex as a developmental abnormality. Margaret Bauman, who'd been trained in children's neurology with us, put together her classic studies of the brain abnormalities in autism. Marty Raff went through the program and became a senior scientist at University College, London, and is still one of their most effective investigators. In sum, one of the most significant excursions toward the periphery of neurology came about through the Kennedy Laboratories and the Shriver Center, both affiliated with the Mass. General Hospital.

RL: *What was going on at the Massachusetts General, itself, at this time?*

RA: At the same time we supported strongly a critical care unit at the Mass. General Hospital for neonates who were in difficulty after birth. And that was set up for the purpose of preventing brain damage, and one of our pediatric neurologists took over the field of neonatology.

Robert DeLong was in children's neurology. I arranged for his first visit to Ecuador, since he had expressed interest in iodine deficiency. He spent a month helping Stanbury in a study of cretinism. He then began to devote himself to the effects of iodine on the nervous system in animals as well as on plant life. He carried out some of his studies in Africa and then began to study cretinism and iodine deficiency in a village in western China. He's now doing the same thing in western Mongolia; he takes time off from his professorship at Duke University, where he went from Mass. General. The work of Bob DeLong has been outstanding. We're all extremely proud of that, and it all came because of that little trip down to Ecuador, paid for by Eunice Shriver; she had given me $20,000 as I remember. (And she had given me $20,000–$25,000 a year for several years, which I used to defray the salary of high school students from minority groups in our laboratories out at the Shriver Center.) When Joe Martin succeeded me as chief of neurology at Massachusetts General, he and I went back to the Kennedy Foundation, and Eunice and Sargent Shriver gave us sufficient funds to endow a new Kennedy Professorship in pediatric neurology at the Massachusetts General Hospital.

RL: *How would you approach the Shrivers for money?*

RA: Well we just pointed out that they'd invested so much and that we had done probably more than any of the other institutions to which they had granted money. We needed to consolidate our programs with a full professorship.

RL: *Was Houston Merritt's support of the development of pediatric neurology in New York similar to your endeavors in Boston?*

RA: We both recognized the importance of pediatric neurology. He himself was never involved in any aspect of developmental neurology or child health.

RL: *You played a big role in the opening up of child neurology and mental retardation studies as branches of neurology.*

RA: Yes. This is a chapter in my life that I feel quite satisfied with.

RL: *What has happened to all that you built on the Fernald campus?*

RA: Unfortunately, there was a strong movement in medical circles in the state to eliminate institutions like Fernald School and to transfer even the more severely affected individuals into homes for ten or twelve residents to make things more pleasant for them. So the population, which was about 1,800, when we first were connected with the school, gradually went down. The most recent census showed that there were only 250 or 300 patients left there. The unions had come in and taken over the staff workers and attendants. They were not working well at all; patients were neglected. So a really superb institution, with gymnasia, with every kind of facility you would want for handicapped individuals, had deteriorated. Of course some of the homes for the patients were run by former workers of state mental retardation field; they could make more money by running a home for ten moderately retarded individuals than they could by staying in the state system. Furthermore, during this period, for the first time, the field of mental retardation was taken over by psychologists and executives, who had no real idea of all these problems.

RL: *I see retarded adults, who are living in these group homes, which you mentioned, and I'm not convinced that they are getting care better than they would have had at a large institution.*

RA: I agree. Some of these homes are inadequate. They don't have a gymnasium; they may not exercise them; they may have actually a less stimulating environment or work privilege. Their religious experiences are cut off very often.

One can set up a state run institution, providing all of the things that such individuals need, with extremely good care. I remember, down in Shreveport, I was taken out to see a state institution for 200 mentally retarded individuals. The director was a pediatrician, who knew every patient there and who saw each one daily. And they had every diagnostic method you could expect to use. It was run very efficiently at relatively low cost. I was full of admiration. So it can be done, if one believes in doing it.

Notes

1. Adams RD. Tribute Mary Efron (1926–1967). *Am J Dis Child* V117, pp 2–3, 1969.
2. Holmes LB, Moser HW, Halldórsson S, et al. *Mental Retardation an Atlas of Diseases with Associated Physical Abnormalities*. The Macmillan Company, New York, 1972, 430 p.
3. Raymond GV, Hugo W. Moser, MD(1924–2007). *Arch Neurol.* V64, pp 758–759, 2007.

3

INVESTIGATION AND IDEAS

Metabolic Diseases

The encephalopathies of organ failure were a neglected area of neurology.

Kinnier Wilson's neurology text of 1940, a three-volume work, was the great synthesis of clinical neurology for the first half of the twentieth century. It had an extensive section on "special forms of toxicosis of the nervous system," but there was no section on the metabolic encephalopathies of organ failure. Aside from Wilson's discussion of deficiency and toxic states, his only other mention of acquired metabolic disease was in the discussion of progressive lenticular degeneration (hepato-lenticular degeneration or Wilson Disease).

Recognizing that knowledge of hepatic encephalopathies was limited and that liver disease was endemic at Boston City Hospital, Ray Adams took advantage of an opportunity. He began to systemically study the clinical and pathological features of the acute and chronic hepatic encephalopathies. Adams analyzed his own extensive material in the light of comprehensive reviews of the relevant literature and thereby wrote definitive treatises on the subject. He analyzed other liver–brain relationships such as that of Wilson disease. Liver disease was only one of the acquired metabolic problems, whose neurology he studied and illumined.

LIVER DISEASE

RL: *Charles Davidson would call you to see his patients with liver disease at Boston City Hospital.*

RA: Yes and that led to a clear differentiation between delirium tremens and the wider range of confusional states, including the one associated with hepatic failure.

About this time I began looking carefully at the brains of patients dying of liver cirrhosis. We had an abundancy of cases. For example, there were ninety-nine cases of liver cirrhosis in 1 year in the Mallory Institute of Pathology. And it was in that material that I observed the widespread hyperplasia of protoplasmic astrocytes with very prominent swelling of the astrocyte nuclei all through the gray matter. Ours was not an original observation. I measured the size of the astrocytes and graphed it. I reported on this finding, giving credit to Scherer and a couple of other German workers, at an international neurological meeting in Paris and later, on an enlarged series, at the American Association for Research in Nervous and Mental Disease. [see Chapter 5]

RL: *I noticed, in reading the proceedings of that meeting, that not everybody accepted your findings.*

RA: No. There was a point of disagreement. Abe Baker claimed that he had studied a large number of cases of cirrhosis and didn't see any glial change, which astonished me after my experience with it. He claimed that there were extensive white matter lesions. But the pictures he showed were of the common artifact in myelin stains; this was the main point of disagreement. But I think subsequent studies have born out the effect of liver coma on the gray matter of the brain with the hyperplasia of protoplasmic astrocytes.

RL: *Was Baker your contemporary?*

RA: Yes. He was a very distinguished neurologist and a founder of the American Academy of Neurology.

RL: *How did you feel when he stood up at this public meeting and commented on your paper?*

RA: Well, no one else in the audience really had any experience. They were surprised that two workers in the same field should have come to such striking disagreement on a common neurologic state. But, at any rate, I persisted in my study of these cases.

Not long after that I was asked by Chester Jones to see a patient, actually a commander in the United States Navy, known to have hemochromatosis. Periodically he would develop a curious tremor. His secretary remarked that the tremor heralded confusion or stupor and that, soon after the appearance of tremor, he would have to go into the hospital. I had not seen this syndrome. Chester Jones, chief of gastroenterology at MGH, said it was not related to liver disease or hemochromatosis because there was no jaundice or ascites. The tremor was so striking, when he entered this state, that I thought it was unique and I took Joe Foley out to see it.

RL: *He was a fellow at Boston City Hospital.*

RA: Yes. I had arranged for him to come to the Boston City Hospital as a Rockefeller fellow, after he got out of the United States Army at the end of World War II.

We noted that the movement was an arrhythmic lapse of sustained contraction. We didn't know what to call this type of curious lapse in posture. Joe Foley knew a Catholic priest, to whom he explained the nature of these lapses. The priest suggested the word "asterixis" to designate it. And that's how that term was introduced into medicine [see Chapter 5 and Appendix J].

After encountering the naval officer with asterixis, we looked over the cirrhotic patients at the Boston City Hospital, Foley and I, and found that those patients, who were going into stupor, frequently showed this. But we also saw that same movement disorder in some of the patients with other metabolic diseases. So it wasn't unique to liver disease. And at a later time, with the aid of Robert Schwab, we got movies of the movement and EMG of the involved muscles and showed that the extent of the movement was determined by the duration of the lapse of contraction. That proved to us that this was a unique neurologic disorder.

RL: *Some people refer to asterixis as negative myoclonus.*

RA: Yes. That's just a way of defining these lapses. I have no quarrel with that, as long as one understands the physiology.

RL: *Does calling it negative myoclonus help you to understand it at all?*

RA: I don't think so.

RL: *Have you ever encountered an experimental model of asterixis?*

RA: No, I don't think we ever tried to reproduce it.

RL: *In 1951 you moved from Boston City Hospital to Massachusetts General Hospital.*

RA: When I returned to the Mass. General Hospital, I was given a set of laboratories just one floor above a metabolic ward of the medical service. It was an ideal arrangement because it enabled me to have easy access to patients with all kinds of metabolic disease.

Along about that time someone in Paris that had found an increase in blood ammonia in liver failure, and Charles Davidson had observed it in some of his cases of hepatic disease. We corroborated this finding in our cases of stupor with liver disease.

About that same time there was a patient that came onto the metabolic ward. McDermott had operated and shunted the portal circulation into the inferior vena cava; the patient, afterwards, became stuporous. We studied him over two or three months and found that, whenever he was fed a high-protein diet, his ammonia level went up, he developed asterixis, then stupor, and coma. When he was fasted, his ammonia levels fell and he brightened up and returned to normal. We found that, when he was given ammonium chloride by mouth, he developed the same syndrome.

This was the first human case of Eck fistula (the fistula being between the portal system and the inferior vena cava). Eck had observed this in animals. And McDermott, who was a very able experimentalist, got interested in Eck fistulae and ammonia. He did a whole series of animal studies, showing that, whenever they would increase the ammonia level for a period of time, the animals would become comatose. I studied the cerebrum in these cases and found that those animals, that were comatose, had hyperplasia of protoplasmic astrocytes.[1] I thought, looking at animals that had liver disease, Eck fistula, or hyperammonemia, I could differentiate them from control cases, using a single Nissl stain of the cerebral cortex. I made a practice of mixing the slides from control animals and those that had hyperammonemia for several days before sacrifice, and I could distinguish them on the basis of the size of astrocyte nuclei in cerebral cortex.

RL: *In routine clinical work, the ammonia level does not reliably correlate with the mental state.*

RA: That's true and it's always been a puzzle. Of course, the arterial blood ammonia has to be measured at the time that the patient is going into coma and not some time later. Analogous is a patient who has come in due to the effects of an extremely low blood sugar and, by the time the blood is drawn, the blood sugar may have returned to normal.

Later we had a series of patients with chronic hepatocerebral degeneration of acquired type, who exhibited a combination of cerebellar ataxia, athetosis, and dementia. They were reported by Monroe Cole and Maurice Victor and myself [see Chapter 5]. We found widespread lesions of the type I've already described, but there was also necrosis of cortex, basal ganglia, and in parts of cerebral white matter. That appeared to be a very distinct disease. It had been reported before by Woerkom in 1911, about the same year that Wilson had reported familial hepatocerebral degeneration. There had been one or two other cases like it, but we had a series and showed that these patients really had chronic liver failure in every instance.

The relationship of acquired hepatocerebral degeneration to Wilson's disease was very intriguing. I had a chance to compare some of our fatal cases of Wilson's disease to this acquired hepatocerebral degeneration. The astrocytic change, which we and others had noted, was present in both diseases, and some of the other cortical lesions were present in both. It would seem that some aspect of Wilson's disease and the acquired hepatocerebral degeneration was quite similar. However, it was very clear that in acquired hepatocerebeal degeneration there was no increase in brain copper, which had been shown, very clearly, to be elevated in Wilson's disease.

Of course, that raised the question as to whether the brain lesions of Wilson's disease are due to copper accumulation. It was thought that they were related to copper because, when the patients were put on BAL, their copper levels declined gradually, as they clearly improved. But whether they improved because of removal of copper in the brain or improvement of some liver function was never clear to us. I don't think, in looking over the more recent literature, that the matter has ever been fully settled.

RL: *Your writing on chronic hepatocerebral disease does propose the identity of its neuropathology to that of Wilson disease. [see Chapter 5]*

RA: Well, the pathology is really quite similar, and it suggests that at least one aspect of the brain lesion in Wilson's disease is the same as that in chronic liver failure without copper being involved. But, there is no doubt that the copper in the brain is increased in Wilson's disease and that reducing copper in the body helps.

RL: *I have the impression that most people assume that Wilson disease is copper toxicity of the brain and don't seem very interested in your findings.*

RA: That's probably true. I can't understand why.

RL: *To the best of your knowledge, has anyone duplicated the chronic hepatocerebral disease in animals?*

RA: I don't think I know, off hand. We never did.

RL: *Do you have any further comment on the astrocytosis in hepatic encephalopathy?*

RA: Of course, it made no sense at all, in patients with hepatic coma, that the main change should be in astrocytes and not nerve cells, cerebral white matter, or a particular ganglionic structure.

HYPOXIA/ISCHEMIA

RL: *I would like to hear about your work on anoxic encephalopathy.*

RA: We had a whole series of patients coming to postmortem examination. Each had been in deep coma and had died with a swollen, necrotic brain after a period of EEG silence. The neuropathologic material of these cases was described by Pierson Richardson. I saw nearly all of the cases. The completely silent electroencephalograms on the same material were described by Robert Schwab.

Harry Beecher, who was professor of anesthesiology at Harvard and chief of the anesthesia service at the Mass. General Hospital, was very interested in defining brain death. Our material had already been published. So he brought William Sweet and myself, a lawyer from Harvard, an ethicist, and himself together to form a committee. He asked me to write the neurological criteria of brain death. [see Chapter 5]

I chose, I think unfortunately, to express the clinical state as a complete unresponsivity to all modes of stimulation—visual, auditory, cutaneous—in a patient who was unable to sustain respirations. We decided that this condition should exist at least 24 hours without other cause for it to be a state of "brain death." Beecher wanted to propose that the condition was equivalent of death due to cardiac-circulatory-respiratory failure. I initially had the notion that complete unresponsivity and areceptivity would include everything, even spinal reflexes. I chose to apply the diagnosis only to the most severe form of this condition, knowing that an error, that permitted the inclusion of any reversible cases, would be most unfortunate. We found in our own material that these criteria held up. In the following year we had about 100 cases dying at the MGH that manifested these criteria after massive cardiac infarct or asphyxiation.

RL: *Once you established the concept of irreversible coma, others suggested modification of the criteria.*

RA: Others have pointed out that we should have specified absence of brainstem reflexes rather than all reflexes.

RL: *What other observations did you make on anoxic encephalopathy?*

RA: In addition to these severe forms there were some others who gradually emerged to what was later called a vegetative state. All of my cases had manifest diencephalic lesions. They had other cerebral lesions too, but some diencephalic damage, without complete destruction, was the common denominator.

One of our patients was a girl who had fallen off a horse and for fourteen months had remained in this state. She was on a neurosurgical service in a nearby clinic. And, amusingly, she was given electric shock by one of the neurosurgeons to see if that would make her more alert and mentally competent. Needless to say, it made her worse, if it did anything.

James Lance, later professor of neurology in Sydney, was working with us for a time. And he and I had a group of four cases, who had developed a diffuse cortical intention myoclonus with definite spikes in the cortex, only during voluntary movement. We referred to this as action or intention myoclonus. The peculiar feature of it was that, if the patient was relaxed, the limbs were quiet. But if he would lift his limb to seize something or point to something, it would involve a very coarse myoclonic jerk, or rhythmic series of them. We didn't have any pathology of this group, but we wrote it up in some detail, and I guess it's sometimes referred to as the Lance Adams syndrome [see Chapter 5]. We assume that there must be cerebellar lesions disinhibiting the cerebral cortex and that it was one of the forms of cortical polymyoclonus. All four of our cases had been hypoxic for a time and then, as they recovered, they were left with this extremely disabling myoclonus.

Toxic Encephalopathy

RL: *What was toxic encephalopathy?*
RA: We had a number of children who were given a considerable amount of intravenous fluid and developed brain swelling and died. We reported this diffuse brain swelling in an article with Gilles Lyon and Philip Dodge in Brain.[2] We didn't know what the basis of the encephalopathy was; we just called it acute toxic encephalopathy contrasting it to encephalitis and other acute diseases of the cerebrum. It was a varied collection of metabolic encephalopathies. The neuropathology was not very specific in this group of children.
RL: *What do you think those cases in your article were? Were they all Reye syndrome, which had not yet been discovered at the time you wrote your article?*
RA: We failed to notice the importance of the rapid enlargement of the liver in one or possibly more cases, which, in retrospect, was Reye's disease. That patient had fatty infiltration in the liver. The others, when we went back later and looked, did not have the typical lipid infiltrate in liver cells. I think that those, without lipid infiltration, had encephalopathy based on a very rapid shift in electrolytes in the child's brain. We also found, in going back over our trauma material in children, that there were a few cases of acute brain swelling and coma. In fact, the only traumatic cases with diffuse brain swelling, that we had at the Boston

City Hospital, had been given a lot of intravenous fluid, probably without proper electrolyte balance.

RL: *Basically brain swelling from too much free water.*

RA: I thought so. And I thought that the child's brain was especially susceptible to the swelling and that acute toxic encephalopathy and the diffuse swelling of trauma all were related to the treatment these children were getting on the pediatric service.

RL: *Did your article on "toxic encephalopathy" have impact on pediatric practice?*

RA: Well, it certainly did at the Mass. General. I don't know how widely it influenced thinking.

RL: *I gather that, at the Massachusetts General Hospital, they changed their method of treatment with intravenous fluid.*

RA: They became very much more careful.

RL: *As Phil Dodge educated the pediatricians at Massachusetts General about your findings, did the incidence of "toxic encephalopathy" decrease?*

RA: I thought that it disappeared.

Notes

1. Referred to in Salam-Adams M and Adams RD. Acquired Hepatocerebral Syndromes. In Vinken PJ, Bruyn GW, Klawans HL (eds.), *Handbook of Clinical Neurology. Vol 5 (49). Extrapyramidal Disorders.* Elsevier Science, Amsterdam, 1986, pp 213–221.

2. Lyon G, Dodge PR, Adams RD. The Acute Encephalopathies of Obscure Origin in Infants and Children. *Brain* V84, pp 680–708, 1961.

Alcoholism

Kinnier Wilson's textbook[1] of 1940 did not recognize delirium tremens as fundamentally an alcohol withdrawal syndrome. In fact, Wilson wrote that distaste for alcohol (cessation of intake) could be a symptom, the first symptom, of delirium tremens. At that time pathophysiologic ideas did not distinguish delirium tremens from alcohol intoxication. Deaths from alcohol intoxication and from delirium tremens were both related to cerebral "edema." Confusion about these entities was also evident in therapeutic recommendations. For delirium tremens, some recommended cerebral dehydration and lumbar punctures.[1] On the contrary, others recommended administering large amounts of intravenous fluid.[2]

Obviously there was poor understanding of what we now know to be manifestations of alcohol withdrawal and what we recognize as signs of alcohol intoxication. Unresolved and undiscovered were the causes of many other neurologic problems seen in alcoholic patients. In discussing Wernicke disease,

Wilson made no mention of vitamin deficiency.[1] Korsakoff psychosis was considered, like "dypsomania" and delirium tremens, to be one of the "alcoholic psychoses." A clear view of these diseases would come only with careful study.

There was ample case material at Boston City Hospital where nearly 40% of men admitted to the medical service were alcoholic. Provided the opportunity of this abundant alcoholism, Ray Adams and Maurice Victor began to systematically study its neurology. Their findings contradicted the opinions of many prominent neurologists.

RA: The studies of alcoholism began at the Boston City Hospital. And the very severe alcoholics, dirty, infected derilects, were being segregated in the cellar of one of the medical buildings, under the most primitive conditions. They were often neglected. Their living conditions were so poor on the alcoholic ward that exposure to infectious diseases was frequent.

At the time Maurice Victor had come to the neurology service after a year of medicine with Max Wintrobe. Upon finishing his three years of neurology training, I urged that he go back onto the medical service for a year to get a better grounding in general medicine. I always felt that one needed a couple of years of medicine before neurology. So Maurice did that, and it was during that year that, together, we became involved in the alcohol problems and the withdrawal syndromes. At the end of that year, he had a series of projects underway. [see Figures 31, 32]

RL: *You concluded that peripheral neuropathy in the alcoholic was due to poor nutrition.*

RA: Maurice Victor and I found, in some 200 cases, that all were nutritionally depleted. We couldn't confirm a direct effect of alcohol on peripheral nerve in any of the patients who were adequately nourished. That became a contentious matter. Derek Denny-Brown thought there was relationship between alcohol intake and peripheral nerve disease. Certainly we couldn't confirm that in our cases.

RL: *Was there any controversy about the cause of delirium tremens?*

RA: Our study of the delirium tremens syndrome included 100 cases, where we had careful measures of the blood alcohol at the time the delirium developed. In every case, the full delirium syndrome had developed at the time when the blood alcohol level was falling. We thought, therefore, that we had indubitable proof that delirium tremens was an alcohol withdrawal or abstinence syndrome [see Chapter 5]. That had been suggested earlier but always had been disputed. For example, Houston Merritt had favored the hypothesis that delirium tremens was due to the direct effect of alcohol. I used to discuss this subject with him in his office; we disagreed.

And then, to make it even more certain, Mendelson and Mello (his wife) undertook a study of prisoners in one of the nearby prisons, wherein they offered a good grade of whiskey to a group of prisoners for a month. (They could drink as much as they wanted. All consented to this with great enthusiasm.) They then withdrew the alcohol, and about a third or more of the prisoners developed typical delirium tremens. Maurice Victor was consultant to them on this study. So, really, the absti-nence syndrome was confirmed experimentally. Later, the study was criticized in the press because the prisoners did not know that they were experimental subjects. But, in those days, it seemed quite all right.

During this time I had looked at a number of brains of patients dying of DTs. Death was usually due to dehydration or lack of proper fluid balance and, some-times, very sudden circulatory collapse. It had been rumored by pathology interns that patients with DTs had a "wet brain." I never could quite understand what "wet brain" was. I decided what they really meant was an increase in CSF around the brain due to brain atrophy. I could find nothing by standard light microscopy with Nissl, myelin, and axis cylinder stain in the cerebral cortex, basal ganglia, and thala-mus in such cases. The lack of clearly defined histopathologic changes was entirely in keeping with the reversibility of the syndrome; after they recovered, patients seemed no worse off than they had been before.

RL: *Can you comment on auditory hallucinosis?*

RA: During this time we came upon the syndrome of acute auditory hallucinosis that had been described in the early German literature. I was not aware of this syndrome before. In this state, the patient, who had been drinking quite a lot, for some days or weeks, would stop drinking and then suddenly go into a state of severe auditory hallucinosis.

It was typified by one patient, a doctor from Florida, who had come to take a course at the Boston City Hospital. He had been drinking all the way to Boston on a train and had registered in a Boston Hotel and then had come over to the Boston City Hospital for the medical course. He had to stop drinking, if he was going to take the course. The next day, when he returned to his hotel, he began to hear voices telling him that he was a scoundrel, a disgrace to the profession, and that he should turn himself in. He was frightened; he changed his room but the voices continued. When he went to the Boston City Hospital the next day, the voices were following him. Frightened, he asked for medical help. They put him in a room in the hospital and called his wife, who came that night. On the next day, he was hallucinating and frightened, trembling. His thinking was clear and lucid. He told us exactly what he'd been doing and where his wife was. I cautioned his wife, when she came, not to leave him alone. But, when I went the following day, he was sitting in his room with the door barred. He'd cut both arms and was letting the blood run in a bucket. (His wife had gone to purchase something in the store.) I was very upset about this, of course. We staunched the flow of blood and put him under observation. He was seen by one of Boston's senior psychiatrists, who verified that this was acute auditory hallucinosis with appropriate emotional reactions and mental clarity. And, in about two weeks, he was normal.

I was very impressed with this syndrome. I had never seen a brain of such a case, and I don't think there was any American literature on it. We then began looking for such patients. Justin Hope and Maurice Victor got interested and collected cases from Boston City Hospital. (Hope had been a Rockefeller fellow in psychiatry on

Stanley Cobb's service at the same time that I was; he may have been the only mulatto in training at MGH at the time.) We followed them along.

Later, I and Maurice Victor found cases at Boston State Hospital, a psychiatric hospital where there resided 150 chronic alcoholics. There were five or six that never stopped hallucinating, but they no longer were concerned about their hallucinosis. We reported that our few cases with chronic hallucinosis were without schizophrenic background [see Chapter 5]. An example was a patient I examined at the Boston State Hospital—a woman who was calm. While she was sitting and chatting with me, I asked her if she heard voices. She said, "NO," but I noticed that she was motioning with her hand to something under the table. When asked about what she was doing, she said she was trying to keep chickens from clucking too much! She was labeled by the psychiatrist as "schizophrenic." But, when we started looking at family and past histories of the group, it turned out that they didn't conform to paranoid or any of the other defined forms of schizophrenia. I don't think any subsequent studies have been done on auditory hallucinosis. I know of no MRI study of such cases.

RL: *Why did you start to study Wernicke disease in alcoholics?*

RA: We began seeing cases in the neuropathology lab. My predecessor in neuropathology at Boston City, Leo Alexander, had reported some cases. We had further cases at the Mass. General. These patients had eye movement disorders. At first they were not testable for orientation and memory; they could not sustain attention. We established, early on, that giving thiamine alone would bring about improvement in this early state. The eye movements could be restored. In one instance, I know, we changed the eye movements to virtual normalcy, except for a little nystagmus, in 2 or 3 hours with intravenous thiamine. And we confirmed that the eye movement problem and other brain stem symptoms were exactly similar to what Wernicke had described in non-alcoholic patients. When they became normally alert, we could detect the memory deficit (Korsakoff psychosis). Establishing the identity of Wernicke disease and the severe Korsakoff psychosis was not original with us.

One of the more interesting aspects of this study came, when Victor and I surveyed all of the patients with alcoholic diagnoses at the Boston State Hospital. We went there one afternoon a week for nearly a year; it turned out that the chronic Korsakoff with some ataxia and nystagmus was the commonest alcoholic diagnosis and that chronic hallucinosis was the next most common.

We persuaded pathologists around Boston to let us have the brains of patients that had been diagnosed as Wernicke–Korsakoff syndrome. And we were able to collect some seventy or seventy-five cases. We had the whole central part of the brain including basal ganglia, thalamus, mid-brain in serial section of more than sixty patients. I reviewed all that material with Victor and Collins [see Chapter 5]. We did find, very clearly, lesions in the mamillary bodies and in the medial walls of the thalamus bordering the third ventricle. (The lesions, in themselves, were of interest because nerve cells could be preserved in the lesions but myelinated axons were damaged.) We had the clinical records, but unfortunately we had not examined these patients ourselves. Because we had cases where there was amnesia but no lesion in the mammillary bodies, we proposed that there was a thalamic, amnesic state as part of the clinical picture of Wernicke–Korsakoff disease.

RL: *Maurice Victor remembered you discovering "alcoholic" midline cerebellar degeneration. He recalled that one day you paused before cutting the cerebellum of an ataxic alcoholic and you said, "I wonder what would happen if we cut it this way?" Then you made a midline, sagittal cerebellar section.*

RA: I had overlooked, early on, the fact that the anterior lobe of vermis and the adjacent parts of the anterior hemispheres was a site of a lesion in the Wernicke cases. I had overlooked it because I had examined the cerebellum in the conventional horizontal plane, that is, horizontally with the brainstem. Once I started removing the cerebellum, as an entity, by first cutting through the anterior and middle and posterior cerebellar peduncles, we were able to slice the cerebellum in the sagittal plane. It was then quite evident that these parts, that I mentioned, were regularly the site of atrophy, cell loss of all the elements of the cortex and a striking gliosis. Also affected were the flocculus and paraflocculus regions of the posterior part of the cerebellum. [see Figure 33]

About that time we also came upon a number of cases that had developed, subacutely, a cerebellar ataxia over a period of two or three weeks. They would become tremulous and extremely ataxic, so that they could really not walk normally. In the course of time we had nine or ten such cases. A review of the literature showed that there had been reference to an ataxia in the alcoholic, but there had been no reports on the pathology. Lhermitte had written about cerebellar ataxia, implying nutrition might be a factor without having put together the pathology. In no French or German case was there a relation between an anatomic lesion and nutrition/alcohol. This series was then worked up with Maurice Victor and one of our fellows, Eliot Mancall. It was published in a fairly extensive monograph [see Chapter 5]. These patients, when followed, gradually improved but they were left ataxic. Indeed, we found that in the Boston State Hospital population there were quite a number that walked very badly, having to hold onto articles of furniture.

Since our patients were in their late 40s, or early 50s, we needed to look at the cerebellum in a series of normal cases of different ages. It turned out that this was quite revealing because there was about a 20–25% loss of Purkinje cells with aging over the last 2–3 decades of life. I encouraged Paul Yakovlev and Angevine to assemble this control material and publish it as an atlas.[3]

RL: *Did your article on alcoholic cerebellar degeneration refer to that control material?*

RA: Yes it did. That was the comparison that we made in writing up that pathology. I think it was a definitive article. The puzzle was whether the cerebellar disorder is a direct effect of alcohol or a nutritional disorder. Favoring the latter etiology was one case, at Mass. General, a woman who was extremely obese. She was put on a restricted diet, and lost a huge amount of weight. She was not given supplemental vitamins. She developed a fairly typical cerebellar degeneration. Also, one of our patients, one who had come into the city hospital without ataxia, after two weeks in the hospital, was first observed to be ataxic. We were quite sure that he had never received alcohol in the hospital. So those cases favored the idea that this was a nutritional deficiency, probably B1 (thiamine) deficiency, but that conclusion was never definitive.

RL: *Were either of those non-alcoholic cases written up?*

RA: No. The one in the Mass. General Hospital, on a diet, did die. We had her cerebellum and that was typical. I mention that in my textbook, when discussing the cause of cerebellar degeneration.

RL: *In your book on Wernicke disease you hypothesized that midline cerebellar disease in the alcoholic was essentially the cerebellar lesion of Wernicke disease.*

RA: Yes, I couldn't distinguish the two. It's highly probable that both the primary cerebellar degeneration of alcoholism and the cerebellar lesion of Wernicke–Korsakoff are the same. However that doesn't explain why the cerebellum seems to be involved severely in some of these cases and not others. So that's a matter that's still to be investigated I think.

RL: *Was there ever difficulty distinguishing the "alcoholic" cerebellar disease from a degenerative disease of the cerebellum?*

RA: One of our cases was the brain of Eugene O'Neill,[4] and he had evidently become quite ataxic toward the later part of his life. How much alcohol he was drinking was disputed. I thought his cerebellum was entirely consistent with residual alcoholic cerebellar disease, and it was included in our study. I knew his psychiatrist, Harry Kozol, quite well. He had been close to the family. I thought that he had indicated (I don't have an exact memory of this.) that O'Neill was a chronic alcoholic. But much later one of the neuropsychiatrists at McLean Hospital went over that material, spoke to O'Neill's wife and tried to document his alcoholism. She said that he hadn't been drinking in the latter part of his life, when the cerebellar atrophy seemed to have taken place. That information was reported in the *New England Journal of Medicine* with E. P. Richardson.[5]

RL: *That interview with O'Neill's wife and the publication of that article occurred many decades after the death of the famous playwright.*

RA: Yes, it was last year. Cerebellar atrophy could have occurred when he was drinking earlier in his life.

RL: *Is O'Neill's brain pictured in your article on alcoholic cerebellar degeneration?*

RA: Yes it is one of the last ones. Bruce Price, who was the main author of the recent article, used the same illustration from our earlier article in making the case that O'Neill's cerebellar atrophy was not alcoholic.

RL: *He argued that it was a special type of degenerative disease.*

RA: The lesions of one of the cortical cerebellar atrophies and the alcoholic cerebellar atrophy, topographically and histologically, are not really different.

One of the amusing examples we came across was that of a patient that Stanley Cobb had seen years before. He was a professor of forensic medicine at Harvard University. He was a heavy drinker, and he had a cerebellar lesion. Cobb had a single section of his brain in the teaching box to show the atrophy of the cortex, and it was labeled as alcoholic cerebellar degeneration for several years. Then the patient's non-alcoholic brother developed the same ataxia! To everyone's embarrassment we had been showing this brain as an alcoholic cerebellar degeneration, and it was probably one of genetic origin.

RL: *Did you do any work on Marchiafava–Bignami disease?*

RA: Corpus callosum degeneration, Marchiafava–Bignami, was a puzzling problem in its relationship to the cortical atrophy of the third layer of the frontotemporal cortex. That those two lesions seemed to go together had been noted by Morel, who was a famous psychiatrist and neuropathologist in Geneva. However, this combination was questioned because one of his cases had the cortical lesion but no corpus callosum lesion! I was puzzled about this because all of the others had both. Michel Jequier and I took an afternoon off, when I was in Lausanne one year, and we went over to Morel's laboratory. Rabinowicz, an ex-fellow of Morel, had access to the slides in storage. (Morel long before had died.) In his case of cortical atrophy "without" corpus callosum lesion, on the edge of one section, there was a tiny bit of corpus callosum. There was a callosal lesion. Thus it was quite clear to us that the lesion, that Morel had described, the atrophy and sclerosis of the third layer of the frontal temporal cortex, was related to Marchiafava–Bignami disease.

In looking at the Marchiafava–Bignami disease—we had several cases (some of them in Lausanne)—the main lesion was in the anterior half of the corpus callosum in the central band of fibers. And I thought—this was quite good evidence—that the third layer neurons in the frontotemporal cortex were those neurons that were connected with commissural fibers of the corpus callosum.

RL: *I gather that the cortical lesions are secondary to the Marchiafava–Bignami lesion in the corpus collosum.*

RA: I thought so, and I was about to write a little commentary on the importance of looking at corpus callosal lesions of other types, traumatic or neoplastic, to see whether there was this atrophy of the third layer of the cerebral cortex.

This lesion, that Morel described, is very striking because usually that third layer of the cortex, on a Nissl stain, stands out very clearly. You know that as well as I. And here these cells are all gone, and in their bed is a prominence of fibrous type astrocytes. So it's an unmistakable lesion, and it must be a lesion that has involved the entire neuron. "Atrophie de troisieme couche" is the term he used for it.

RL: *So would you look in the areas of frontal lobe or temporal lobe that are at the level of the corpus callosum lesion?*

RA: Yes. Look there in a case with clear corpus callosum involvement of some duration and see if there's cell loss.

We had one patient, at the Massachusetts General Hospital, an auto mechanic, who was a heavy alcoholic. He had developed bifrontal syndrome. Afterwards, when abstinent, he cleared mentally but was unable to release his grasp on tools because of the prominence of his grasp reflexes. He died about a year and a half later, and we examined his brain. Peirson Richardson at first observed no abnormality in the corpus callosum. I urged that we cut further slices in the anterior part of the corpus callosum, and then was seen a gray zone in the center of the corpus callosum; it was just reduced to a thin line, the residual lesion of Marchiafava–Bignami disease.

RL: *Please comment on dementia in the alcoholic.*

RA: The question was did the alcoholic dementia represent merely a state of chronic Korsakoff or was it something more than that. We thought that the main problem in the Korsakoff disease was memory with a few other subtle changes. Despite the fact that the ventricles of the chronic alcoholic were enlarged, we really could not establish the existence of a generalized, diffuse impairment of mental function, different from Korsakoff. That was and is a very controversial topic.

Courville, one of the first to write about cortical changes in the alcoholic, reported alteration in the density of staining of the neurons. I could not convince myself that the changes that he illustrated were anything more than artifact due to postmortem changes and to handling of unfixed tissues.

Torvik, who had worked with us in neuropathology and became chief of neuropathology at Oslo University, looked through their alcoholic dementias there. He found Wernicke lesions in each case. He too was not impressed by any change in the cortex or white matter. We never could settle that in our material. The person who has done some of the most careful neuropathologic studies of alcoholism is Harper, who is a neuropathologist in Australia. I talked to him, when I was visiting professor at the University of Western Australia. Recently he has thought that there were very subtle electron microscopic changes in the cortex. He's a reliable observer. That matter, I believe, is still unsettled. The findings are interesting and need validation.

Of course, when you throw a net over the chronic drunkard you have a very peculiar population of patients; they have all sorts of things wrong with them. They are frequently very severely depleted nutritionally; they frequently have head injuries etc. So, it isn't an easy material to interpret. The volumetric change (enlargement of the ventricles) in the alcoholic has no clearly established pathologic basis in our material.

RL: *When you wrote the article about central pontine myelinolysis, you argued very effectively that the stereotyped location and the symmetry of the lesion indicated that there must be some type of metabolic or chemical cause. Eventually your analysis was proven correct.[6]*

RA: Yes.

RL: *Do you remember being taught that concept or do you remember reading that concept or do you remember developing that idea from your own experience?*

RA: No. I think the idea was generally accepted that a very symmetric involvement of the medullated fibers often would have some type of metabolic basis. That was a general concept pretty widely accepted.

RL: *I cannot find that written about in Wilson's neurology textbook or in Spielmeyer's pathology book. Was it something you might have learned from Kubik?*

RA: No. I think there were examples of other diseases, in kernicterus for example.

RL: *I know there were many examples. I am asking whether anyone had made the generalization?*

RA: Probably not too clearly.

RL: *I am thinking that you may have made the generalization without even thinking too much about it.*

RA: Well, it's hard to say. It's hard to know where you get ideas.

The intense study of Adams' and colleagues led to a clear classification of the neurologic manifestations of alcoholism. By the first edition of *Principles of Neurology* (1977) they had categorized the neurologic disorders seen in alcoholism as follows:

1. Alcohol intoxication
2. The abstinence or withdrawal syndrome
3. Nutritional diseases
4. Diseases of uncertain pathogenesis (alcoholic myopathy, Marchiafava–Bignami disease etc.)
5. Hepatic encephalopathies

This classification has required only little modification over the subsequent three decades. To each of the five categories, Adams and Victor added important new information and analysis. This classification is used repeatedly by others who write about the neurology of alcoholism.

Notes

1. Wilson, SA Kinnier. *Neurology*. Edward Arnold & Co., London, 1940, 1838 p.
2. Cecil RL, Loeb RF. *A Textbook of Medicine*. W.B. Saunders, Philadelphia, 1951.
3. Angevine J, Mancall E, Yakovlev P. *The Human Cerebellum an Atlas of Gross Topography in Serial Sections*. Little Brown and Company, Boston, 1961.
4. Black S. *Eugene O'Neill: Beyond Mourning and Tragedy*. Yale University Press, New Haven, 1999.
5. Price BH, Richardson EP. The Neurologic Illness of Eugene O'Neill—A Clinico-pathological Report. *N Engl J Med* V342, pp 1126–1133, 2000.
6. Laureno R. Central Pontine Myelinolysis Following Rapid Correction of Hyponatremia. *Ann Neurol* V13, p 232, 1983.

Memory

At mid-century, little was known about the anatomical basis of memory. A *Textbook of Clinical Neurology* by Nielsen, who was very interested in cerebral localization, included interesting discussion of the localization of lesions in aphasia, agnosia, apraxia, and other disorders.[1] However, when Nielsen mentioned traumatic amnesia or Korsakoff psychosis, he offered no information on their anatomical basis. In the 1950s, interest in memory was stimulated, when neurosurgeons observed amnesia in patients with bilateral medial temporal lobe lesions. In non-surgical cases (bilateral posterior cerebral artery occlusion or inclusion body encephalitis), bilateral medial temporal lobe lesions were also associated with amnesia. Since the hippocampus is a prominent feature of the medial temporal lobe and since it was affected in these diseases, damage to the hippocampal formation was considered to be the basis of the amnesia.

By the decade of the 1950s, Raymond Adams and colleagues had long been studying Wernicke disease. They recognized on clinical and pathologic grounds, the unity of Wernicke disease and Korsakoff psychosis, that is, the concept that the amnesia (Korsakoff psychosis) was a persistent manifestation of the disease in some of the patients who had earlier experienced the confusion, ophthalmoplegia, and ataxia of Wernicke disease. Thus, the study of Wernicke lesions in the brains of those with and without memory loss provided an opportunity to seek the anatomic basis of memory loss in these amnesia patients. [see Figure 34]

RL: *In* Principles of Neurology *you originally used the term, "amnestic syndrome," but in recent editions you have preferred the term, "amnesic syndrome."*

RA: Well, "amnesic" is the proper word. "Amnestic" also is used in another context in medicine—refers to past history, the "amnestic" data.

RL: *You found that the amnesia in the Wernicke–Korsakoff syndrome is due to medial thalamic lesions and can occur when there are no lesions of the mamillary bodies. Was this analysis accepted? [see Chapter 5]*

RA: The mammillary sparing was contested by Brion. But it certainly was suggested by our cases. And a thalamic form of amnesia was later found in other diseases. The medial dorsal nuclear lesions of thalamus must have affected the thalamic connections of the hippocampal-fornical system.

RL: *How did you conclude that?*

RA: Well, because by then there had been clear evidence, in other diseases, that hippocampal and adjacent lesions could cause the same amnesic defect as the thalamic lesions in Wernicke disease.

RL: *You showed pathologic evidence of hippocampal lesions in amnesic patients with Herpes simplex encephalitis.*

RA: This form of inclusion body encephalitis causes widespread destruction all through the medial and inferior parts of the temporal lobes.

RL: *Do these amnesic patients realize that their memory is defective?*

RA: Korsakoff cases lack insight. If they were aware of any memory deficit, they did not appreciate the degree of the problem. In trying to recollect things that had happened recently, they would not recognize at all that they had completely misplaced them in time.

RL: *You and Miller Fisher wrote a monographic article on transient global amnesia. [see Chapter 5]*

RA: This was a syndrome of episodic memory loss with retrograde amnesia. There was preserved alertness and capacity to perform other elaborate mental activities during the episode. They seemed normal in other respects. In other words it was not a state of confusion, as seen in an epileptic attack. It was unlikely to have been a transient ischemic attack because none of our patients ever had a stroke or developed one in subsequent years.

RL: *Do you recall any of your cases?*

RA: Our first case was the wife of the dean of a medical school, who brought her to me. They had been at their summer place. It was their practice to get up in the morning to go for a swim in the cold north shore water. She set the breakfast table. When they returned from the swim, she had no memory of having set the table or having gone for the swim. Her memory for the day before was virtually nil. He called me and brought her to the Massachusetts General Hospital that afternoon and by then she was completely recovered. She did not remember the episode or the events of the preceding hours. That was our first case, several years before our publication.

Fortunately, most were highly intelligent professional people. There were three or four physicians. One was a headmistress of a very prominent girl's school in Boston. She had three short episodes after swimming in the Boston harbor. One was a banker who, having no memory at all, was able to go through documents and find errors.

Striking was the case of the brilliant head of our cancer institute at Massachusetts General. He had agreed to give a discourse on the origins of industrial medicine to some reporters. They came to his summer home in Cape Cod, and he talked for about an hour, giving a very coherent and excellent account of the subject, and they all got up and were leaving. As they went out the door, he turned to his son, who was a physician, and his wife, and he said, "Who are those people and what were they doing here?" They were quite alarmed; his son made him lie down. He began moving his arms and legs around, asking if he'd had a stroke. They gave him a shot of whiskey and reassured him. He looked at his son and said, "Well what in the hell are you doing here?" His son had come down three days before, and they had chopped wood together on the previous afternoon. He had a complete memory gap for that period. By nightfall he was well. He lived for several more years without any sign of cerebrovascular disease.

Actually, one of our psychiatrists had an episode. He was interviewing a patient in his office when the attack started. The patient recognized that he was not making sense and immediately called his wife. His wife took him to Logan Airport, to pick up his daughter, where he met an old friend with whom he carried on a correct conversation. Then, at MGH, Pierson Richardson talked to him and found that he could do intricate calculations, but a few minutes later he could not remember having done that. I saw him in this; it lasted about 6 hours.

RL: *When I asked you about your childhood, you said that, "When you are in late years, early memories fade." However, most neurologists emphasize that the most recent memories are disproportionately lost.*

RA: Yes. There is retention of distant memories. The events and faces and episodes of childhood in general are held better than the memories of what you had for breakfast yesterday. That has always caught the fancy of people. However, the earliest memories also are progressively effaced with age.

RL: *Is there good literature on the loss of earliest memories?*

RA: I don't think so. I haven't seen careful studies, and it's hard to think of a way of doing it. I have the impression that a five-year-old has memories from age two, but that when he is twenty-five, he does not have memories going back to the second year. My evidence is very subjective. There are incidents from the first seven years of my life that I retain, but certainly, the detail of memories from age three or four is gone.

Adams and colleagues produced two seminal works on memory. One was the study of Wernicke–Korsakoff syndrome. The other was the monographic article on transient global amnesia.

Victor Adams and Collins's monograph on Wernicke disease, a systematic study of 245 cases, 82 with postmortem examination, allowed correlation of lesion location and the presence of amnesia. Although some doctors had considered the mamillary body lesions the cause of amnesia, Adams et al. found that the mammillary bodies could be prominently affected in the absence of amnesia and that amnesia was consistently correlated with involvement of the dorsal medial nuclei of the thalamus. From this investigation they demonstrated that amnesia could occur in bilateral medial thalamic lesions just as it could in bilateral medial temporal lobe lesions.

This concept of thalamic amnesia has been confirmed by the study of other diseases, especially bilateral thalamic infarction without any temporal lobe disease.[2] Further confirmation has come with experimental thalamic lesioning.[3]

This concept, diencephalic amnesia, has stimulated further thought and investigation. Horel has argued that the thalamus is connected to the temporal lobe by a "temporal stem" of white matter. He proposed that these connections to the thalamic memory area are the site of the amnesia producing injury in medial temporal lesions. His proposal that the eye catching hippocampus is not the critical temporal lobe structure for memory is supported by evidence from animal experimentation.[4]

During the years that Miller Fisher and Adams were collecting their cases of transient global amnesia, the disorder had been observed elsewhere. In one brief article in an obscure journal, Bender gave a good overview of the clinical syndrome in one paragraph; most of the three-and-a-half page article dealt with discussion of possible etiologies.[5] Fisher and Adams gave the entity its accepted name in their definitive study. This idiopathic syndrome is now the source of renewed interest. With diffusion-weighted magnetic resonance imaging (MRI) there is new opportunity to seek a physiological correlate for the transient memory loss. This method offers the investigator a great advantage, the ability to obtain sequential images in vivo. There are indications that one may find transient signal abnormalities in the hippocampi of such patients. Recently a flurry of such reports has appeared, only one of which is noted here.[6] One anticipates that new MRI sequences and improved sensitivity of MRI scanning will bring new information about this disorder.

Notes

1. Nielsen JM. *A Textbook of Clinical Neurology*. Paul B. Hoeber, Inc., New York, 1951.
2. Graff-Radford N, Tranel D, Van Hoesen G, et al. Diencephalic Amnesia. *Brain* V113, pp 1–23, 1990.
3. Zola-Morgan S, Squire LR. Amnesia in Monkeys after Lesions of the Medi-Dasal Nucleus of the Thalamus. *Ann Neurol* V17, pp 558–564, 1985.
4. Horel JA. The Neuro Anatomy of Amnesia: A Critique of the Hippocampal Memory Hypothesis. *Brain* V101, pp 403–445, 1978.
5. Bender MB. Syndrome of Isolated Episode of Confusion with Amnesia. *J Hillside Hosp* V5, pp 212–215, 1956.
6. Bartsch T, Alfke K, Deuschl G, et al. Evolution of Hippocampal CA-1 Diffusion Lesions in Transient Global Amnesia. *Ann Neurol* V62, pp 475–480, 2007.

Cerebrovascular Diseases

When Ray Adams was a psychiatry fellow, the first edition of Kinnier Wilson's textbook of neurology was published. In the section on stroke, Wilson devotes the same amount of space to hypothesized cerebral arteriospasm as he does to cerebral embolism. (At the time, vasospasm was often invoked to explain cerebral infarctions for which no vessel occlusion was found at autopsy.) Much of Wilson's brief discussion of embolism relates to air embolism, fat embolism, and infectious diseases. Through the 1940s and 1950s, the importance of cerebral embolism and cerebral arteriospasm in the cause of stroke remained unclear to many authorities.

Between 1942 and 1946 Adams studied 1,400 brains at the Mallory Institute of Pathology. He made the first good clinicopathologic report on occlusion of the anterior inferior cerebellar artery. With cases from Boston City Hospital and Massachusetts General Hospital (MGH), Adams and Charles Kubik wrote the standard clinicopathologic article on basilar artery occlusion; this paper brought Ray Adams international recognition. Some of these occlusions were atherothrombotic, and some were embolic. He gradually concluded that there was no mystery about the brains with recent infarctions with no demonstrable vessel occlusion at autopsy. Often there was a cardiac disease as the likely source of embolism in these cases. It seemed reasonable that the embolus had lysed before death and autopsy. He saw no reason to invoke vasospasm to explain these cases. Surveying his experience with the neuropathology of stroke, he published a three-part review of cerebrovascular disease.[1] The organization of that paper shows the roots of his subsequent textbook chapters on this subject. There are tables on syndromes caused by occlusion of various brain arteries, the frequency of different vascular diseases of brain, the distribution of arterial thromboses, and the sites and causes of cerebral embolism. He argued that cerebral embolism had been underestimated as a cause of stroke.

When he began to attract fellows in neuropathology, he often directed them to the study of cerebrovascular diseases. With Jan Cammermyeyer, who came from Oslo, he wrote a clinicopathologic study of the neurology of thrombotic thrombocytopenia purpura (Moschowitz disease) and a clinicopathological analysis of neurological disorders resulting from surgery on the neck and thorax (see Chapter 5). With Henri Vander Eecken, who came from Belgium, he studied border zones and the surface collaterals of major cerebral arteries (see Chapter 5). In 1949, C. Miller Fisher came from Montreal to be Adams' fellow at Boston City Hospital; cerebral embolism became a focus of their investigative collaboration.

RL: *C. Miller Fisher was your fellow.*

RA: Yes. When he came to work as a fellow in my lab at the Boston City Hospital he was just full of ideas, a new one every few months. He was fascinated with heart muscle fiber. He had all kind of ideas about how that should be studied. And he got interested in the carotid artery, which we couldn't examine at the Boston City Hospital. The undertakers wouldn't allow it. When he went back to Canada to Montreal General Hospital, he was able to put together the first really good study of the internal carotid artery.

RL: *Tell me about your investigation of cerebral embolism.*

RA: Miller was fascinated with all aspects of neuropathology; he'd never been exposed to it. We started looking at the cerebral infarcts that we couldn't find any vascular basis for. There was a suggestion that vascular spasm might be the cause. But that didn't satisfy us. And so we looked at all of the vascular lesions in about 800 brains in succession in 1949. As a cause of infarction, we found that there was most commonly either a demonstrated embolus or auricular fibrillation, which could be the basis of an embolus, even though we couldn't find it in the brain. There might be embolic occlusion in the kidney or the intestine or elsewhere. But in some of these cases we could not find the embolus in the brain, even though we knew the patient was having embolic disease. When Miller and I presented our data showing that cerebral embolism was frequent, other neuropathologists ridiculed the idea. [see Chapter 5]

RL: *Miller Fisher told me that, during his second month as your fellow, he cut nine brains in one day; three had hemorrhagic infarction. When he reviewed the hospital charts, he found that all of these three patients had atrial fibrillation, which could have given rise to cerebral embolism. [see Chapter 5]*

RA: Well, we thought that the hemorrhagic infarction must have been due to occlusion at one time, after which the embolus either had disintegrated or moved to distal parts of the infarct. And I took pains to make blocks through the infarct, looking for fragments, sometimes finding them, oftentimes not. We used to discuss this daily almost.

RL: *You and Fisher?*

RA: Yes, and Vander Eecken and the other fellows. When we looked carefully at this material, it turned out that in those cases, where we could not find the embolus, about a third of them had all through the cortex a large and extensive hemorrhagic infiltration. That was always closer to the heart than the main softening of the brain, which could be pale or anemic. We decided that hemorrhagic infarction was due to a migratory embolism.

We wrote this material up, in extenso, and presented it at the American Association of Neuropathologists [see Chapter 5]. It was received with considerable skepticism. We had claimed that embolism was the main type of stroke, either proven or inferred. A number of neuropathologists disclaimed that. And we stated that extensive hemorrhagic infarction was due to transient occlusion of the arterial system by a migrating embolism. This paper was written up and sent to the American Journal of Pathology and they refused it. And so we just set it aside. And about forty years later, someone was editing a book on embolism and asked if we would send that paper to them! Essentially the same paper finally was published in that book on embolism. [see Chapter 5]

RL: *Miller Fisher says that you wrote the original manuscript. It sounds like you were intimately involved in the early observation about the hemorrhagic transformation of the proximal portion of the infarct.*

RA: Yes. Going back in the German literature (Miller did most of that), there was reference to the fact that hemorrhagic infarction was sometimes seen in stroke. But it had not been worked out in detail in terms of migratory embolism.

RL: *So that was original with you?*

RA: I think so—with Miller and me.

RL: *Miller Fisher told me that the concept of migratory embolism finally explained those cerebral infarcts, for which there was no vessel occlusion found at autopsy and thereby disproved the prevalent theory that vasospasm was responsible for such lesions.*

RA: The general pathologists at the Brigham Hospital and others[2] had suggested that vascular spasm was the cause.

RL: *Were you and Vander Eecken the first to analyze surface collaterals of the arteries of the brain?*

RA: Cohnheim and later Beevor had noticed that occlusion of major arteries produced infarcts that were less than the extent of the arteries' territory of supply, as if there might be some overlap. We verified that by injecting Schlesinger solution into cerebral arteries; all the major cerebral arteries had end-to-end anastanoses on the surface and in the sulcal system of the brain. [see Figure 35]

RL: *On becoming Bullard Professor in 1954, you asked Miller Fisher to join you at Massachusetts General Hospital. Had you been impressed with his performance as your fellow or with his work after he went back to Montreal?*

RA: Both. I offered a position to Miller Fisher due to his clinical skill and his interest in vascular diseases. I thought that all vascular cases should be seen by a neurologist. Up to that time, neurology and medicine were vying with each other to keep such patients off of their services.

RL: *When you wanted Miller Fisher to set up a service for vascular disease, was there any precedent for such a neurological service?*

RA: I don't remember. It seemed logical to me. After Miller came, nearly always, one or two research fellows would come and work with him; they were outstanding.

RL: *Your 1953 article on vascular diseases of the brain[3] has a classification of cerebrovascular disease which foreshadows that of the ad hoc Committee of the National Institute of Health which was published later, in 1958.[4]*

RA: Bailey, the head of the institute of neurology asked several people, myself, Miller, and others to write a classification.

RL: *Miller Fisher told me that you and he basically wrote the whole document for the committee.*

RA: Miller and I were the only ones that had looked at the brain in vascular disease. The others only had a speaking knowledge.

RL: *Unlike your earlier classification, that NIH document includes the term "transient ischemic attack."*

RA: Fisher is to be credited on the matter of transient ischemic attack. The idea of Denny-Brown was that these were due to episodes of low blood pressure. That didn't prove to be the case. Fisher and I dropped the blood pressure of a patient having many attacks and could not reproduce the attack.

Late in the twentieth century the American Heart Association vigorously involved itself in the field of stroke. The motivation was the hope that therapy for stroke could be enhanced in the way that treatment for occlusive coronary artery disease had been advanced by thrombolytic medicine and interventional procedures. Half a century earlier the American Heart Association had likewise plunged into the realm of stroke, the impetus being the apparent success of anti-coagulant medicine in the treatment of coronary artery disease. Enthusiastic about therapy but uninformed about cerebrovascular disease, the cardiologists were "searching for facts prior to initiation of a program for clinical investigation of various therapeutic procedures."[5] As a result, a series of conferences were held in Princeton, New Jersey, on the subject of stroke. (Eventually the National Institute of Neurological Disease and Blindness came to support and the American Neurological Association to co-sponsor the conferences, whose transactions were published as books.) At the first conference Raymond Adams was selected to explain the pathology of cerebrovascular disease.[5] Questions came from startled conference participants about Adams' observations on the frequency of cerebral embolism. At the second conference Dr William T. Foley of Cornell referred to "Dr. Adams' thesis, which was revolutionary three years ago; that embolic phenomena to the brain are a common finding. We used to think perhaps only four or five percent of strokes were due to emboli and Dr. Adams thought the number was nearer 30 to 35 percent. Large autopsy series have now borne this out."[6]

At the first of these Princeton conferences there was also controversy about Adams' categorization of stroke into three different categories, hemorrhage, pale infarction, and hemorrhagic infarction, and his correlation of hemorrhagic infarction with reperfusion of the proximal part of the infarction after distal migration of embolic fragments. Specifically Dr Zimmerman, neuropathologist at Columbia University, disagreed.[5]

Disagreement about Adams' ideas related to cerebral embolism was not new. In 1951 Fisher and Adams had presented their analysis of this subject to the American Association of Neuropathologists' meeting; their ideas were greeted with skepticism. In fact the American Journal of Pathology twice rejected their complete paper on the subject. Fisher put the article aside because he had become involved in studying the carotid artery. Adams continued to propound their ideas about embolism.[3] [see Figure 36]

In Boston there were believers. The ad hoc committee, which recommended Ray Adams to be the Bullard Professor of Neuropathology at Harvard, wrote in its report that "The field which he had perhaps investigated most intensively is that of vascular disease, in which he has made a real contribution. He has brought orderliness into this subject. By exploitation of a combination of chemical and pathological methods, he has attempted to determine some of the mechanism of apoplexy. This grew out of a series of studies of hemorrhagic infarction of the brain that not only brought order into a previously confused subject but put the histology of cerebrovascular disease on a dynamic basis." (see Appendix)

Elsewhere, however, skepticism persisted. In 1955, the venerable *Textbook of Medicine* by Cecil and Loeb (Ninth Edition) continued to state that in "encephalomolacia" one fails to find the thrombosis in only a small percentage of cases.[7] Likewise the 1954 *Principles of Internal Medicine* (Harrison et al.) stated that embolism was the cause of only 5% of cerebral infarctions.[8]

However, in the 1958 edition of *Principles of Internal Medicine*, Adams, himself, was given charge of the sections on neurologic diseases. He and his co-authors brought clarity to the subject of stroke for the student, the internist, and the neurologist.[9] His 47-page chapter on cerebrovascular diseases included the about-to-be-published, classification of cerebral vascular diseases. He distinguished pale from hemorrhagic cerebral infarction and offered explanation for the association of hemorrhagic infarcts with cerebral embolism. The chapter included a table and ten drawings illustrating different aspects of ischemic stroke and relevant anatomy, a spectacular expansion of and advancement in exposition on cerebrovascular disease. This chapter made stroke, its basic concepts and its details, comprehensible; it served as the basis for the chapter on stroke in all future editions of *Principles of Internal Medicine* and eventually for the stroke chapter in Adams' *Principles of Neurology*. Having passed the test of time the rejected article on cerebral embolism was finally published nearly four decades after it was rejected (see Chapter 5)! At the same time the invention of cross-sectional brain imaging allowed in vivo demonstration that hemorrhagic infarction was associated with cerebral embolism and that bleeding occurred, not at the time of the stroke, but after a latency of hours or days.[10] As a result the present-day neurologist has the opportunity to confirm the concepts of Adams and Fisher in his or her daily work.

Notes

1. Adams RD, Cohen ME. Vascular Disease of the Brain. *Bull New Eng Med Cent* V9, August pp 180–190 and October pp 222–230 and December pp 261–273, 1947.

2. Hicks SP, Black BK. The Relation of Cardiovascular Disease to Apoplexy. *Am Heart J* V38, pp 528–536, 1949.

3. Adams RD, Vander Eecken HM. Vascular Diseases of the Brain. *Ann Rev Med* V4, pp 213–252, 1953.

4. Ad hoc Committee. A Classification and Outline of Cerebrovascular Disease. *Neurology* V8, pp 185–216, 1958.

5. Wright IS, Luckey EH. *Cerebral Vascular Diseases*. (Transactions of a conference held under the auspices of the American Heart Association). Grune and Stratton, New York, 1954, 163 p.

6. Wright IS, Millikan CH. *Cerebral Vascular Diseases*. (Transactions of the Second Conference held under the auspices of the American Heart Association). Grune and Stratton, New York, 1958, 224 p.

7. Cecil RL, Loeb RF. *A Textbook of Medicine* (9th edition). WB Saunders Co., Philadelphia, 1955.

8. Harrison TR, et al. *Principles of Internal Medicine* (2nd edition). The Blakeston Co., New York, 1954.

9. Harrison TR, et al. *Principles of Internal Medicine* (3rd edition). McGraw Hill, New York, 1958.

10. Laureno R, Shields R, Narayan T. The Diagnosis and Management of Cerebral Embolism and Hemorrhagic Infarction with Sequential Computerized Cranial Tomography. *Brain* V110, pp 93–105, 1987.

Infectious Diseases

Raymond Adams entered neurology when infectious diseases were treated with horse serum, arsenic, mercury, and surgical drainage. His contributions to this field were many. He was able to study abundant syphilitic material from the pre-penicillin era. He was able to systematically categorize the clinical and pathological manifestations of that disease and to place them in temporal relationship. Having characterized syphilis as a chronic meningitis, he studied the pathology of acute bacterial meningitis and was able to place the meningitides in conceptual relationship.

In viral diseases, his clinicopathologic correlations provided facts, where others had provided speculation. He proved, what Charles Symonds had hypothesized, that the encephalitis, which rendered its victims amnesic, had damaged the medial temporal lobes. He disproved, what Ramsay Hunt had hypothesized, that the main damage in zoster related facial palsy was in the geniculate ganglion.

RL: *What motivated you to take up the subject of subdural empyema?*

RA: The Massachusetts Eye and Ear Infirmary had entire wards full of patients with ear infections. As a resident in neurology, I was called there frequently to consult on patients with mastoiditis, who were suspected of having some type of intracranial complication. There was an astonishingly high mortality. Charles Kubik and I examined, post mortem, a number of patients. Each had developed headache, high fever, and acute unilateral cerebral symptoms, which had been misdiagnosed as brain abscess. We found that they had no brain abcess; they had cerebral compression by subdural empyema. We thought it would be worth writing about these cases in order to clearly differentiate empyema from brain abscess, clinically and pathologically [see Chapter 5)

RL: *Would that distinction have affected the management?*

RA: Yes. At that time, the common practice was to delay operation on brain abscess on the assumption that time would allow encapsulation of the abscess. I had seen a patient, who, while the surgeons were waiting, had died of a subdural empyema. It should have been drained through a burr hole. Subdural empyema was a more fulminant condition than brain abcess, in which focal signs were more slow to evolve. Once we had the clinical picture firmly in mind we made a clinical diagnosis in two or three cases of subdural empyema that were successfully drained. We satisfied ourselves that, by early operation, subdural empyema was a perfectly treatable condition.

Pathologically it was rather interesting to observe a pyogenic infection lodging on the external surface of the arachnoid causing only a reactive change in the cerebrospinal fluid. We showed very clearly that the empyema was nearly always localized to one part of the subdural space. Often you would see a pial vein, where only the outer half of the vein wall showed endothelial reaction and contained a thrombus. In the underlying cortex, there were varying degrees of ischemic change, which you would not see underneath a subdural hematoma. This ischemic change, in the brain of patients with subdural empyema, was the basis, we thought, of the seizures, reversible hemiplegia, and other focal neurologic signs.

RL: *You said that Charles Kubik could remove the entire brain with the dura intact. What was the advantage of that?*

RA: Others had surely reported dural and subdural inflammation. But by cutting through the dura, and taking out the brain in the usual way, they would lose anatomical relationships. So Kubik thought that it would be worthwhile to do this in order to preserve the anatomical relationships between the dura and arachnoid.

RL: *Can you tell me about your collaboration with Houston Merritt on the study of neurosyphilis?* [see Chapter 5]

RA: He and I worked closely. I attended his neurosyphilis clinic once a week, and we wrote several articles together. We finally collaborated on a book on neurosyphilis; I did the pathology and helped with the clinical side. Harry Solomon, Professor of Psychiatry at the Boston Psychopatic Hospital, was a collaborator, but his other duties allowed little time for it.

RL: *Why was Solomon involved?*

RA: In Merritt's clinical work he was aided by Solomon in the treatment of general paresis. Solomon was in charge of neurosyphilis at the Boston Psychopathic Hospital and always provided us malarial parasites for treating paretic neurosyphilis. He and Merritt became good friends, and they decided to collaborate on a book on neurosyphilis. I was added as third author. The book was published just as penicillin was found to be the first safe treatment of neurosyphilis. Before that we were still using neo-arsphenamine and bismuth.

RL: *You say that Solomon provided you with malarial parasites?*

RA: Yes. The only treatment for general paresis at the time was hyperthermia. We had a certain benign malaria strain that we repeatedly injected in our patients. We would use fresh blood from a previously injected patient to inject the next. It was a way of causing repeated episodes of hyperthermia.

RL: *Was this injection intravenous?*

RA: Yes. We would induce malaria and let them have chills, usually series of about ten. After several fevers we treated the patient with quinine.

RL: *Were you convinced that this therapy was beneficial?*

RA: Yes! There was no question about that. And, of course, everyone was very excited about it.

RL: *The diagram from your book on neurosyphilis you've continued to use in your Principles of Neurology.* [see Figure 37]

RA: Yes. The diagram relating the various types of neurosyphilis was by Merritt and myself. The idea emerged during evening discussions. The underlying idea was that all forms of neurosyphilis were products of a chronic meningitis—actually the most chronic form of human meningitis.

RL: *Had anybody else recognized chronic meningitis as the common denominator of neurosyphilis?*

RA: Dattner, a New York syphilologist had recognized the chronic meningitis. He had a wide experience with this aspect of the disease. I was influenced by his writings. Syphilologist, Earl Moore, at Johns Hopkins made some excellent contributions on syphilis in general and also substantiated the occurrence of early meningitis. And he appreciated the temporal relationships of the different forms of neurosyphilis.

RL: *You say you met with Merritt in the evening.*

RA: I would go to Merritt's home and have dinner with him and his wife and then stay on 2 or 3 hours writing some part of the book or editing what we had written. And, of course, there were continuous discussions of aspects of the disease.

Merritt, himself, was fully conversant with the ideas and general principles of neuropathology. He had spent a sabbatical in Spielmeyer's laboratory.

RL: *As far as I can tell, that diagram was your synthesis. It wasn't a common conception previously.*

RA: Yes. I thought that this diagram properly expressed the relationship of meningitis to the other forms of neurosyphilis. Earl Moore observed that the meningitis didn't appear, until some months or a year after the inception of the syphilitic infection. Only occasionally it would flare rapidly as an acute symptomatic meningitis.

We noted that the vascular lesions tended to appear later, when the meningitis became more chronic. It was then called meningovascular disease of syphilitic type, with a clear Heubner's endarteritis and thrombosis.

If the process remained very chronic, detectable only by CSF examination at five years after the inception of syphilitic infection, then gradually there would emerge one of the other late forms, general paresis (syphilitic encephalitis) or still later, tabes dorsalis or combined tabo-paresis. Along the way there could be an isolated optic neuritis, unilateral and then bilateral, or a myelitis, either a meningomyelitis related to chronic spinal meningitis or a meningo-vascular disease of spinal cord with infarction. So I thought that all these manifestations of neurosyphilis were congruent as an elaboration of a basic meningeal process.

RL: *Your diagram doesn't show gumma.*

RA: Well, it turned out that we no longer had such cases. In the 1700s and 1800s syphilis was often fatal. Its malignancy diminished through time. Gumma was quite prominent early on, when syphilis was introduced into Europe. I looked through all of the files of the Mallory Institute of Pathology, and there was not a single gumma of the nervous system that had been recognized. And I didn't have one in the ten years of neuropathology that I supervised. So it had become increasingly rare. By the time that Merritt and I were studying syphilitic syndromes, they were more benign than they were in 1900. Indeed, by then, the human organism had become so adapted to the treponema pallidum that, if a person did not have chronic meningitis and if there was no symptom of aortitis, it meant that he probably would never develop one of the late forms of syphilis. If the CSF became normal within five years after the infection, the chance of developing a late form of neurosyphilis was 1/100.

RL: *Please comment on the medications that preceded penicillin.*

RA: The older forms of treatment of syphilis, arsphenamine, neoarsphenamine, bismuth, mercury—those were only partially effective and needed to be given over a period of months to a year. It's forgotten, I think, that no one really knew whether those treatments, themselves, were more dangerous than having the more benign forms of syphilis (i.e. a case without neurosyphilis or aortitis).

Thus, an experiment was undertaken by our public health service, to study a group of untreated patients. They took a group of syphilitics, who didn't have neurosyphilis and left them untreated to see if they did as well or better than those treated (viz. the older forms of therapy). Actually this was a wise and thoughtful plan. It was the only way you'd be able to evaluate the potential dangers of the therapies under these conditions.

RL: *Can you tell me about the adverse effects of treatments used before penicillin was available?*

RA: Some would have skin rashes; others liver injury, kidney disease, loss of teeth. Tryparsamide, a form of arsenic, had to be introduced intrathecally; it would often cause temporary damage to the spinal cord. I remember having to give it as a resident in medicine at Duke University. There was a syphilis clinic of about 200 patients in an evening, from 7 to 9 p.m. They came for their intramuscular shots of bismuth or neoarsphenamine. If they had neurosyphilis they would get intrathecal tryparsamide. They would often have headache and stiff neck, and were full of complaints.

RL: *In Betty Banker's neuropathology laboratory we studied a patient, who, despite documented treatment for neurosyphilis, had residual Argyl Robertson pupils. At autopsy we could not find any pathological correlate for the abnormal pupils.*

RA: It was probably the inadequacy of your neuropathology. The question is: where is the lesion for the Argyl Robertson pupil? At first it was thought that it must be due to midbrain disease, selectively affecting the fibers that cause pupillary reaction to light, but sparing fibers that are responsible for pupil constriction on near vision. Merrill Moore and Merritt in Boston wrote a paper to that effect. I disagreed with Merritt. I thought the lesion was peripheral, the best evidence being that, in a diabetes, you can see the same thing (light-near dissociation). The lesion is probably in the distal part of the third nerve or the ciliary ganglion in the orbit.

RL: *We did not examine those structures.*

RA: Therefore you probably were missing the pathology.

RL: *I have a patient in the hospital with paranoia due to neurosyphilis but with little cognitive problem. Have you seen one like that?*

RA: I had a patient, a doctor who was brought in because he was acting peculiarly, was changed in personality and we didn't twig to the fact that he had neurosyphilis right away. While we were fiddling around, trying to decide what to do, he'd made about $200,000 in the stock market. Everyone was laughing about it. He was in touch with his stockbroker every morning. He wasn't demented, but he certainly had an abnormal spinal fluid.

RL: *Comment about syphilitic lightning pains.*

RA: Bill Caviness was working here in Boston at the Memorial Hospital, and he had a patient that had radicular lightning pains in a given area of his leg. He persuaded this fellow, who was suffering severely, to undergo operation on a ganglion (the pain was within the confines of one spinal root). I think Walter Wegner removed the offending root and ganglion. He gave half of it to me. The spinal nerve was normal but the nerve root itself was clearly involved. There was damage to the posterior root fibers all through, right up to the surface of the cord. I made sections for cell stains and silver stains that showed many large periphytes (probable regenerative axons from ganglion cells); the ganglion was otherwise intact. Bill Caviness knew that Castro was visiting the Rockefeller Institute in New York. Castro had written the definitive paper on dorsal root ganglia; it's in one of those three volumes of Penfield.[1] Bill took my sections down and showed them to Castro. He studied them for a few minutes and said, "This is typical tabes." My unproven hypothesis was that the periphytes may have somehow caused the lightning pains. I hadn't seen a case like that. Nor had I seen a case, where I could associate the root lesion with a given set of symptoms.[2]

RL: *We are looking at your book on neurosyphilis. Here's a picture of the cauda equina showing the thin gray posterior roots and normal anterior roots. It's the opposite of what you see in ALS, in which the anterior roots are atrophic.* [see Figure 38]

RA: That's right.

RL: *Can you comment further about tabes dorsalis?*

RA: It was known that tabes affected the dorsal roots and would cause ataxia and pain and that the roots were involved in meningeal inflammation. We found that the root disease could be at any point along that dorsal root, as long as it was within the leptospinal meninges. That had been the source of much controversy for a long time—whether the tabes lesion was in the dorsal columns or the dorsal root and, if dorsal root, whether it was at root entry zone or more peripherally. Erroneously, Spielmeyer had taken the position that the lesion in the posterior columns was primary. Castro had argued correctly that the cord degeneration was due to posterior root inflammation.

RL: *Later you studied the pathology of bacterial meningitis.*

RA: With the syphilitic meningitis, of course, most of our pathologic material was subacute or chronic. Even in the children with neurosyphilis we felt that it was very chronic. Having studied chronic meningeal disease, I naturally thought that it would be very instructive to look at the acute phases of meningeal disease in bacterial meningitis.

Influenzal bacillus meningitis was not responding well to the antibacterial treatments that were then available. They were using immune serum. Through our laboratories, we had cases that had lived for one or two or three days only and some who, with antiserum and various modes of treatment, were living up to three months. So these cases provided acute and subacute material that we never really saw in the neurosyphilitic series. It was obvious that the main changes were going on in the pia, though the arachnoid could be involved to a lesser extent. There was always some extraarachnoid subdural involvement, but that was prominent mostly in children. We could trace the earliest stages of this reaction to the bacillus into the perivenous system of the pia. Virchow–Robin spaces were crowded with inflammatory cells. From there polymorphonuclear leukocytes would migrate into the subarachnoid space and to some extent into the arachnoid. Gradually the exudate in the pia would change from polymorphonuclear cells to lymphocytes and mononuclear cells. Interestingly, the acute phase of that polymorphonuclear reaction included a lot of early (juvenile) polys with rather primitive nuclei. In a later phase we observed reacting fibroblasts. Virtually all of the lesions in the brain looked ischemic.

RL: *Was there similarity between the pathologies of syphilitic and influenzal meningitis.*

RA: I thought that that was the main reason for writing that paper on bacterial meningitis [see Chapter 5]. The most chronic influenzal bacillus meningitis duplicated the Heubner's endarteritis of syphilis; there were inflammatory cells in the subendothelial area as well as in the adventitia, as you would see in neurosyphilis.

RL: *Was the pial predominance of inflammation in influenzal meningitis similar to syphilis?*

RA: Yes.

RL: *This is the paper about herpes simplex (inclusion body) encephalitis. [see Chapter 5]*

RA: Maurice Victor was called to see a case of acute simplex encephalitis in an elderly man, who looked exactly like he was having delirium tremens. The patient was trembling and hallucinating and confused. Maurice said to be sure and get a history of his alcohol intake because this looked like a typical DTs. The patient sank into coma and died, and he proved to have temporal lobe encephalitis. I thought that the case strongly suggested that the abnormality in DTs was in the temporal lobes, because the clinical phenomena were so similar.

I had a number of fairly rapidly fatal cases of an encephalitis with this very interesting and peculiar anatomical topography. All had intranuclear inclusion bodies as well. The pattern was very striking, medial temporal or inferior temporal, sometimes extending upward towards the Sylvian fissure, and regularly extending posteriorly up over the corpus callosum into the cingulate gyri, and sometimes extending anteriorly into the orbito-frontal area. It was a strikingly peculiar distribution; it seemed almost unique. Moreover, it was a devastating type of encephalitis because the brain could become quite necrotic and the patient could die in three or four days. The etiology was not known. The inclusions indicated it was probably viral.

RL: *What was your paper's contribution?*

RA: We added to the distribution of the gross pathology and the clinical picture and emphasized the uniformly devastating effect on memory. We showed that it is one of the most common sporadic forms of encephalitis in the States.

RL: *Could further pathologic study of this disease be useful?*

RA: There has not been a continuous serial section study of the olfactory nerve filaments, olfactory bulb, etc.

RL: *I would like to turn to herpes zoster. Tell me about the case of Ramsay Hunt syndrome that you described.*

RA: At Boston City Hospital we had a superb case of zoster with facial weakness, the Ramsay Hunt syndrome. The patient had a hematologic disease and died after one month from a ruptured spleen. The patient was already recovering from his facial weakness when he died. Derek Denny-Brown and I carried out the postmortem examination. We were able to dissect out the seventh nerve and the geniculate ganglion from the temporal bone. I think it was the first anatomical study of a case of Ramsay Hunt Syndrome, where the facial nerve had been demonstrably involved. Ramsay Hunt had never examined the geniculate ganglion.*

At the C^2 C^3 levels there was also intense ganglionitis and there was posterior and anterior root involvement, and the posterior horns of the spinal cord showed a poliomyelitic type lesion. This and other of my cases of zoster established the pattern as one of unilateral, multisegmental poliomyelitis in the spinal cord and medulla with inflammation in the roots, posterior more than anterior, and less so in the peripheral nerve. Of course, at that time, no one had been able to isolate the zoster virus; that was done later over at Harvard Medical School.

RL: *This is a drawing done by you in the Bulletin of the New England Medical Center.*

RA: Yes.

RL: *It appears that you are showing the topography in herpes zoster, demonstrating that the ganglion and the spinal nerve, the posterior root and some of the spinal cord are inflamed with relative sparing of the anterior root.*

RA: Well, the anterior root can be affected a little bit. There can be paralysis, as you know.

RL: *You witnessed the emergence of the concept that there could be slow viral infections, such as subacute sclerosing panencephalitis (SSPE).*

RA: Van Bogaert of Belgium really put it on the clinical map. He suspected a viral cause. Greenfield wrote to Van Bogaert and borrowed his case material. Greenfield simply did H & E stain on Van Bogaert's material and revealed inclusion bodies in the brainstem nuclei. Van Bogaert had used only Nissl stain, which did not show the inclusion bodies.

RL: *Tell me about your early experience with progressive multifocal leukoencephalopathy.*

RA: The first time I'd seen it, at the Mass. General, was in the patient with lymphocytic leukemia. The medical service had diagnosed lymphocytic invasion of the brain. I hadn't observed anything like it. I had felt that the clinical picture represented something unique, but I didn't know what it was. I was astonished to see, in Karl Erich Astrom's section of the brain lesions, that the pathology was strikingly demyelinative and that there were abnormal astrocytes with multiple bizarre mitoses and oligodendrocytes with inclusion bodies. That was unique in his and my experience. Byron Waksman saw the material and noticed the inclusions; he was the one who proposed that it might be a viral infection. It started us on the trail of a series of similar cases that were dying at the Mass. General. Karl wrote it up and Pierson Richardson joined in the publication. I did not add my name to it. [see Chapter 5].

---

*Ramsay Hunt had hypothesized that geniculate ganglion damage was the basis of the facial palsy. Adams found, in his case, that the obvious disease was in the seventh cranial nerve itself.

RL: *Is there room for more research on PML?*
RA: The experimental transfer of PML has not yet been accomplished.

Ray Adams' contributions to infectious diseases were many. Important for diagnosis and therapy was his demonstration that subdural empyema had different presentation and required different and more urgent therapy than brain abscess. Important in clinicopathologic correlation were his study of facial paralysis in herpes zoster and his paper about amnesia in inclusion body encephalitis. His main contribution to conceptualization of infectious disease was the systematic exposition of meningitis in its spectrum from acute to chronic. His writings on all of these subjects are as worth reading now as they were half a century ago.

Unfortunately these papers attract little attention today. The extraordinary advances in antibiotic and anti-viral medication properly dominate the field of infectious diseases. However, modern experts in infectious disease know less pathology than their predecessors. As a result they sometimes make uninformed statements about these conditions. They would benefit from the study of these classic pathologic works.

Notes

1. Penfield W (ed.). *Cytology and Cellular Pathology of the Nervous System*, 3 *Vols*. Paul B. Hoeber Inc., New York, 1932, p 1280.
2. Caviness W, Adams R, Pope A, Wegner W. The Role of the Dorsal Root Ganglia in the Production of the Lancinating Pains of Central Nervous System Syphilis. *Trans Am Neurol Assoc* V74, pp 60–64, 1949.

Demyelinative Diseases and Neuro-immunology

The fact that inflammatory ,demyelinative, allergic disease can affect the central nervous system (e.g., multiple sclerosis) or peripheral nervous system (e.g., Guillain–Barré syndrome) is a standard teaching of the current era. When Ray Adams entered neurology, these ideas had not been well formulated or widely accepted. A *Textbook of Medicine* by Cecil and Loeb (1951) listed many theories about the cause of multiple sclerosis: deficiency of trace elements, brucellosis, virus, coagulation disorder with venular thrombosis, transient repeated vaso-constriction, emotional disturbances, and others including allergic mechanisms. In his textbook (1940) Kinnier Wilson wrote that the primary hypotheses about the cause of multiple sclerosis were microbial, viral, and chemical. Ray Adams would play an important role in moving neurology from this confusion, to the modern concept of auto-immune causation for these diseases.

At Boston City Hospital Ray Adams had already been studying a demyeli-native disease, acute necrotizing hemorrhagic encephalopathy. However, two

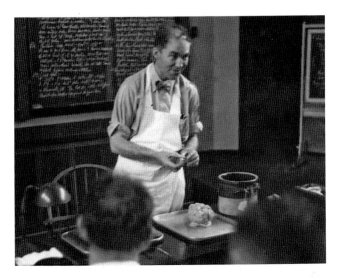
Raymond D. Adams at brain cutting conference in the Mallory Institute of Pathology at Boston City Hospital.

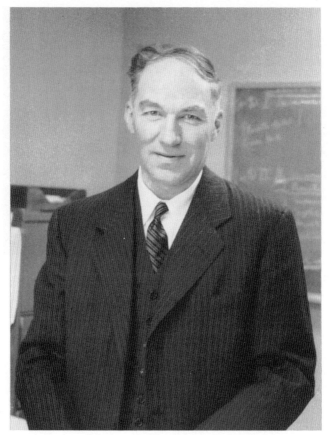

Figure 1 Raymond D. Adams at Massachusetts General Hospital.

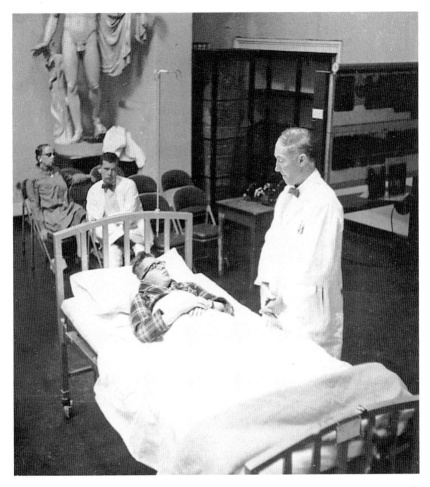

Figure 2 Raymond D. Adams interviewing a patient during Neurology Grand Rounds at Massachusetts General Hospital.

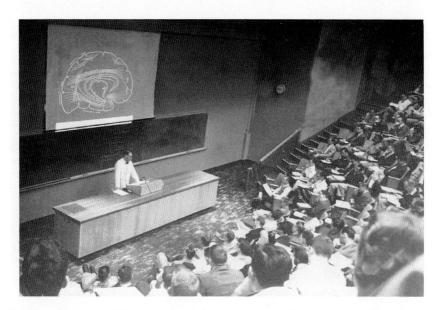

Figure 3 Raymond D. Adams lectures to students in his neuropathology course at Harvard Medical School.

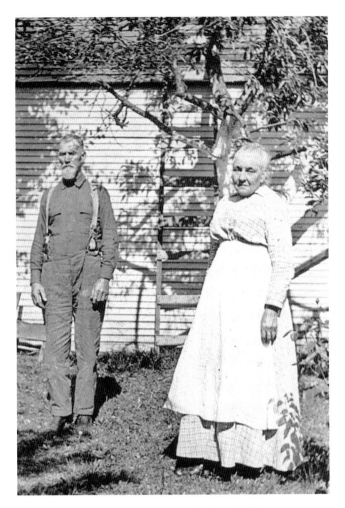

Figure 4 Maternal grand parents of Raymond Adams in Oregon.

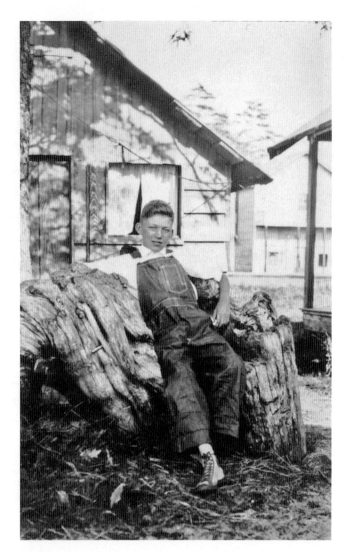

Figure 5 Raymond D. Adams.

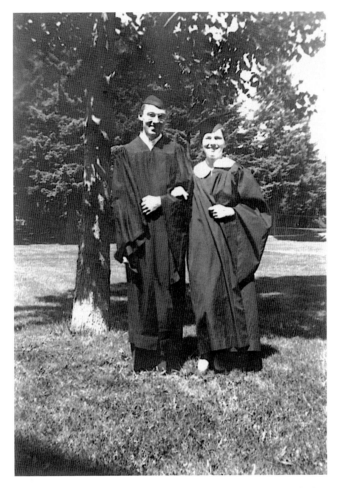

Figure 6 Raymond D. Adams with his bride, Margaret Elinor Clark, at the Sixth Commencement at University of Oregon, 1933.

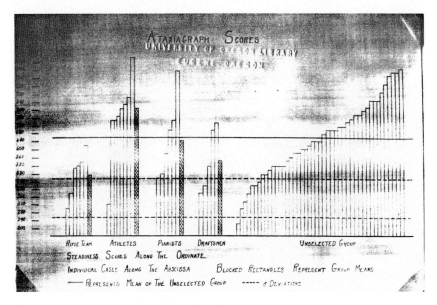

Figure 7 Bar graph from Master's thesis of Raymond D. Adams. The ataxia graph scores of the Rifle Team are better than the other groups. The blocked rectangles show the mean score for each group.

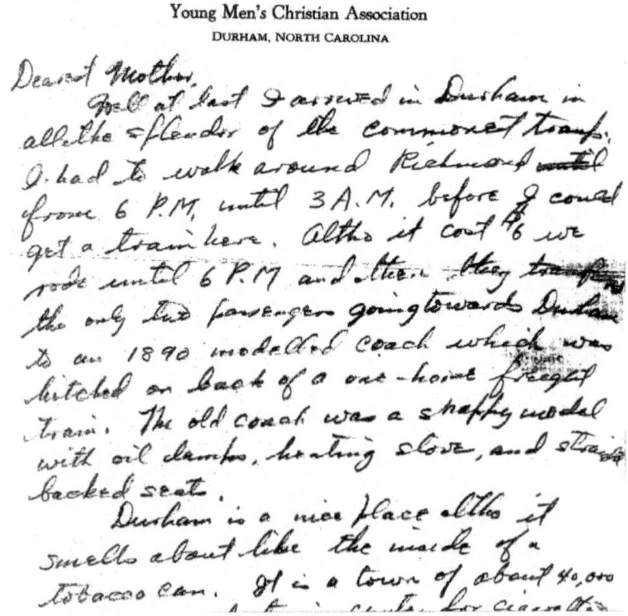

Young Men's Christian Association
DURHAM, NORTH CAROLINA

Dearest Mother,

Well at last I arrived in Durham in all the splendor of the commonest tramp. I had to walk around Richmond ~~until~~ from 6 P.M. until 3 A.M. before I could get a train here. Altho it cost $6 we rode until 6 P.M. and then ~~they transf~~ the only two passenger going towards Durham to an 1890 modelled coach which was hitched on back of a one-horse freight train. The old coach was a shabby model with oil lamps, heating stove, and straight backed seat.

Durham is a nice place altho it smells about like the inside of a tobacco can. It is a town of about 40,000

Figure 8 Letter written by Raymond Adams after arriving in Durham, North Carolina.

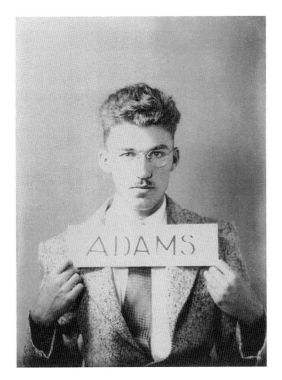

Figure 9 The medical student on arrival at Duke University. Several students wore the same jacket for their photographs.

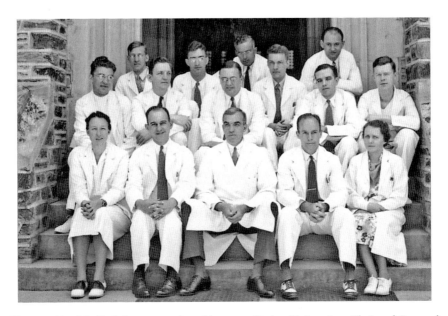

Figure 10 Medical interns and residents at Duke University. Chair of Internal Medicine Dr Hanes is front and center. Adams is in the second row, *far left*. Behind him is George Harrel (see Figure 11).

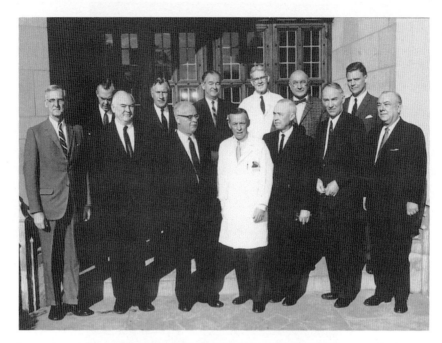

Figure 11 Advisory Committee to Duke University includes distinguished alumni such as Adams, *front row, second from right*; and George Harrel, *front row, far left* (see Figure 10). Harrel became the dean of the medical school in Hershey, Pennsylvania. *Front row third from left*: Houston Merritt.

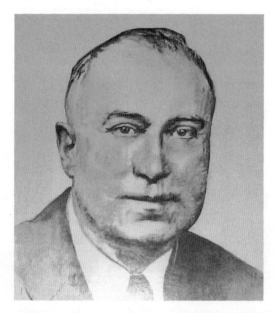

Figure 12 Robert Graves, who taught Adams how to do the neurologic examination at Duke.

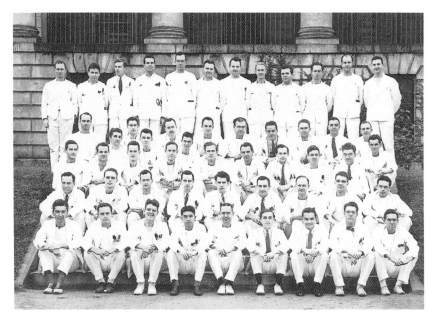

Figure 13 Massachusetts General Hospital interns and residents. Ray Adams is in the third row, *far right*, with tie and eyeglasses, 1938–1939. Note the absence of women, a difference from the Duke photograph (see Figure 10).

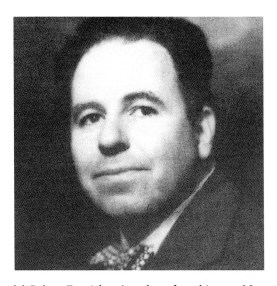

Figure 14 Mandel Cohen, Ray Adams' teacher of psychiatry at Massachusetts General Hospital.(Courtesy of Dr Anne Cohen.)

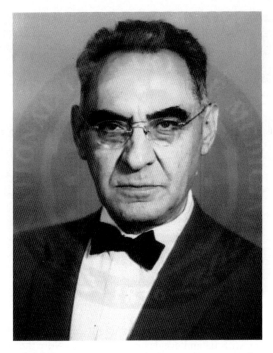

Figure 15 Eugen Kahn, who taught Ray Adams psychiatry at Yale.

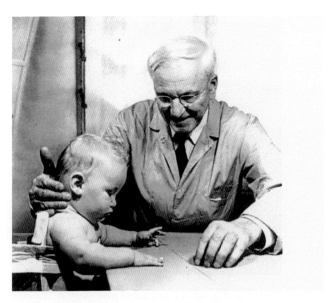

Figure 16 Arnold Gesell, who had important influence on Adams at Yale.

THE ROCKEFELLER FOUNDATION

49 WEST 49th STREET, NEW YORK

THE MEDICAL SCIENCES
ALAN GREGG, M.D., DIRECTOR
ROBERT A. LAMBERT, M.D., ASSOCIATE DIRECTOR

CABLE ADDRESS:
ROCKFOUND, NEW YORK

March 3, 1939.

Dear Doctor Adams:

I was disappointed not to see you when you were here. We are so accustomed to have our fellows call whenever they are in the city that it never occurred to me that you would pass through New York twice without dropping in, particularly since the question of your plans for next year were under discussion. On receipt of a note from Doctor Diethelm on the 23rd that you had visited the Payne Whitney Clinic two days before I tried in vain to locate you. From the New York Psychiatric Institute I learned that you called there on the 22nd but that in the absence of Doctor Nolan Lewis you went away without meeting any one else. May I suggest in this connection that you should never hesitate, in the absence of the chief, to ask some one else to show you over an institution. There is a lot of good work going on at the Institute which I am sure you would have been interested to see, though I do not think at this stage of your training it is the place you would choose to spend a year.

Since you were in Durham last Friday and presumably back in Boston on Monday, I am wondering if you stopped in Philadelphia

Figure 17 Portion of letter from Rockefeller Foundation, March 3, 1939.

During past two years in Boston I proved to be a better than average neurologist but a rather poor psychiatrist, whether from lack of interest or aptitude I dont know. The men with whom I have worked urge me to continue to work in neurology rather than psychiatry. When this vacancy at Harvard occurred Stanley Cobb recommended two people for the job – Charles Aring, of Cincinnati, and myself. Since Aring could not leave he recommended that I take the position. His argument was that in another 18 mo. – which is the duration of the appointment – I could become a first class neurologist, begin several research problems which could be continued in subsequent years, and be more valuable to Duke as a result of this.

Figure 18 Portion of Adams' letter to Dr Hanes, February 11, 1941.

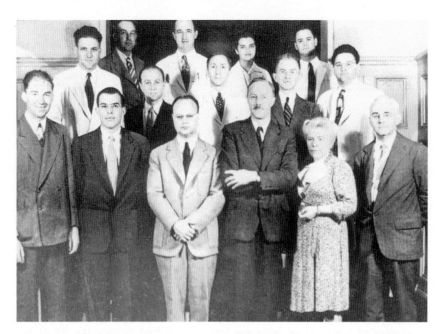

Figure 19 Neurology staff of Boston City Hospital, 1944–1945. *Front row, left to right*: R. D. Adams, Charles Brenner, Houston Merritt, Derek Denny-Brown, Alexandra Adler, William Lenox; Second row: Freddy Homberger, A. Friedman, Ira Ross, Paul Yakovlev, R. Ravven; Top row: Ed Cole, Avery Weisman, Frances Bonner, Daniel Sciarra.

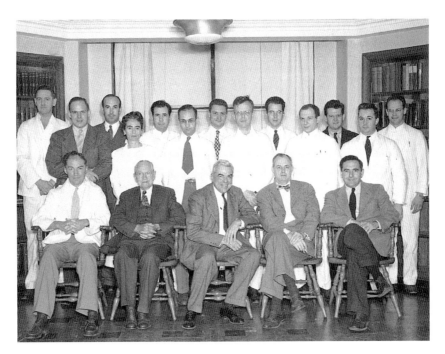

Figure 20   Mallory Institute of Pathology staff. Front row: Raymond Adams, Timothy Leary, Frederic Parker, Kenneth Mallory, Stanley Robbins; Third row: *second from left* is C. Miller Fisher, Adams' fellow in 1949.

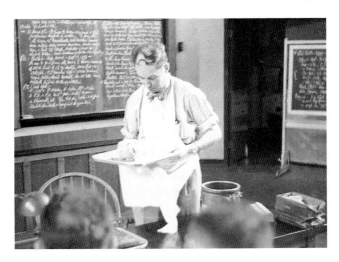

Figure 21   Raymond D. Adams preparing for brain cutting conference at Mallory Institute of Pathology, which was connected by a tunnel to Boston City Hospital.

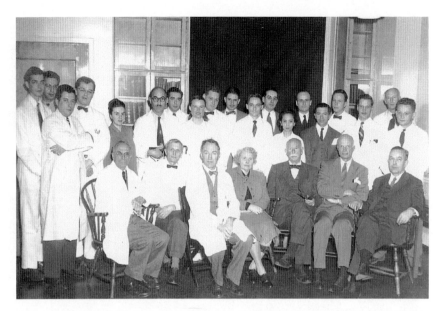

Figure 22 Raymond D. Adams on his return to Massachusetts General Hospital as neurology chairman in 1951. *Front row, left to right*: Stanley Cobb, Charles Kubik, Raymond Adams, Madeline Brown, and James Ayer. *Second row, right to left*: Al Heyman, E. P. Richardson. In front of bookcase to left are Robert Schwab and Maurice Victor.

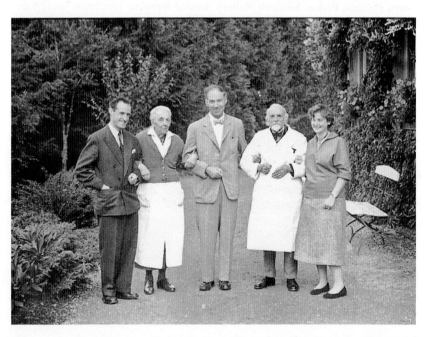

Figure 23 Ray Adams visits the laboratory of Oskar and Cecille Vogt. Shown in the garden with Adams' former fellow Henri Vander Eecken and his wife. Vander Eecken later became chairman of neurology at the medical school in Ghent.

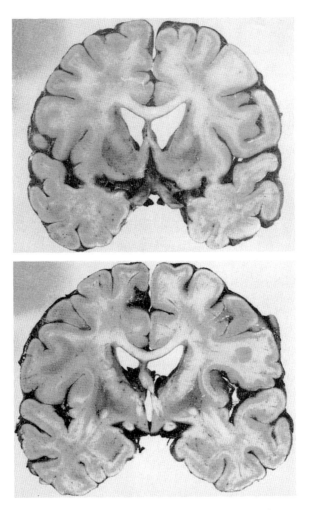

Figure 24 During his sabbatical, Ray Adams studied his cases of striatonigral degeneration with van Bogaert. Pictured here is one of the brains from their joint publication. The caudate and putamen are very atrophic on these two slices. (Reproduced by permission from the *Journal of Neuropathology and Experimental Neurology*.)

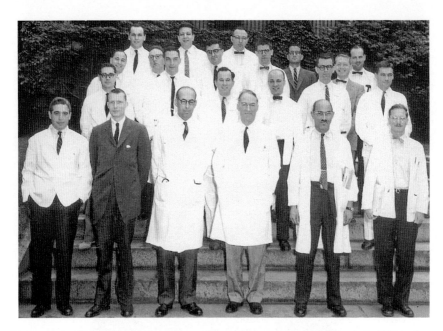

Figure 25 Neurology Department, Massachusetts General Hospital. This photo shows residents who started in the 1950s. *Front row* (faculty), *left to right*: M. Victor, P. Dodge, C. Miller Fisher, R. D. Adams, R. Schwab, E. P. Richardson. *Second row*: B. Arnason, D. Drachman, P. McHugh, G. Winkler, R. T. Johnson, B. Konigsmark. *Third row*: M. Cole, I. Zeiper, B. Behari, A. McPhedran, A. Pollack, E. Picard, A. Weiss. *Fourth row*: B. McLeroy, H. Moser, B. Flynn. (Thanks to Richard Johnson for providing the names.) *Note*: From this group of residents came the chairmen of departments of neurology at the University of Chicago, Johns Hopkins University, and the University of Massachusetts, the chairman of Psychiatry at Johns Hopkins University, the director of the Kennedy Krieger Institute at Johns Hopkins, and the director of a family medicine program.

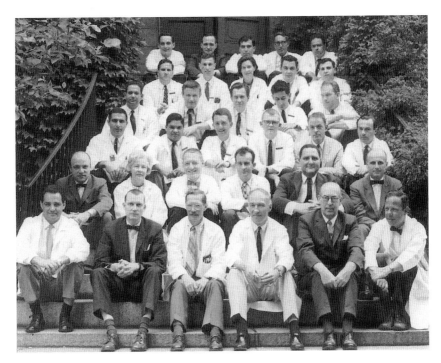

Figure 26 Neurology Department, Massachusetts General Hospital, a sample group photograph from the 1960s. *Front row, left to right*: Byron Kakulas, Phillip Dodge, E. P. Richardson, R. D. Adams, C. Miller Fisher, Pierre Dreyfus. *Second row*: G. Winkler, Dr Scholl, E. Picard, H. Webster, D. Poskanzer, V. Perlo. *Third row*: (unknown), Dr Pant, (unknown), J. R. Baringer, A. Asbury, (unknown). *Fourth row*: (unknown), Donald Price, Verne Caviness, (unknown), (unknown). *Fifth row*: all unknown. *Sixth row*: unknown except T. Chase (*second from right*). (Thanks to H. Webster for providing the names.) *Note*: At least six persons seen in this photo became department chairmen elsewhere.

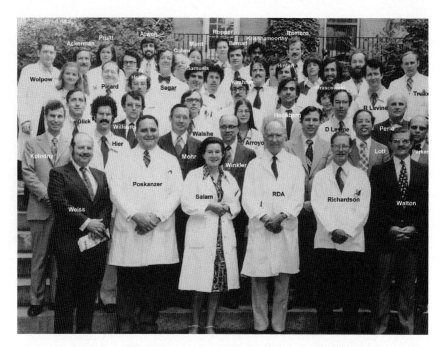

Figure 27 Neurology Department, Massachusetts General Hospital, a sample group photograph from the 1970s. Dr Adams stands next to his wife Maria Salam. Apparently visiting is his ex-fellow, John Walton. Dr Adams' teacher of psychiatry, Mandel Cohen, is near the rear, *left of center*. Many of the pictured members of the faculty and resident staff had distinguished careers. For example, Allan Ropper and Martin Samuels became authors of Adams and Victor's *Principles of Neurology*. (Thanks to Allan Ropper for providing the names.)

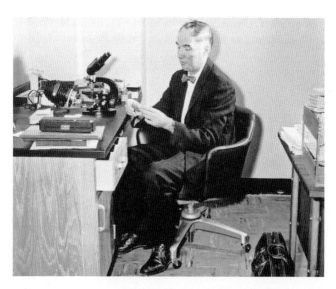

Figure 28 Raymond Adams at his lab in the Warren Building at Massachusetts General Hospital, 1957.

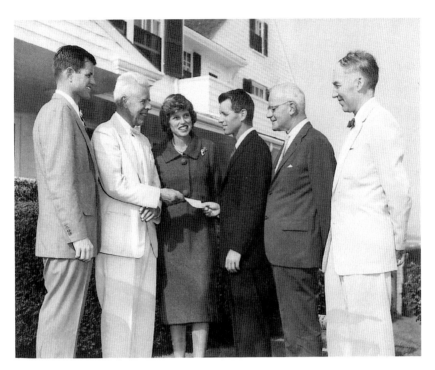

Figure 29 Presentation of the check for development of the Joseph P. Kennedy, Jr. Laboratories for Research on Mental Retardation from the Joseph P. Kennedy, Jr. Foundation. *Left to right*: Edward M. Kennedy, Francis C. Gray, Chairman of the Board of Trustees of Massachusetts General Hospital, Mrs Robert Sargent Shriver, Jr (Eunice Kennedy Shriver), Vice President of Kennedy Foundation, Robert F. Kennedy, President of Kennedy Foundation, Dr Dean A. Clark, General Director of the Hospital, and Dr Raymond Adams. On this occasion in 1959, Adams commented, "Three major objectives will be pursued at the Kennedy Laboratories. First we will attempt to improve the care of infants and children with diseases of the nervous system; second to aid in the education of students and physicians, particularly those who aspire to teaching and research in pediatric neurology; third, to investigate the cause, treatment, and prevention of diseases of the nervous system of infants and children." The laboratories were dedicated in 1962 with Dr Raymond Adams as director. Nowhere else had there been conceived such an ambitious program to advance pediatric neurology.

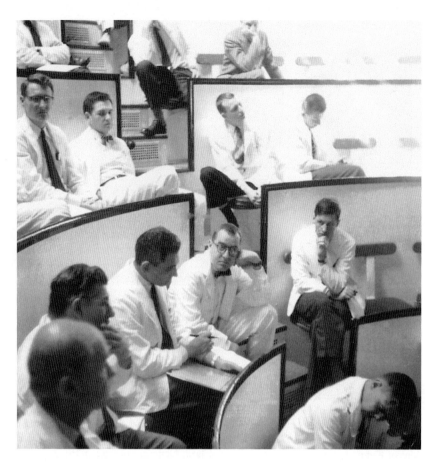

Figure 30 Residents and staff in the Ether Dome in the 1950s. Guy McKhann (*front row with bowtie*) would leave for Stanford to develop pediatric neurology, Peter Huttenlocher (*across the aisle*) would leave for the University of Chicago to head pediatric neurology, and Phil Dodge (*in plaid tie above Huttenlocher*) would leave for Washington University to head the Department of Pediatrics.

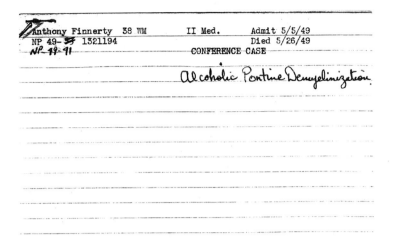

CC: Hearty drinking recently.
PH: Heavy drinker for " 28 years" with intermittent sprees.
D.T.'s twice before.
PI: On spree for 2 weeks. Unable to eat 3-4 days. Evening pta
got the shakes, began to see "impossible things".
PE: T 102, P 130, R 45, BP 90/60. Dehydrated, signs of consol-
idation over LLL. Tremulous, fluctuating awareness with per-
iods of irrelevent speech and agitation. Reflexes OK except
KJ and AJ absent bilat. Toes↓↓.
Lab: Urine 1 plus alb. Hgb. 12.5, WBC 11000, 96% polys. Hinton
neg, NPN 55 to 27, CO2 58, Cl 101. Bl. cult.- pneumoc. type V.
Throat swab same.
Course: Started on penicillin 200,000 u q2h. Pt. became deler-
ious soon after adm. phys. and remained so until 5/10, when he
seemed to have improved very slightly. Because of slow reso-
lution of pneumonia, was started on aureomycin 5/9. 5/10-
Difficulty talking and swallowing, but very ill. More alert.
5/12- Moves arms and legs well. 5/14- Moves extremities less
well. 5/15- Unable to swallow but can close his mouth. 5/16-
Absent sensation throughout, but corneals present. 5/17- Pt.
able to follow commands to close and open eyes, does not respond to painful stimuli. Fundi normal. Pupils- rr and e, react to light. EOM ok. V- Conreals equal, sluggish; no evidence that he feels pinprick. VII- no facial movements. X- un-
ab;e to speak or swallow. XII- unable to protrude tongue.
Motor flaccid quadriplegia. Reflexes- biceps and triceps present
the rest absent; toes↑↑. 5/19- Much as before; slight movements of rt. arm and leg in response to strong supraorbital
pressure.

Reflexes

	B	T	W	K	A	Pl.
L	⧺	⧺	⊦	→	+	o
R	⧺	⧺	+	+	+	↑

5/20- Limitation of upward gaze. Deviation downward of rt. eye
on looking to L. Respirations irreg. Other observations as before. 5/24- Reflexes can be elicited, brisker on rt. Left lung
appears atelectatic. 5/26- Death.
LP: 5/17- IP 65, clear colorless, 1 lymph, TP 24, CG 0011221000,
no growth.

Figure 31 On interesting autopsy cases Adams would keep 5″ × 7″ index cards of clinical information along with the microscopic slides. This case, from 1949, he presented at
a conference as "pontine demyelinization" in an alcoholic. After he had collected a total
of four cases of this entity, he, ten years later, wrote the classic article seen in Figure 32.

Central Pontine Myelinolysis

*A Hitherto Undescribed Disease Occurring in Alcoholic and
Malnourished Patients*

RAYMOND D. ADAMS, M.D.; MAURICE VICTOR, M.D., and ELLIOTT L. MANCALL, M.D., Boston

In the course of our studies of the neuropathology of alcoholism, which were begun at the Neurological Unit, Boston City Hospital, and have continued in the laboratories of the Neurology Service, Massachusetts General Hospital, two of us (R. D. A. and M. V.) observed three, perhaps four, cases in which the myelin sheaths of all the nerve fibers in the central part of the basis pontis had been destroyed in a single, large, symmetric focus. The nerve cells and axis cylinders were spared for the most part, and the blood vessels were patent and unaffected. There were no signs of inflammation in or near the lesion. The disease had occurred on a background of alcoholism and malnutrition; in the two cases with the largest lesions, it had manifested itself clinically by a pseudobulbar palsy and quadriplegia, leading to death in about 13 and 26 days. In the other two cases there were no symptoms referable to the lesions, presumably because of their small size.

The disease which is to be described does not resemble any of the known varieties of demyelination. It is unique both in its distribution and in the apparent character of the pathologic process and resulting morbid change. We have searched the medical literature in order to determine whether or not this condition was known to other neuropathologists but have failed to discover a

single case of this type. These considerations have encouraged us to present our cases in some detail and to attempt an analysis of the main features of this disease.

Report of Cases

CASE 1.—*A chronic alcoholic entered the hospital with lobar pneumonia and delirium tremens. His symptoms were improving when, over a two-day period (9th to 11th hospital day), he developed flaccid quadriplegia, weakness of the face and tongue, and inability to speak and swallow. Death ensued on the 22d hospital day, and postmortem examination disclosed a symmetric destruction of the myelinated sheaths of the basis pontis, with relative intactness of the nerve cells and axis cylinders.*

A 38-year-old man was admitted to the Second (Harvard) Medical Service of the Boston City Hospital on May 5, complaining of tremulousness and hallucinations, of recent onset. The patient was a confirmed alcoholic who had been drinking steadily for many years. In addition, there were intermittent periods in which he would greatly increase his alcoholic intake, and twice in the past, after such an episode, he had been hospitalized for delirium tremens.

For two weeks before his final illness the patient had been drinking particularly heavily, and in the last three or four days of this period he had been unable to eat and vomited several times. On the day before admission he became very tremulous and began to see "impossible things." He feared that he was losing his mind and asked for protection from the police, who, in turn, brought him to the hospital. The patient also gave a history of a recent cold, with cough and pain in the left chest.

On admission to the hospital the patient appeared seriously ill. He was dehydrated; his respirations were rapid and gasping, 45 per minute; the temperature was 102 F, pulse 130 per minute, and blood pressure 90/60. The important physical findings were in the lower lobe of the left lung, where dullness to percussion, increased bronchial breath sounds with egophony, and fine inspiratory rales were detected. Although the patient was restless

Received for publication Feb. 13, 1958.

From the Neurology Service, Massachusetts General Hospital, and the Department of Neurology-Neuropathology, Harvard Medical School. This study was supported in part by a research grant, M-767 (c), from the National Institute of Mental Health, National Institutes of Health, U. S. Public Health Service.

Figure 32   Front page of the article on Central Pontine Myelinolysis. The case documented in Figure 31 is Case 1 in the article. One of the four patients he reported was not alcoholic. (Reproduced by permission from *Archives of Neurology and Psychiatry* 81(2): 154–172. Copyright © (1959) American Medical Association. All rights reserved.)

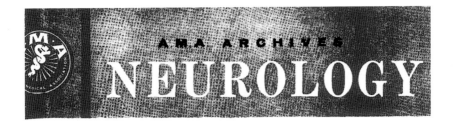

A Restricted Form of Cerebellar Cortical Degeneration Occurring in Alcoholic Patients

MAURICE VICTOR, M.D.; RAYMOND D. ADAMS, M.D., and ELLIOTT L. MANCALL, M.D., Boston

Introduction
Clinical Observations
The Natural History of the Disease
Clinical and Pathological Case Reports
A Quantitative Estimation of the Changes in the
    Cerebellar Cortex
Comment
  A. Clinical Features
  B. Nature and Significance of the Pathological
        Findings
  C. Clinical and Pathological Correlation
  D. Etiological Considerations
  E. Review of the Medical Literature
  F. Spontaneously Occurring Cortical Cerebellar
        Degenerations in Animals
  G. Restricted Cortical Cerebellar Degeneration
        in the Alcoholic Patient—a Clinical-Patho-
        logical Entity
Summary and Conclusions

Introduction

The relationship of cerebellar cortical degeneration to chronic alcoholism has been a controversial matter for many years. There are now several published accounts of a cerebellar syndrome in alcoholic patients, but these are purely clinical, and one has no way of ascertaining the nature of the pathological changes and of deciding

Submitted for publication June 29, 1959.
Present address (Dr. Mancall): Department of Neurology, Jefferson Medical College, Philadelphia.
This work was aided in part by a research grant (M-767C) from the National Institute of Mental Health, U.S. Public Health Service.
From the Neurology Service, Massachusetts General Hospital, and the Departments of Neurology and Neuropathology, Harvard Medical School.

whether they differed in any way from the other known types of cerebellar atrophy. Isolated, pathologically verified instances of primary cerebellar degeneration have been described in alcoholics, but, in general, the pathology has been incompletely described and the etiological relationship to alcohol has not been critically studied.

In the course of our own studies on the effect of alcohol on the nervous system, we have made clinical observations on a group of 50 patients, all of whom were undoubted and severe alcoholics and were afflicted with a remarkably uniform cerebellar syndrome. This syndrome was characterized, in almost every instance, by an ataxia of gait and of the legs, with relatively little involvement of the arms, speech, and ocular motility and, in the majority of cases, by an evolution over a short period of time, followed by years of stability. In seven of these patients a complete postmortem examination of the nervous system was made. Essentially, the lesion consisted of degeneration, varying in severity, of all neurocellular elements of the cerebellar cortex, particularly the Purkinje cells, with a striking topographical restriction to the anterior and superior aspects of the vermis and of the hemispheres. In addition to these seven patients, a similar cerebellar lesion was discovered in four others, in whom there had been a history of severe alcoholism but no indication of cerebellar

Figure 33   Front page of the article on nutritional cerebellar degeneration in the alcoholic. (Reproduced by permission from *Archives of Neurology* 1(6): 579–688. Copyright © (1959) American Medical Association. All rights reserved.)

THE WERNICKE-KORSAKOFF SYNDROME

and Related Neurologic Disorders Due to Alcoholism and Malnutrition

SECOND EDITION

MAURICE VICTOR, M.D.
Professor of Medicine (Neurology)
Dartmouth Medical School
Distinguished Physician of the Veterans
  Administration at White River
  Junction, Vermont

RAYMOND D. ADAMS, M.D.
Bullard Professor of Neuropathology,
  Emeritus
Harvard Medical School
Senior Neurologist and
Formerly Chief of Neurology Service
Massachusetts General Hospital
Director Emeritus, Eunice K. Shriver
  Center
Boston, Massachusetts

GEORGE H. COLLINS, M.D.
Professor of Neuropathology and
  Neuropathologist
State University of New York
College of Medicine and Health Science
  Center
Syracuse, New York

F. A. DAVIS COMPANY ● Philadelphia

Figure 34   Front page of edition two of the book on Wernicke disease.

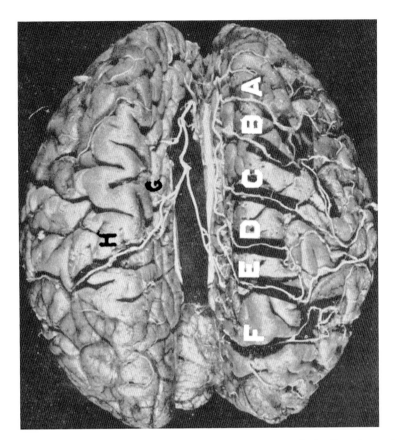

Figure 35 From the study of surface collaterals of the brain which affect the territory infarcted when a vessel is occluded. Injection of the right middle cerebral artery shows anastomoses with the right anterior cerebral and also with the left anterior cerebral artery and thence the left middle cerebral artery (H). (Reproduced by permission from the *Journal of Neuropathology and Experimental Neurology*.)

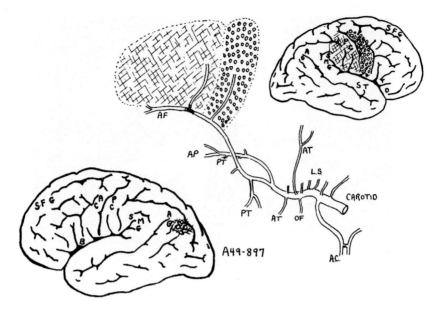

Figure 36 Hemorrhagic infarction due to cerebral embolism. Drawing to show that the hemorrhagic area (*circles*) is proximal to the embolic fragment, which has moved distally. Distal to the embolus, the infarct is not bloody (*cross hatched*). (Reproduced by permission of the *Journal of Neuropathology and Experimental Neurology*.)

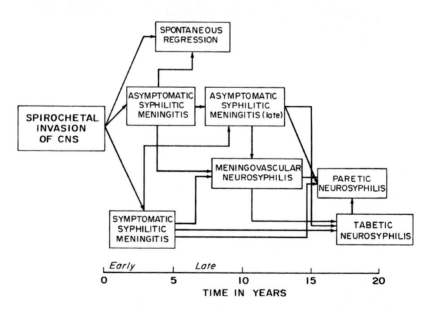

Figure 37 Neurosyphilis conceptualized in a diagram indicating the fundamental process (meningitis), the chronology, and the relationships of different types of parenchymal involvement. (Reproduced by permission of The McGraw-Hill Companies from Adams, RD and Victor, M, *Principles of Neurology*, 1977.)

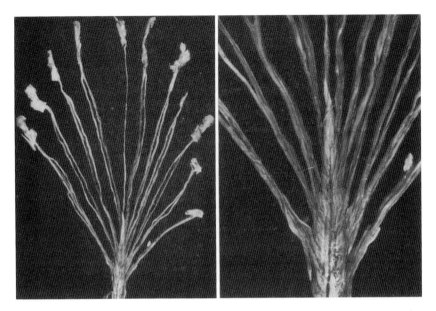

Figure 38 Photograph of cauda equina showing atrophy of dorsal roots in tabetic neurosyphilis.

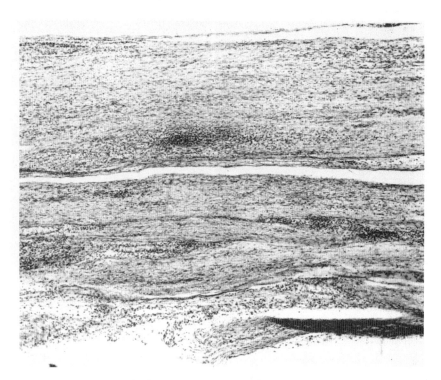

Figure 39 Experimental allergic neuritis in the guinea pig sciatic nerve. Areas of infiltration by inflammatory cells are evident. (Reproduced by permission of the *Journal of Neuropathology and Experimental Neurology*.)

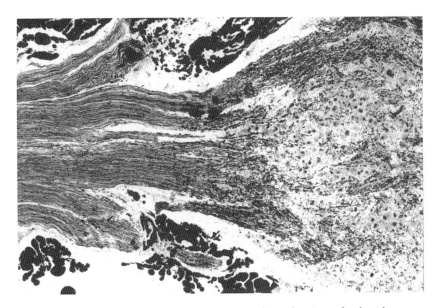

Figure 40 Diphtheritic polyneuropathy causing demyelination of a dorsal root ganglion and sparing the nearby spinal nerve. (Reproduced by permission of the *Journal of Neuropathology and Experimental Neurology*.)

POLYMYOSITIS

BY

JOHN N. WALTON
M.D., M.R.C.P.

First Assistant in Neurology, King's College, University of Durham, in the Royal Victoria Infirmary, Newcastle upon Tyne. Late Nuffield Foundation Fellow in Neurology and Neuropathology, Harvard Medical School and Massachusetts General Hospital, Boston, Mass., and King's College Travelling Fellow in the Neurological Research Unit, the National Hospital, Queen Square

AND

RAYMOND D. ADAMS
M.D.

Bullard Professor of Neuropathology, Harvard University and Chief of the Neurological Service, Massachusetts General Hospital, Boston, Mass.

E. & S. LIVINGSTONE LTD
EDINBURGH AND LONDON
1958

Figure 41 Title page of book on polymyositis. (Reproduced by permission of Elsevier from *Polymyositis* by John Walton and Raymond D. Adams, Churchill Livingstone, 1958.)

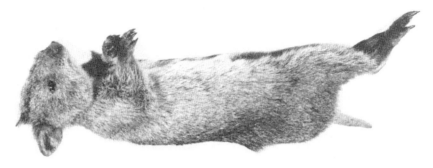

Figure 42   Paralyzed quokka with myopathy due to vitamin E deficiency.

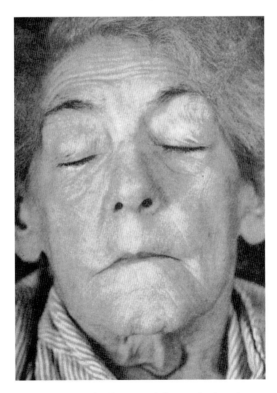

Figure 43   This patient with oculopharyngeal dystrophy is trying to open her eyes.(By permission of Dr Raymond Adams.)

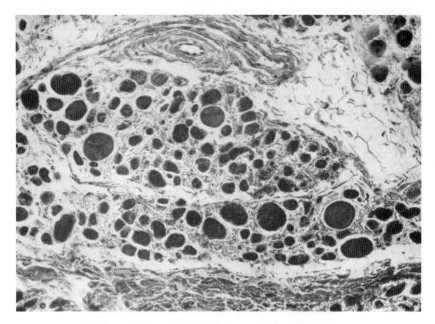

Figure 44 Cross section of muscle biopsy from Adams' patient with congenital muscular dystrophy shows variation in muscle fiber size

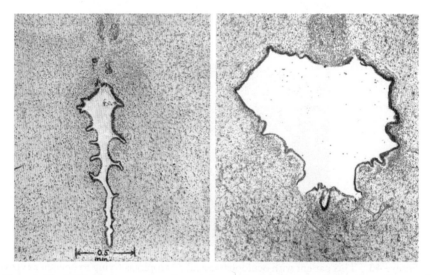

Figure 45 Hereditary aqueductal stenosis on the *left* compared to a normal control acqueduct on the *right*.

SYMPTOMATIC OCCULT HYDROCEPHALUS WITH "NORMAL" CEREBROSPINAL-FLUID PRESSURE*

A Treatable Syndrome

R. D. Adams, M.D.,† C. M. Fisher, M.D.,‡ S. Hakim, M.D.,§ R. G. Ojemann, M.D.,¶ and W. H. Sweet, M.D.‖

BOSTON, MASSACHUSETTS, AND BOGOTÁ, COLOMBIA

THE term *hydrocephalus* refers to distention of the cerebral ventricles, usually as the result of obstruction somewhere along the pathway of the cerebrospinal-fluid circulation. *Occult* indicates that enlargement of the ventricles has occurred after union of the cranial sutures, and hence the head remains of normal size. Hydrocephalus is said to be noncommunicating or obstructive if the blockade of circulation is in the ventricular system and communicating or nonobstructive if there is a normal patency of the pathways from the ventricular system to the lumbar subarachnoid space. Its causes are numerous and include tumors encroaching on the ventricles, carcinomatosis of the meninges, aqueductal atresia or stenosis (as a result of tumor or ependymal gliosis), the Arnold–Chiari and other malformations, meningeal fibrosis after spinal anesthesia, bacterial meningitis and subarachnoid hemorrhage from saccular aneurysm, head injury or intracranial operations. And there are, in addition, a certain number of patients in whom the cause of the blockade of the subarachnoid space cannot be ascertained. In most cases, regardless of the cause or type of hydrocephalus, the cerebrospinal-fluid pressure is elevated (200 to 600 mm.). If the condition develops acutely, it is usually accompanied by headache, vomiting, papilledema and obtundation; if the mode of onset is slower, these symptoms may be absent.

*From the Neurology and Neurosurgical services, Massachusetts General Hospital, and the Departments of Neurology and Surgery (Neurosurgery) Harvard Medical School, Boston, and the Neurosurgical Service, Military Hospital and the Neurology Department, National University, Bogotá, Colombia.

Supported, in part, by the Harrington Fund, Harvard Medical School.

†Bullard Professor of Neuropathology, Harvard Medical School; chief, Neurology Service, and neuropathologist, Massachusetts General Hospital.

‡Assistant professor of neurology, Harvard Medical School; neurologist, Massachusetts General Hospital.

§Associate professor of neurology, National University; chief, Neurosurgical Service, Military Hospital, Bogotá, Colombia; formerly, research fellow in neurology and assistant in neuropathology, Harvard Medical School.

¶Instructor in surgery, Harvard Medical School; assistant in neurosurgery, Massachusetts General Hospital.

‖Associate professor of surgery, Harvard Medical School; chief, Neurosurgical Service, Massachusetts General Hospital.

Reprinted from the *New England Journal of Medicine*
273:117-126 (July 15), 1965

Recently, two of us (S.H. and R.D.A.)[1] reported the clinical findings in adults who had a chronic symptomatic hydrocephalus with a "normal" cerebrospinal-fluid pressure (180 mm. or less). Of greater importance, neurosurgical shunting procedures resulted in a remarkable restoration of neurologic function, amounting to a cure. The point of emphasis was the mechanism of "normal-pressure hydrocephalus." The present communication describes our 3 most striking clinical examples of occult hydrocephalus and normal cerebrospinal-fluid pressure in which the improvement after a shunting procedure was most dramatic. After having become helplessly demented, the patients regained full mental function as the result of a shunt that reduced the "normal" pressure to even lower levels. Here, the focus of attention will be on the clinical manifestations and the diagnostic and therapeutic aspects of the syndrome.

The clinical picture in chronic, symptomatic occult hydrocephalus, which is the principal topic of the present communication, is a disabling dementia with psychomotor retardation. The importance of recognizing this condition lies in the opportunity it affords of rescuing from oblivion at least a few of the vast number of middle-aged or elderly patients now labeled as having senile dementia or "cerebral arteriosclerosis." Furthermore, it is our impression that a familiarity with some of the details of the clinical and pathological state may result in a better understanding of all forms of hydrocephalus as well as a number of other conditions in which a meningeal cyst or a local dilatation of ventricle may become symptomatic in the face of "normal" cerebrospinal-fluid pressure.

The case histories presented below summarize but a part of the recent clinical experience of the Neuro-

---

Figure 46   Front page of the article on normal pressure hydrocephalus. (Reproduced by permission from the *New England Journal of Medicine*: Adams, RD et al. Symptomatic Occult Hydrocephalus with "Normal" Cerebrospinal Fluid Pressure. V273, pp 117–126. Copyright(1965) Massachusetts Medical Society. All rights reserved.)

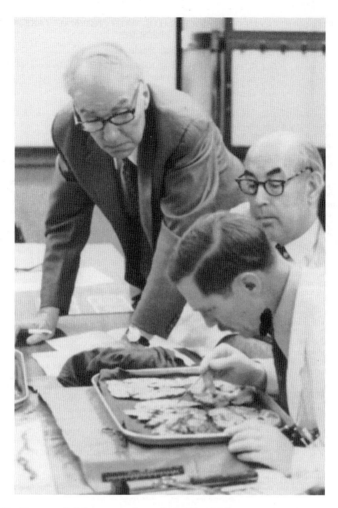

Figure 47 Raymond Adams *standing*, C. Miller Fisher *seated*, as E. P. Richardson inspects brain slices.(Reproduced by permission of Dr Jonathan Trobe)

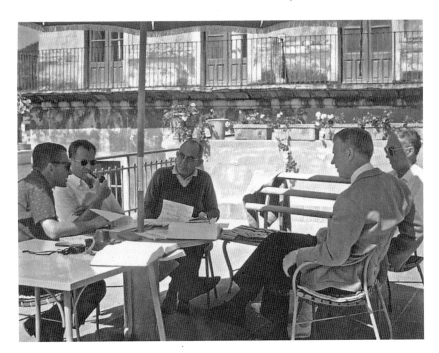

Figure 48 Editors of *Principles of Internal Medicine*. *From left to right*: Ivan Bennett, Maxwell Wintrobe, Tinsley Harrison, George Thorn, Raymond Adams. Adams is dressed to play tennis. The missing editor William Resnik probably took the photograph. Planning for an upcoming edition was done on group trips to desirable locations in Europe and the Caribbean.

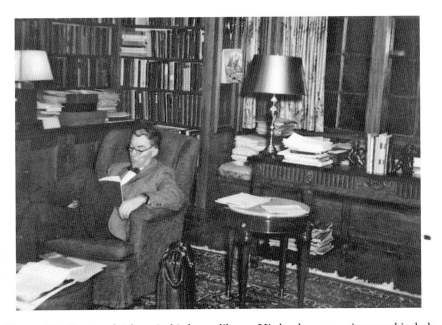

Figure 49 Raymond Adams in his home library. His books were written at this desk in long hand on yellow pads. He would nap in the easy chair, after coming home, and then write for hours. He moved from this home in Milton after a 1977 house fire.

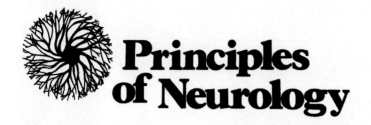

Principles of Neurology

RAYMOND D. ADAMS, M.A., M.D.
Bullard Professor of Neuropathology, Harvard Medical School
Chief, Neurology Service and Director of The Joseph P. Kennedy, Jr.,
Memorial Laboratories, Massachusetts General Hospital, Boston; Director,
Eunice K. Shriver Laboratories, Fernald School, Waltham, Massachusetts.
Médecin Adjoint de L'Hôpital Cantonal, Lausanne, Switzerland.

MAURICE VICTOR, M.D.
Professor of Neurology, Case Western Reserve University, School of
Medicine. Director, Neurology Service, Cleveland Metropolitan General
Hospital, Cleveland.

McGRAW-HILL BOOK COMPANY
A Blakiston Publication
New York   St. Louis   San Francisco   Auckland   Bogotá   Düsseldorf
Johannesburg   London   Madrid   Mexico   Montreal   New Delhi
Panama   Paris   São Paulo   Singapore   Sydney   Tokyo   Toronto

Figure 50 Title page of the first edition of *Principles of Neurology*. (Reproduced by permission of the McGraw-Hill Companies from Adams, RD and Victor, M, *Principles of Neurology*, McGraw-Hill Book Company, 1977.)

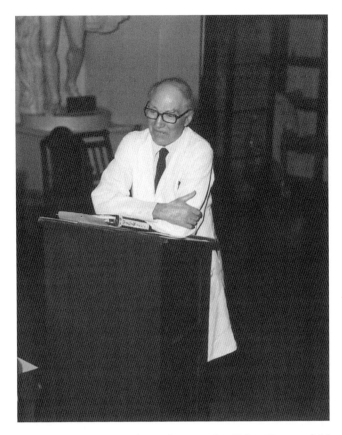

Figure 51 Raymond Adams at the podium in the Ether Dome of Massachusetts General Hospital.

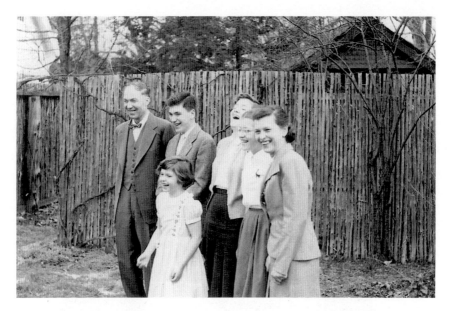

Figure 52 Adams family in the 1950s in Milton Massachusetts. *Front row*: Sarah Ellen; *Second row*: Raymond Adams, John William, Mary Elinor, Carol Ann, and Margaret Elinor Adams.

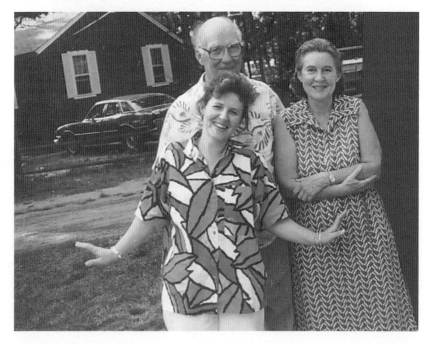

Figure 53 Raymond Adams with Maria Salam and her daughter Nina (Antonina) Salam. Ray and Maria married in 1974.

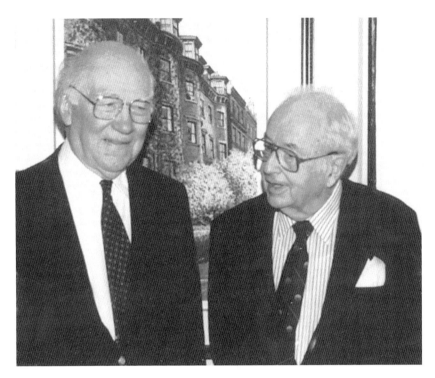

Figure 54 Raymond Adams and David Cogan, who was "one of my favorites." Pictured at a reception in honor of the great neuro-ophthalmologist after his retirement from Harvard.

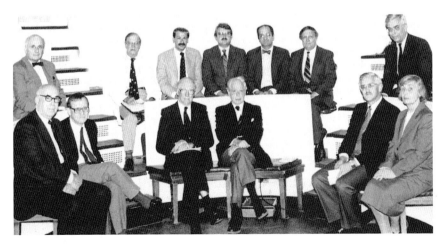

Figure 55 The Ether Dome was nearly full for the scientific session honoring Maurice Victor and Betty Banker about the time of their retirement from their positions in Cleveland. *Front row, from left to right*: C. Miller Fisher, Andrew Engel (Banker's co-editor of *Myology*), Raymond Adams, Maurice Victor, Joseph Martin (Adams' successor as chair and Bullard professor), and Betty Banker; *Second row*: Vincent Perlo, E.P. Richardson, James Anthony, Robert Shields, Robert Laureno, Charles Brausch, Richard Johnson.

HISTOLOGY AND HISTOPATHOLOGY OF THE NERVOUS SYSTEM

Compiled and Edited by

WEBB HAYMAKER, M.D.
and
RAYMOND D. ADAMS, M.D.

CHARLES C THOMAS · PUBLISHER
Springfield · Illinois · U.S.A.

Figure 56 Title page from two volumes, which Adams edited after his retirement from his chairmanship. This successor work to Penfield's volumes exceeded 2,500 pages. (From Haymaker, W and Adams, RD. *Histology and Histopathology of the Nervous System*, 1982. Courtesy of Charles C. Thomas Publisher Ltd., Springfield, Illinois.)

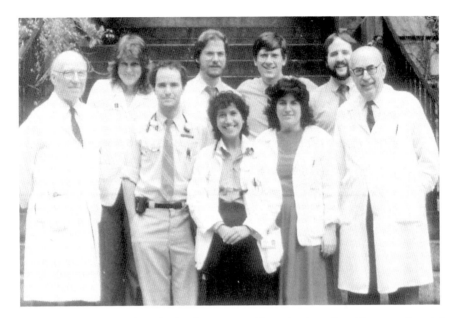

Figure 57 Photograph with the first year residents in the 1980s. *First row, from left to right*: Raymond Adams, John Barlow, Nancy Newman, Karen Kerman, C. Miller Fisher; *Second row*: Stasha Gorminak, Lennart Mucke, Jonathan Horton, Charles Duffy. (Thanks to Jonathan Horton for providing the names.)

HARVARD MEDICAL SOCIETY

TUESDAY, NOVEMBER 10, 1959, at 8:00 p.m.
AMPHITHEATRE D, HARVARD MEDICAL SCHOOL
DR. RAYMOND ADAMS, Presiding
STUDIES IN CLINICAL NEUROLOGY

1. MULTIFOCAL LEUCOENCEPHALOPATHY: ITS NATURE AND MEDICAL IMPLICATIONS
     E. P. Richardson

2. ACUTE TOXIC ENCEPHALOPATHY IN INFANTS AND CHILDREN
     Philip Dodge

3. TRANSIENT GLOBAL AMNESIA
     C. Miller Fisher

ROBERT E. GROSS   ALBERT E. RENOLD   G. E. ERIKSON
Program Committee, H. M. S.

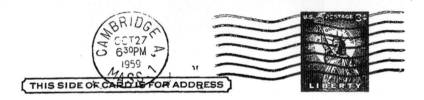

Dr. Raymond DeL. Adams
320 Adams St.
Milton 86, Mass.

Figure 58 Postcard announcing a session with Raymond Adams presiding. He arranged a program of presentations on current projects by three of his colleagues from Massachusetts General Hospital. Adams was involved in observing or describing all three of these important clinical entities.

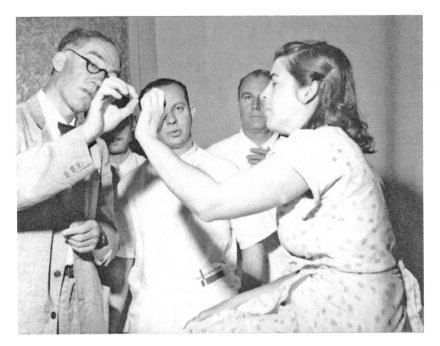

Figure 59 Raymond Adams examines a patient when he was visiting professor in Cuba circa, 1959.

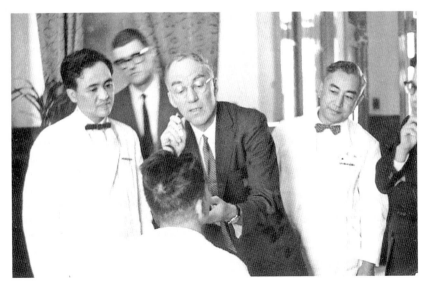

Figure 60 Raymond Adams examines a patient, probably in Guam, 1962.

Neurology of Hereditary Metabolic Diseases of Children

Raymond D. Adams, M.A. (Hon.)
M.D., D.Sc., M.D. (Hon.)
Neurology Service
Massachusetts General Hospital
and Eunice K. Shriver Center
Department of Neurology
Harvard Medical School

Gilles Lyon, M.D.
Chief of Neuropediatrics
University of Louvain (UCL)
Medical School (Brussels)

● **Hemisphere Publishing Corporation**

Washington   New York   London

McGraw-Hill Book Company

New York   St. Louis   San Francisco   Auckland   Bogotá
Guatemala   Hamburg   Johannesburg   Lisbon   London
Madrid   Mexico   Montreal   New Delhi   Panama   Paris
San Juan   São Paulo   Singapore   Sydney   Tokyo   Toronto

Figure 61   Title page of this book, a product of his years of studying the patients at Fernald School and Shriver Institute. Written after Adams' retirement as chairman. (Reproduced by permission of the McGraw-Hill Companies. From Adams, RD and Lyon, G. *Neurology of Hereditary Metabolic Diseases of Children*, McGraw-Hill Book Company, 1982.)

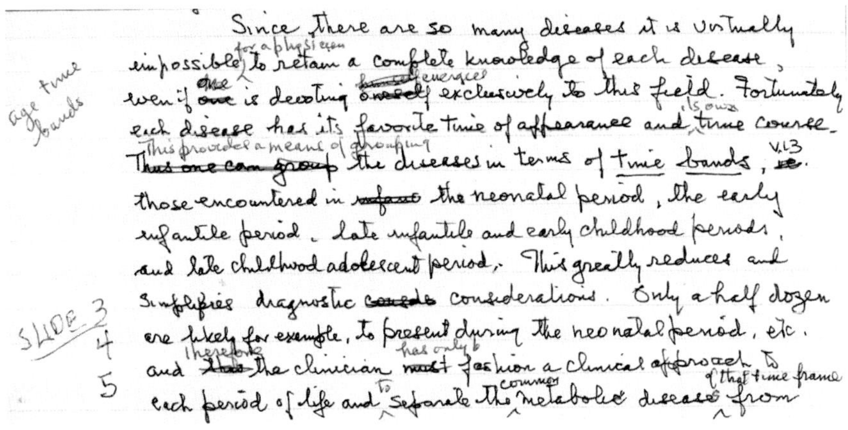
age time bands

Since there are so many diseases it is virtually impossible for a physician to retain a complete knowledge of each disease, even if one is devoting his energies exclusively to this field. Fortunately each disease has its favorite time of appearance and its own time course. This provides a means of grouping the diseases in terms of time bands, viz. those encountered in the neonatal period, the early infantile period, late infantile and early childhood periods, and late childhood adolescent period. This greatly reduces and simplifies diagnostic considerations. Only a half dozen are likely for example, to present during the neonatal period, etc. and therefore the clinician has only to fashion a clinical approach to each period of life and to separate the common metabolic diseases of that time frame from

SLIDE 3
4
5

Figure 62 Notes in preparation for a lecture on hereditary metabolic disease.

Reprinted from *Journal of Neurosurgery*,
1950, Vol. VII, No. 5, pages 421-439

ACUTE DEGENERATIVE CHANGES IN ADENOMAS OF THE PITUITARY BODY—WITH SPECIAL REFERENCE TO PITUITARY APOPLEXY

MILTON BROUGHAM, M.D., A. PRICE HEUSNER, M.D.,
AND RAYMOND D. ADAMS, M.D.

*Neurological Unit and Neurosurgical Service, Boston City Hospital, and Department
of Neurology, Harvard Medical School, Boston, Massachusetts*

(Received for publication February 13, 1950)

DEGENERATIVE changes in pituitary adenomas and their attendant clinical manifestations occur not infrequently yet they have been mentioned in only a few of the more complete descriptions of these tumors. These changes usually consist of small hemorrhages and areas of necrosis with "cyst" formation, reparative fibrosis and sometimes calcification. Some writers relate such lesions to the apparent arrest of acromegaly or to the rapid development of dyspituitarism. However, in most instances these degenerative changes are regarded as unimportant findings without precise relationship to symptoms and without significant effect on the growth of the adenoma.

In the routine examination of the brains of individuals who have died unexpectedly we have several times discovered tumors of the pituitary gland in which widespread necrosis and/or extensive hemorrhage had occurred. Clinically, these changes were associated with a sudden onset of neurological symptoms such as ophthalmoplegia, blindness, stupor or coma and they have resulted in death within a few hours to days. Extensive lesions of this type have seldom been described. In fact, a review of the literature disclosed only 5 cases showing similar symptomatology and pathological findings. The following cases are presented, therefore, in order to call attention to these severe retrogressive pituitary lesions.

REPORT OF CASES

Case 1. (B.C.H. 115140, A 44-421) This patient, a 65-year-old negro, was hospitalized because of epigastric pains of 7 weeks' duration. Investigation revealed nothing of importance except a low blood pressure (100/70) and a slight reduction of blood chlorides. A diagnosis of adrenal insufficiency was made and treatment with sodium chloride and desoxycorticosterone was instituted.

On the night of the 16th hospital-day the patient complained of severe frontal headache, and the next morning he was found semicomatose. Temperature was 105°F. and the neck was very stiff. The right pupil measured 6 mm., the left 4 mm. and neither reacted to light or on convergence; there was a complete right ophthalmoplegia. No other abnormal signs were elicited. CSF was xanthochromic and under a pressure of 180 mm.; it contained 155 RBC, 55 neutrophilic leucocytes and 295 lymphocytes/c.mm.; total protein 182 mg., and sugar 55 mg./100 cc.

On the 21st hospital-day there was definite improvement in that the patient was able to respond to simple questions. However, he remained confused and the

Figure 63 First page of paper describing pituitary apoplexy. (Reproduced by permission of the *Journal of Neurosurgery*.)

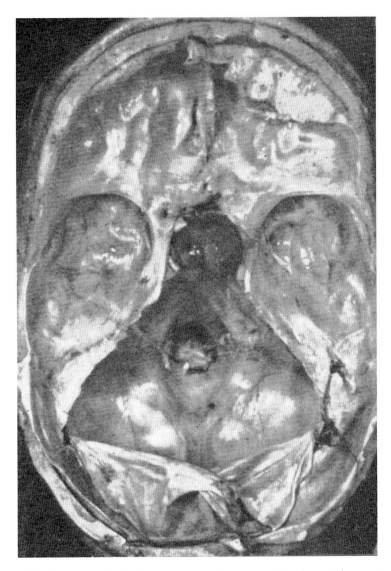

Figure 64 Hemorrhagic pituitary tumor in situ pictured in the article on pituitary apoplexy. (Reproduced by permission of the *Journal of Neurosurgery*.)

JOURNAL OF THE ROYAL SOCIETY OF MEDICINE   Volume 98   December 2005

The long shadow of cerebral localization

Saad Shafqat

J R Soc Med 2005;**98**:549

In 1995, during my first week as a neurology resident at Massachusetts General Hospital, I had the privilege of meeting the late Raymond Adams. He was an established octogenarian by then, but the years had made no difference to his air of professionalism and academic authority. His reputation was made in the 1950s and 1960s, when he developed Boston as a major centre of clinical neurology. Among other things, he is immortalized through a famous textbook that has appeared in multiple editions.

Our meeting took place at a clinical conference in which I was required to present a case. He was a demanding clinician, and my neurological examination did not meet his standards of thoroughness. Despite my best efforts, I could not remove the look of displeasure from his face. I defended myself, invoking time efficiency and what not, but Dr Adams was unforgiving. 'You can't rush a neurological examination,' he said. 'A proper one takes three days.'

Dr Adams was, of course, echoing a mindset that goes back to the very foundations of neurology. In 1875, Jean-Martin Charcot had delivered a series of lectures to the Paris Medical School on cerebral localization, laying out a method that sought clinical alliance between pathological cerebral lesions and clinical signs in living patients. He was already much more than a professor by then, his profile and personality was compared to Napoleon and Caesar. He was also well into a legendary career at the Salpêtrière Hospital that would enshrine him as the father of neurology.

The method of cerebral lesion localization became the founding pillar of neurology as a clinical discipline. It is a powerful diagnostic tool that permits reasonably accurate spatial localization of a lesion within the nervous system without resort to technology. The benefits are obvious. The problem, unfortunately, is that lesion localization became an end in itself.

It is the element of theatre. A well-conducted localization exercise enables a formidable display of clinicoanatomic mental gymnastics that can leave impressionable medical students and trainees gasping. In no other specialty are clinical examinations performed in front of large audiences. They are called 'demonstrations', but to an external observer they have all the elements of a freak show. It is also a very visible activity that creates an impression that its practitioners are involved in very busy and important work. Burdened by these distractions, the line connecting lesion localization to patient therapeutics and functional outcomes became obscured.

Admittedly, the deck was always stacked against neurologists. The brain is a complex organ that is slow to yield its secrets, and without the benefit of imaging technology the clinical process does not get very far. But certainly neurologists did themselves no favours when they got seduced by lesion localization and pursued it for its own sake.

It was the advent of CT and MR scanning that finally liberated neurology from these shackles. Indeed, in the early days of brain imaging, it was commonly said that now that neurologists can see the lesion on a scan, they would have nothing to do. It was a joke—but only just. Such was the hold of lesion localization on the practice of neurology and on the perceptions it had created among professionals from other disciplines.

Modern neurology, thankfully, has finally emerged from this distracting influence. Over the last three decades, efficacious treatments have become available for the majority of neurological diseases, including epilepsy, migraine, Guillain–Barré syndrome, Parkinson's disease, multiple sclerosis, and ischaemic stroke. This revolution came about by keeping clinical outcomes foremost through the integrated application of basic research, drug development, biotechnology and clinical trial methodology.

And what about the extended neurological examination? With the availability of tissue-plasminogen activator as thrombolytic therapy for acute ischaemic stroke, even 3 minutes is a luxury, let alone 3 days.

Associate Professor of Neurology, Aga Khan University Medical College,
Karachi 74800, Pakistan

E-mail: saad.shafqat@aku.edu

549

Figure 65   Article referring to the "late Raymond Adams" with annotations by Adams. See Appendix K. (Reproduced by permission of the Royal Society of Medicine Press, London)

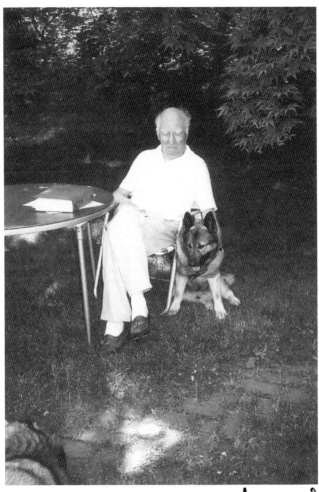

Raymond Adams

Figure 66 Raymond Adams in retirement with Omi, his favorite of his Norwegian Elkhound triplets. (When he was raising his four children, the family usually had two or three dogs adopted from the dog pound. A favorite of his was Smokey. He was survived by his last dog, Reggie (Regina), a Corgi.)

unexpected occurrences truly turned Ray Adams' focus to demyelinative disease. The first was the death of experimental neuropathologist, Raymond Morrison. He had been collaborating with an immunologist, who, in order to carry on their work, needed help with neuropathology. Secondly, Adams was recruited to move to the MGH, which arranged for his salary to be funded by the Multiple Sclerosis Society.

Ray Adams studied human autopsy material and compared the findings in human demyelinative diseases to those of the animal disease, resulting from injection of central nervous system myelin (experimental allergic encephalomyelitis). Thereby, Raymond Adams systematically built support for the allergic hypothesis of multiple sclerosis and allied conditions. Later, Adams and colleagues injected animals with peripheral myelin, which produced inflammatory demyelinative disease in peripheral nerves. The clinical and pathological findings in this experimental allergic neuropathy resembled those of humans with acute inflammatory polyneuropathy (Adams' term for Guillain–Barré syndrome). The cumulative evidence, Adams argued, pointed to an immune mechanism for acute polyneuropathy in humans. This synthesis was a great advance on the uncertain teachings of the day.

RL: *How was your ninth Adams' day at Shriver Institute?*

RA: It was interesting. It was on demyelination, mainly multiple sclerosis.

RL: *After listening to the presentations, have you any new thoughts about multiple sclerosis?*

RA: No. I pointed out to them that the common lesion in all of the inflammatory demyelinative diseases is perivenous (Dawson type) perivascular cuffing and para-adventitial demyelination, with the lymphocyte being the initial actor in the drama, followed by mononuclear cells, which appear simultaneously with demyelination. They seemed in agreement with that concept.

RL: *How did you come to study this subject?*

RA: I had become interested in neuroimmunology by the chance acquaintance of Byron Waksman. He had been working with Raymond Morrison, who was a neuropathologist at Mass. General. About 1947 Morrison started a study of the immunology of demyelination. Morrison died. Waksman, a brilliant immunologist, knew very little about neuropathology. He brought some of Morrison's animal slides to me at the Boston City Hospital; we looked them over together and formed a friendship and working relationship. So, when I moved back to the Mass. General, we decided to work together.

RL: *Waksman had been working with Morrison on an experimental allergic encephalomyelitis, an animal model, introduced by Rivers at Rockefeller Institute.*

RA: Yes, Rivers had published in 1935. Then Abner Wolf and an immunologist at Columbia had shown, that by mixing myelin with the wax of tubercle bacilli and mineral oil, so called Freund's adjuvants, that they had an antigen, very much more potent than myelin alone for producing brain and spinal cord lesions. That work was published, I believe, in 1947 or 1948, and Raymond Morrison published his findings in 1947. I began reviewing the material of Morrison, after he died, probably in 1949, and then continued, when Waksman joined our neurology Department at MGH. (It was also understood that, when I came back to MGH, I would take an interest in multiple sclerosis, since I was being paid by an MS fellowship.)

In 1954, in order to keep me at Mass. General, they gave me a new floor of laboratories in the building that was just going up. I thought it worthwhile to set up a division of neuro-immunology.

RL: *Were there many places that had a division of neuro-immunology?*

RA: I don't think there was any one place in the country; possibly there could have been a laboratory for this in Abner Wolf's neuropathology department in Columbia.

I assigned to Byron Waksman about a half of the floor of laboratories for a division of neuro-immunology. We had one room where animals were autopsied and another room for technicians to do the staining procedures. There was a room for Waksman and another room where I could work. I spent about 3 hours a morning over in that laboratory for several years. I was given very much instruction by Byron Waksman in immunology, and I think I helped him in the understanding of pathology.

A number of noteworthy things happened during this period. Waksman and I had the idea that there ought to be a way of refining the myelin component that was antigenic. About that time I had established a friendship with Jordie Folch-Pei, who was director of McClane Biochemistry Institute. He had isolated a substance called proteolipid protein, which he'd extracted from myelin. His associate, Marjorie Lees, was able to purify it. So we decided to take the different refined products of myelin and see if they were antigenic. Of the various myelin components, only the proteolipid seemed to be an effective antigen [see Chapter 5]. Finally, we got it to the point where as little as two gamma, injected in the foot of a rabbit, would produce an encephalomyelitis. We tried to get Folch to produce other fractions of myelin, but Jordie Folch-Pei was very rigid about his work and would give us nothing that was worth testing, except proteolipid.

Waksman was very interested in the mechanism whereby the injected antigen led to the damage of the myelin sheath. It turned out that the antibody, that was produced and was in the blood of the injected animal, did not correlate at all well with the lesions. From this finding Waksman deduced that the lesions were cell-mediated. We went on, Byron and I, to the study of the lesion in different animals. It turned out that the guinea pig, the mouse and the rabbit did not respond in the same way to this antigen. In the guinea pig, for example, injection of the central nervous myelin would induce both peripheral nerve, spinal cord, and brain lesions. Whereas, in the rabbit, injection of the central myelin would induce brain and spinal cord lesions and few peripheral nerve lesions. [see Chapter 5]

Because of my interest in peripheral nerve I had urged Byron Waksman to make extracts of the peripheral nerve myelin and to inject it with Freund's adjuvants, and that material produced, clearly, an acute inflammatory polyneuritis. We discovered that, if we used the antigen from the peripheral nerve of the rabbit, we produced only peripheral neuropathy. That work was duplicated several times in a large series of animals. I think it was the first clear demonstration of an experimental, non-infective, inflammatory, demyelinative polyneuropathy. We pointed out the similarity of that to the so-called Landry–Guillain–Barré syndrome, which I thought was also a hypersensitivity to the myelin antigen. That work, I think, held up pretty well and was probably a worthwhile discovery. [see Chapter 5 and Figure 39]

It was during this time also that Charles Kubik and I decided to look at all of the pathological material of multiple sclerosis and other demyelinations that had come through the neuropathology laboratory.

RL: *Did he have a lot of these cases on file?*

RA: Yes. He did all the stains himself. We looked through all that material, going back to about 1930.

RL: *Here is an illustration in your article on the morbid anatomy of the demyelinative disease.*

RA: There are some nice cortical lesions there. In some of our cases the lesion went right through gray matter and left the neurons untouched.

RL: *Was it original with you that there can be loss of axons in lesions of multiple sclerosis?*

RA: No, Dawson, the Scot, was aware of that, as I remember. There is nothing original about that.

RL: *In the late 1990s, authors reported the axonal loss in multiple sclerosis, as if it were a new discovery.*

RA: Yes, but of course they don't always read the literature. It was quite evident, if you look at a series of lesions of different ages, that one stage affected myelin and another stage affected the myelin and axis cylinder. In the third, more advanced stage, all supporting structures are affected. And you probably have seen that. In looking over a brain with multiple sclerosis, you occasionally will see one or two cavitating lesions and all the rest in various stages of demyelination.

RL: *Do you consider the Devic's disease as one variety of multiple sclerosis?*

RA: My impression was that it was different because of the extensive necrosis of the spinal cord. It's more like acute hemorrhagic leukoencephalitis. But it may overlap with MS.

RL: *Currently some neurologists argue that Devic's is a separate disease from multiple sclerosis.*

RA: Well, certainly I had one convincing case, in which there was widespread necrosis of gray and white matter, destroying several segments, in the spinal cord, which was reduced to meningeal membranes. The patient must have had a cerebral lesion at the time of the spinal cord disorder because the patient had had seizures and hemiplegia temporarily. At autopsy year later there were typical demyelinative lesions all throughout the brain.

RL: *So your case was an instance of ongoing multiple sclerosis, in the course of which there was an intense attack of optic nerve and spinal cord disease, which resembled an episode of Devic's.*

RA: Yes.

RL: *I have autopsy material on an identical case.*

RA: Well it's worth working those up very carefully and reporting them because I don't think it's widely known.

RL: *Are all of these demyelinative diseases related?*

RA: I think there is a relationship between all of these diseases. All of them, basically, in their acute phase, are inflammatory demyelinations.

RL: *Here is your article on acute necrotizing hemorrhagic encephalopathy. How do you distinguish this disease from acute multiple sclerosis?*

RA: By its hemorrhagic character. And there's a histologic difference too. In the vessels there is fibrin exudation, and there is necrosis, which you don't see in acute MS, usually.

I had been very interested in hemorrhagic leukoencephalitis, having had four cases of that disease provided by friend, a pathologist at Boston University. We called it, as had others, the Hurst disease. There was a striking inflammatory reaction involving venules and small vessels with little hemorrhages and widespread myelin injury and perivascular and meningeal inflammation.

Byron Waksman and I decided to see if, by injecting the Freund's adjuvants with myelin and then injecting the toxin of the meningococcus, we could convert the experimental encephalomyelitis to a hemorrhagic encephalomyelitis. I thought that the meningococcus toxin would allow the inflamed vessels to exude fibrin, which is found in all of our hemorrhagic leukoencephalitic cases. This did happen, more or less. The meningococcus toxin, produced some injury to the small arteries and veins, which allowed fibrin to exude into the vessel wall. This does not happen in experimental allergic encephalomyelitis induced without meningococcus toxin. But even with the meningococcus toxin we did not get the widespread necrosis of the Hurst disease. At least this study brought that disease into possible connection with the post-infectious encephalomyelitis. [see Chapter 5]

RL: *With the advent of electron microscopy came new insight into experimental allergic neuritis.*

RA: Yes, Karl Eric Astrom, worked on the earliest lesion in experimental allergic neuritis. He found that the lymphocytes in the venules of the nervous system first would begin to move peripherally in the circulation and then attach themselves to an endothelial cell in the vein. They would then pass right through the endothelial cell, not between endothelial cells. The endothelial cells would engulf the lymphocyte and, when it came out on the other side in the perivenous space, it would be a little bit enlarged and would be joined very quickly by a mononuclear cell. Later, the mononuclear cell would become active as the myelin sheath was broken down by the lymphocytes. [see Chapter 5]

RL: *That was in peripheral nerve.*

RA: That was peripheral nerve, but we suspected that the same was happening in the demyelinative disease of the spinal cord and brain.

RL: *Can you think of any other diseases, where lymphocytes pass through the cells of the wall of the venule? When inflammatory cells appear in a cerebral infarction, do they pass through the cytoplasm of the venule endothelial cells?*

RA: I don't know the answer to that.

RL: *What else did you do with Waksman?*

RA: Waksman and I also took the trouble to look carefully at the lesion of measles encephalomyelitis. The measles virus, injected with Freund's adjuvant, produced the demyelinative type of lesion; we compared that with direct infection in the brain by the measles virus. I thought there was a striking difference between the two lesions. The perivenous and para-adventitial demyelination was unique to the allergic inflammatory myelin breakdown disease. Whereas the direct viral encephalitis did not show this perivenous distribution at all. [see Chapter 5]

RL: *What became of Byron Waksman?*

RA: Byron and I were very close. I tried to get him promoted to full professorship at Harvard. The head of microbiology had a grudge against Byron and blocked it. So Byron resigned and went to Yale as professor. Waksman was talented in every way, quick and accurate in writing up his experimental finding.

RL: *Can you think of a disease outside the nervous system, in which, analogous to relapsing and remitting multiple sclerosis, there is multi-focal damage by a cell-mediated immune process, which comes and goes?*

RA: Well, Hashimoto's thyroiditis and necrotizing colitis are certainly examples of that.

Today there is general acceptance of Adams' basic ideas about these diseases. Fundamentally unchallenged are his description of the inflammatory lesion in multiple sclerosis, his description of the inflammatory lesion in acute polyneuropathy and the concept that the immune system is somehow involved in the pathogenesis of these two diseases.

Current therapies and experimental treatments for multiple sclerosis include corticosteroids, the immunomodulatory medications and antibodies targeting one or another aspect of the immunologic response. Current therapies for Guillain–Barré syndrome include plasmapheresis and gamma globulin, each of which is aimed at affecting the immune response. The entire field of neuro-immunology grew out of the study of these diseases and the related experimental models. Raymond Adams, his collaborators, and his former residents were among the leaders in establishing autoimmune disease as an important concept, a paradigm shift in neurology.

As late as 1957 the concept met resistance. For example, Adams was challenged during a discussion of the interrelationship of demyelinating diseases. It was said that many diseases cause patches of demyelination and that a grouping of demyelinative diseases may not be meaningful. The skeptic was a prominent neuropathologist at Columbia University. Adams' unflinching response:[1]

Dr Zimmerman, I believe that it is too easy for us to conclude that there are so few ways the nervous system can react that one cannot distinguish diseases one from the other. To me this seems to be a repudiation of a fundamental principle in pathology. I do not think anyone would disagree with you that patches may occur in the nervous system in which the tissue appears pale in a myelin stain and that this alteration might be due to a number of different disease processes. In fact, every one of the attributes that I listed in Table I could be attacked and rejected as the criterion of any particular disease. But what becomes of great significance in neuropathology is a combination of tissue changes and their temporal sequence; and both positive and negative findings are of importance. The fact that lesion after lesion in these demyelinative diseases may be observed without vascular occlusion becomes as important as the perivenular relationship. And to find a combination of four or five tissue changes may stamp a process with remarkable specificity. One of the most interesting and difficult assignments for the neuropathologist is to delineate the essential changes and place them in meaningful sequence. Once that is accomplished the lines of profitable study become more clear to the experimental neuropathologist or anyone else working in this field.

Note

1. Kies MW, Alvord EC. *"Allergic" Encephalomyelitis*. Charles C. Thomas Springfield, IL 1959.

Peripheral Nerve Diseases

Textbooks, published during the early years of Ray Adams' career, show that knowledge of peripheral neuropathy was limited. The discussions of terminology were pre-modern. Nielsen's textbook (1951) argued for using the term, neuritis nonspecifically, rather than limiting its use to inflammatory disease.[1] A *Textbook of Medicine* (1951) stated that the term "neuropathy" was preferable to the word "neuritis" for noninflammatory nerve diseases. However, in the text, this book complied with the common practice of interchangeable use of these terms.[2]

Thinking about nerve pathology was in a primitive state. Nielsen's book stated that, "changes in syphilitic, lead, arsenical, alcohol, diphtheritic and leprous polyneuritis are ultimately the same as those in which a nerve has been divided."[1] Classifications of polyneuropathy were similarly ripe for advancement. Generalized neuritis was divided by causation into the following groups: bacterial toxins (including gonococcus), viral (i.e., acute febrile polyneuritis), chemical, metabolic (including gout), vascular (including thromboangiitis obliterans), hypertrophic, and undetermined.[2]

The studies of Raymond Adams and his students would advance our knowledge of nerve pathology and would transform this classification and its subcategories.

RL: *Was peripheral nerve well studied, when you entered the field of neuropathology?*

RA: Well we hardly ever looked at nerve. It was usually removed by the general pathologist, one or two pieces of nerve from someplace very accessible to the prosector. Unless there was something very striking, like a tumor, nerve was seldom even mentioned in the autopsy report. There was almost nothing being written about the pathology of nerve from The Mallory Institute of Pathology until we started our neuropathologic studies.

Neurologists, here and there, had looked at nerve, when the patient had clear and unmistakable polyneuropathy of some kind. That was usually done in a separate institute, and the whole line of study was dictated by a clinical syndrome, already recognized. But there was not any place where there was a general study of peripheral nerve.

RL: *Did the neuropathology textbooks of Greenfield and Spielmeyer deal with peripheral nerve?*

RA: Spielmeyer, no: except that he commented on the roots of the spinal cord in tabes. Greenfield's book, up to that time, hadn't been written.

RL: *How did you begin to study peripheral nerve pathology?*

RA: I started becoming interested in peripheral nerve disease through my association with Derek Denny-Brown. When he first arrived in Boston, he was curious about immersion foot, a condition noted during the first war years. German submarines were sinking American and other ships. Survivors, having been in a boat with their feet in water, would develop a painful neuropathy in the toes and feet. It had been looked at by Dorothy Russell and Blackwood but had not been studied carefully enough. One had very little information about hours and temperatures. So Denny devised an apparatus, whereby cat peripheral nerve, the sciatic I believe it was, would be enclosed in a chamber, the walls of which had circulating cold water. He could keep the water at different temperatures for different periods of time. When he would keep it down as low as 4°C for an hour, there would be necrosis. And the nerve would lose its conductive capacity. If the cold exposure was very brief, 15 minutes, that didn't happen. I was given the job of studying the lesion with him. I found that there was destruction of myelin and Schwann cells and even endoneurial fibroblasts. Because the small vessels, veins, venules, and arterioles were occluded, we concluded that it was a circulatory difficulty. Later there was Wallerian degeneration, distally, if the animal was permitted to live.[3]

Thus introduced to an experimental lesion that produced Wallerian degeneration, I became interested in peripheral nerve disease. Roy Swank had come from Montreal and was working at the children's hospital in Boston. He had worked on thiamine deficiency in pigeons, and he knew about the newer work on B vitamins, ones other than thiamine and nicotinic acid—i.e. panthothenic acid, pyridoxine (vitamin B6), and riboflavin. Max Wintrobe and his group had shown that you could produce peripheral nervous system change with deficiency of pantothenic acid and pyridoxine, and Roy Swank wanted to reproduce that. We made swine deficient in either panthothenic acid or vitamin B6; all the other vitamins were supplied in generous amounts. And in both groups of animals there was gradual development of peripheral neuropathy clinically. The B6 animals also had seizures. And my job was to look at these lesions in different phases of development. I found that there were definite lesions in the peripheral nerve, starting distally and moving more proximally, and alterations of the dorsal root ganglia, with some loss of cells and some swollen nerve cells, and later lesions in the posterior roots and posterior columns. The lesions with both deficiencies looked about the same as far as we could tell [see Chapter 5]. We really did not much more than verify what Max Wintrobe had found. This study made me very much aware of the importance of study of peripheral nerve and the necessity of really examining the peripheral nervous system.

RL: *You also studied diphtheria.*

RA: It was about this time that we had six cases of a fatal dipththeritic polyneuropathy in our alcoholic patients at the city hospital. They had died of myocardiopathy. In looking at our cases, we found a striking demyelinative lesion in the dorsal roots, spinal ganglia, and adjacent anterior root. It was strictly a demyelinative lesion with macrophages and no significant degree of inflammation, as far as we could tell. These were a few of the best-studied cases of diphtheritic polyneuropathy.

RL: *Here is your article with Miller Fisher on diphtheritic polyneuritis [see Chapter 5]. This caption says "sensory ganglion and adjacent spinal nerve to demonstrate localization of pathologic process. There are abundant fatty macrophages within the ganglion and not in the spinal nerve only 4mm away." So the photo demonstrated the selective vulnerability of the ganglion in this disease. [see Figure 40]*

RA: Yes. Strangely, at that time there was only one other person, in Germany, who had recently written about diphtheria. Going way back, there were countless papers showing slight alterations (artifacts in large measure) of nerve cells in the spinal cord, but they had never looked at the nerve roots and ganglia of the nervous system.

Later, when I went to the Mass. General Hospital, Waksman and I decided to try to reproduce it in animals with a mixture of toxin–antitoxin. We could reproduce the lesion quite satisfactorily and could trace the toxin into peripheral nerve within 10 hours after subcutaneous injection. Yet the diphtheritic polyneuropathy would not occur until much later. It looked to us as though this was a pure toxic, noninflammatory effect. It did something to the nerve that would cause it to begin to lose function several days to weeks after the toxin had arrived in the nerve. [see Chapter 5]

RL: *You talked about the nerve root involvement that you saw in diphtheria and you talked about the radiculitis that you found in syphilis. We spoke earlier about your article on herpes zoster, which also affects nerve roots. Is it correct to summarize your findings as follows: in diphtheria you found a noninflammatory demyelinative process of nerve root and ganglion; in syphilis you found an inflammatory process of the posterior but not anterior root, sparing the ganglion; and in zoster you found an inflammatory process of roots, ganglion, and spinal cord?*

RA: That's right. And, as you know, zoster usually affects two or three or more dorsal root ganglia on one side and there can be a paralysis on one side at that segmental level.

RL: *Please comment on acute inflammatory polyneuropathy.*

RA: At the BCH I was able to do a fairly complete autopsy of a case of acute, intense polyneuropathy. Because the spleen was enlarged and there were enlarged nodes, I called it "infective." I think that was a misnomer because we never found any infective organism. It was a very complete study; there were intense lesions of inflammatory type all through the peripheral nervous system.[4]

Later, I realized that we were seeing the same lesion as was found in Landry–Guillain–Barré Syndrome. Arthur Asbury and I looked through all of our material on this disease, all the fatal cases, of Landry–Guillain–Barré syndrome of the inflammatory type at the Mass. General. I think our paper was probably the first complete study of that disease [see Chapter 5].

Interestingly, Webb Haymaker and Kernohan of the Mayo Clinic had written an earlier paper, looking at the lesions in the dorsal roots and anterior roots, but they didn't have nerves. Theirs were Armed Forces Institute cases. They had received the spinal cord but not nerves, and they didn't see much in the way of lesion. They postulated some process other than inflammation. Ours was a far more complete study. We probably had a case or two where there was very little inflammation, but, of course, our cases died at varying intervals of time after the onset. I am sure that we did not see a purely axonal form of the disease, such as was described fairly recently.

RL: *What other peripheral nerve diseases did you study?*

RA: Michelsen and I had two cases of a striking hypertrophic polyneuropathy with huge nerves developing in the neck; there was varying sensorimotor loss. Earlier, it had been thought that, this was von Recklinghausen's disease. But it turned out, when we went through biopsy material carefully, that this was localized inflammatory disease with striking regeneration. These cases were very chronic; they lasted months. There have been a few other cases in the literature like this.

And it brings us right to the point of the regenerative lesions in nerve. Of course, everyone knows about the pseudo-neuromas that form, after nerve has been cut, with a meshwork or scar of regenerating axons all through the connective tissue of the neuroma. But there can be also these enlargements of nerve with increased connective tissue and regenerating fibers that are fairly diffuse over a distance of several centimeters. Webster and I and others had made a study of the Schwann cell overactivity and its role in the formation of the onion bulb. We thought the overactivity and generative capacity of the Schwann cell with fibroblasts formed that circular structure that we interpret as a hypertrophy of nerve.[5] Later P.K. Thomas wrote a very good paper on recurrent demyelination as a factor favoring formation of onion bulbs.

RL: *You told me that you have developed concepts of peripheral nervous system disease.*

RA: Yes. As a consequence of all these studies, I formed certain concepts of peripheral nerve disease. One was that almost every disease of the peripheral nerve, and now there are forty to fifty of them demonstrated, need to be more carefully studied.

Another point: you'd think that it would be very simple to differentiate these diseases on the basis of pathologic change, the various combinations of Gombault demyelination and Wallerian degeneration, various types of injury with regeneration, and various types of inflammatory reaction. Actually you also differentiate these diseases on the basis of the topography of the disease. You determine the topography by looking at the whole peripheral nervous system, the terminals and the sensory endings, the whole extent of the nerve, the roots, the ganglia, the autonomic ganglia, and the central connections. And it is the topography that has really defeated most pathologists. They seldom will take out all of the tissues that are needed for proper study of the peripheral nervous system.

And then the last point: from the study of these many diseases one can conclude that there are phases of disease, when there is functional change before there is demonstrable structural change. The study of the peripheral nervous system is a field that still is worth cultivating.

RL: *When you say functional change, you mean that a chemical lesion of nerve may precede a structural lesion.*

RA: Yes, a functional disorder, a metabolic or toxic difficulty, prior to the appearance of physical alternations of myelin or axon. In that I have the least good data. It deserves to be proved.

RL: *In which diseases were you able to take out the nervous system from the nerve root down to the nerve terminal?*

RA: Well, any one we wanted to. We wouldn't do it that completely. We would get nerves, centrally and peripherally and sometimes in between, and we could take out the spinal cord if we wanted to. The only restriction was that it took time, and frequently the undertaker would be after us. I remember when Denny-Brown and I were trying to get out the geniculate ganglion. It took us about 3 hours with rather dull tools, a blunt chisel and a hammer, to chip away the petrous bone.

RL: *This was in the herpes zoster case.*

RA: Yes. The autopsy was taking so long that the diener tried to force us out. The diener told us to get the hell out of there; he didn't care if we were professors or what we wanted to call ourselves. He wanted to go home.

RL: *Did Denny-Brown defer to the diener?*

RA: No. Denny-Brown told him off.

The classification of "neuritis," in the Cecil–Loeb textbook of 1951,[2] can be used to see the impact of Raymond Adams and his colleagues. The category of bacterial toxins was clarified by his study of diphtheritic polyneu-ropathy in humans and animals. Furthermore his data showed that "alcoholic" polyneuropathy was due to nutritional deficiency. The category of viral dis-ease was transformed; he showed that acute polyneuropathy was allergic rather than viral in cause. He advanced the metabolic category by documenting ure-mic polyneuropathy. The vascular category was transformed; Miller Fisher, his former fellow, showed that thromboangiitis obliterans did not exist. The hypertrophic category was clarified.[5] The idiopathic grouping was dimin-ished by his demonstrating that some polyneuropathies were due to multiple myeloma.

Comparing Adams' own classification of polyneuropathies to his predeces-sors is also revealing. By 1962 he had taken on the neuropathy section in the Harrison textbook of medicine.[6]

He split the neuropathies into two categories, localized and general-ized. The latter, the polyneuropathies, he divided into those due to poisons, deficiency states, inflammatory states, vascular disease, familial disease, and idiopathic causes. For a twenty-first century reader the categories and subcate-gories are much more familiar. By 1966 his analysis of neuropathy had again advanced; there was a multidimensional categorization including temporal, clinical, and pathological features, an important advance in thinking.[7]

Notes

1. Nielsen JM. *A Textbook of Clinical Neurology*. Paul B. Hoeber, Inc., New York, 1951.

2. Cecil RL, Loeb RF. *A Textbook of Medicine* (8th edition). W.B. Saunders Company, Philadelphia, 1951.

3. Denny-Brown D, Adams RD, et al. The Pathology of Injury to Nerve Induced by Cold. *J Neuropathol Exp Neurol* V4, pp 305–323, 1945.

4. Parker F, Adams RD. An Unusual Case of Infective Polyneuritis with Visceral Lesions. *N Engl J Med* V237, 976–983, 1947.

5. def Webster H, et al. The Role of Schwann Cells in the Formation of "Onion Bulbs" Found in Chronic Neuropathies. *J Neuropathol Exp Neurol* V26, pp 276–299, 1967.

6. Harrison TR, Adams RD, Bennett IL, et al. *Principles of Internal Medicine* (4th edition). McGraw Hill Book company Inc., New York, 1962.

7. Harrison TR, Adams RD, Bennett IL, et al. *Principles of Internal Medicine* (5th edition). McGraw-Hill Book Company Inc., New York, 1966.

Muscle Diseases

As Ray Adams entered neurology, the field of muscle disease was uncultivated and the field of muscle pathology was barren. Wilson's textbook of neurology (1940) discussed the pathology of the dystrophies in a brief paragraph with-out photo or drawing of the histologic features. Wilson stated that spinal cord lesions are "not unusual" in dystrophy. Polymyositis and dermatomyositis are discussed, under the heading, "Toxi-Infective Myositis." Again, there were no photographs or drawings of the histology.

Ten years later there was little progress evident. Nielsen's neurology text-book (1951) makes no mention of polymyositis or dermatomyositis clinically or pathologically. The *Textbook of Medicine* by Cecil and Loeb (1951) had its sections on muscle disease written by doctors of internal medicine. Mus-cle diseases were classified into three categories, parenchymotous myositis, myopathies, and interstitial myositis. Polymyositis is mentioned only as fol-lows: "polymyositis hemorrhagica is probably a form of dermatomyositis but it differs from the usual form of this disease in that there are hemorrhages in the muscles and into the skin." As for the muscular dystrophies it was stated that although "classification serves a useful purpose in some instances, progressive muscular dystrophy may be considered as a clinical and pathological unit in which the various types are distinguished by no fundamental differences."

Although there were classical fine descriptions of various dystrophies, the science of the field, especially its pathology, had not advanced. No book on muscle pathology had appeared since the beginning of the twentieth cen-tury. Ray Adams found himself in a leading institute of pathology, where no pathologist was interested in muscle. He found himself in a neurology depart-ment where Denny-Brown was interested in muscle and its physiology. Not surprisingly, Ray Adams found muscle disease and pathology a field ripe for investigation.

RL: *Were you interested in muscle disease during your year as a neurology resident at Massachusetts General Hospital?*

RA: Not at all. Indeed, I don't think we had dystrophic cases at all. They were looked after by internists or pediatricians.

RL: *Was the field of muscle pathology developed, when you turned to neuropathology at Boston City Hospital?*

RA: In fact there was very little in pathology of muscle. There had been an excel-lent book, written by Lorenz in 1904, with a lot of diagrams.[1] The pathology was discussed in many of the diseases, polymyositis, dermatomyositis, syphilis of mus-cle, tuberculosis, lots of work on inflammation, on diseases that were not very often seen any longer in our generation. But it was a scholarly presentation. From that time on there was a hiatus in the study of muscle.

There was no one in Mallory Institute of Pathology who had an interest in mus-cle. It was common practice to take two or three muscle specimens in each autopsy and, only if they saw an obvious abnormality, they would make note of it. Then we began to receive muscle biopsies, and they came directly to my laboratory around 1945–1950. I realized that I didn't have any good reference except the Lorenz book. And so I began to assemble cases. Usually they were biopsies from patients with neuromuscular disease.

Carl Pearson, one of the pathology residents, I encouraged to collect all of the data we had on muscle and to put together a teaching monograph, that would be a reference for our own residents. We finally decided to write a book on muscle. After we had it finished, I showed it to Derek Denny-Brown, and he was furious.

Denny was quite irritated that we were doing this because he had been interested in the EMG of muscle and always looked upon muscle as his province. So I invited him to join us, which he did. And he hastily made some observations in animal on denervation atrophy and on muscle lesions and contributed substantially to that monograph. It was finally published. I guess it was the first monograph on the pathology of muscle since Lorenz's time; it was well received. [see Chapter 5]

RL: *There must have been some volume of case material that stimulated you to make these organized observations.*

RA: Yes. When we began talking about muscle pathology in conferences, we received more and more biopsies. So the material grew.

RL: *Did you study inflammatory muscle disease?*

RA: Yes, it was quite clear that a lot of disease was being lost there. For example, I accidentally discovered the first example of a toxoplasma in a myocyte, in an endomysial cell.[2] That patient had fever and slight liver trouble and had a number of other symptoms. In three or four years we had quite a collection of material. There was a fair number of inflammatory diseases, mostly idiopathic or combined with skin lesions.

When I went over to the Mass. General, I found, in just two or three years, a large number of cases of polymyositis and dermatomyositis, that we were able to biopsy and treat with steroids. John Walton, now Lord Walton, joined as a fellow. He came to our department because of our muscle book. He thought he would learn more about the pathology of muscle. He put all that material together; there were about eighty-five or more cases of this type of idiopathic inflammation. And we wrote a small monograph [see Chapter 5] on that particular category of disease and offered a classification that included cases in relation to cancer and in relation to connective tissue disease with and without skin lesions. That came out in about 1954 or 1955, just after Walton went back to England. When he went back to England, he found that, at the National Hospital at Queen Square, there was not a single case of polymyositis or dermatomyositis in their neuropathology files for the prior twenty years or so. [see Figure 41]

RL: *I gather they weren't biopsying or autopsying them.*

RA: Well, they weren't recognizing them.

RL: *Did Walton work on other projects?*

RA: When he was with us, there was a controversy going on about whether a dystrophic fiber, if injured, would regenerate. Derek Denny-Brown had insisted that a dystrophic fiber had impaired capacity to regenerate. So we decided, in both the cases of progressive muscular atrophy and dystrophy, that we would injure the muscle a couple or three days before the biopsy was taken, and then take the biopsy on the edge of the injured site. We'd inject a little alcohol to injure the muscle, with the patient's consent. It would cause a little irritation but not much. We found that in the normal cases, and in the dystrophic cases, there was the same regeneration of endomysial cells and connective tissue around the fiber. That convinced us that, whatever the abnormality was in dystrophy, it was not reflecting itself in altered regeneration after direct injury; it had some other basis.

RL: *What was the importance of that study?*

RA: It turned attention to aspects of the dystrophic fiber other than response to injury. When a muscle is cut in a biopsy, as you probably know, many of the fibers are thrown into an intense contraction, wherein they reduce their length by a third or a fourth. And if you make a transverse section through a contraction band, the sarcoplasm has a hyaline appearance; it seems swollen. It was very striking in cases of Duchenne muscle dystrophy; I mistakenly thought that was an artifact. It turned out that that probably was something peculiar to that form of dystrophy. I believe Walton was the one who pursued that. And later, when Engel at Mayo Clinic showed in Duchenne that the abnormality was in the sarcolemma or sub-sarcolemmal dystrophin, it seemed that the "contraction bands" were probably a reflection of that pathology. I think that I overlooked the importance of that in Duchenne dystrophy. We showed it but misinterpreted it. In later editions we acknowledged that.

RL: *What did Walton do after leaving Massachusetts General Hospital?*

RA: Strangely, he was not accepted very well at National Hospital, Queen Square. He spent a year there. They are rather restricted in their staff, and he was not supported. He returned to Newcastle and set up a muscle institute, a muscle dystrophy center, the first one in England. He obtained funds and built a laboratory and had a group of very distinguished workers. Wally Bradley was one; there were others. He also established a muscle dystrophy society of England. So he pursued muscle disease and, I think, was one of the leaders in the world in that field through his retirement.

RL: *You also had connections with Australia.*

RA: Mercy Sadka, who had been a resident with us, was an Oxford graduate from Australia, Perth. Hers was a Jewish family that had migrated through Eastern Europe, during periods of persecution, and settled in Perth. She spent three years with us, did pathology for a year. She was well trained. When she went back to Australia, she was very much rejected by the male neurosurgery group.

One of the medical students, Byron Kakulas, brought her a section of muscle that he felt was diseased. It was from an animal, called the quokka, a marsupial that was being domesticated for laboratory use (it's like a kangaroo). And after a few months it wouldn't hop. She asked him to do a complete autopsy on one of these animals and to send the muscle tissue to me. I had just been looking at Dr Pappenheimer's work on muscle in vitamin E deficiency; it was exactly the same lesion as seen in his vitamin E cases, scattered muscle fiber necrosis, changes in the adventitia, and reactive macrophages. I wrote back and then sent Kakulas out to Rottnest Island, where the quokka lives. He measured vitamin E in the normal animals and then in the laboratory animals and found that the laboratory animals were deficient in vitamin E. There was great excitement about vitamin E deficiency being the possible cause of muscular dystrophy, but it turned out to be unrelated to human dystrophy.

RL: *But it was the cause of the animal disease.*

RA: Yes. They gave vitamin E to the domesticated animals and cured them. About the same time I received this quokka material, I received a biopsy specimen from a weak kangaroo at the Frankfurt zoo, and it had the same lesion. So it looked as though vitamin E deficiency was occurring in experimental animals and in captured animals.

Byron Kakulas then decided, after he graduated, to come to our department in Boston. He worked in neuropathology exclusively; he didn't work on the neurology service. We studied the quokka lesion more completely [see Chapter 5] and, later, when he returned to Perth, Australia, he became a professor of neuropathology and later, dean of a medical school in Western Australia. He also founded the Australian muscle dystrophy society. He obtained funds from families of muscle dystrophy cases and others in Perth and built an institute, which is a huge affair now. He is doing very important work in muscle and has trained quite a few people in neuropathology. In fact, the two professors of neuropathology in Sydney and Melbourne were pupils of his.

When Byron Kakulas was with us, I had a patient, adolescent with a distal weakness of the legs. Biopsy showed intranuclear inclusions in muscle fibers plus an inflammation. That was the first case of inclusion body myositis [see Chapter 5]. We reported that with Fred Samaha who was, at that time, in charge of our diagnostic neuromuscular laboratory, and I sent a piece of the muscle to our EM lab; it was lost. So we never got the EM on that material. When the patient kept getting worse, I showed the case to John Walton, who was visiting. He suggested that we give him steroids, which made him worse. He finally died with extensive muscle disease, almost quadriplegic.

RL: *Please comment about oculopharyngeal dystrophy.*

RA: The students showed me a case of an elderly woman who had an ocular and pharyngeal progressive atrophy, and one of the students looked up the family. It turned out to be a member of the same family that E. Willis Taylor, professor of neurology at Mass. General, had reported in the New England Journal of Medicine as a bulbar atrophy. I thought that peculiar. We biopsied the masseter muscle or pharyngeal muscle (I forget which), and it was a dystrophy. And so we reported that as an oculopharyngeal dystrophy, the first reported cases [see Chapter 5]. The family, it turned out, was from Canada. There were more than 300 descendants of one Canadian immigrant, going back four or five generations. Now it's quite well demonstrated, and it is one of the classic dystrophies with its own genealogy and enzymatic change. [see Figure 43]

During this period I thought that it was worthwhile to study the biometrics of muscle atrophy. Of course, the motor unit atrophy, characteristic of denervation, was easily demonstrated by this method. In experimental animals we had shown that denervation reduced muscle fiber size around 75% within four months of the time of nerve fiber loss, and that disuse atrophy reduced it only 20–25% after some months. With DeReuck from Belgium and with others, who worked in the lab, we were able to verify these volumetric changes.[3]

RL: *Comment on congenital muscular dystrophy.*

RA: We, also, with Betty Banker and Maurice Victor, discovered a form of congenital muscle dystrophy [see Chapter 5]. There had been no recording of that before, as far as I knew. [see Figure 44]

RL: *The baby had arthrogryposis.*

RA: In our autopsy material it was quite clear that arthrogryposis could be the result of either a muscle disease or a spinal cord disease or possibly a peripheral nerve disease. If it was in the spinal cord, it was often combined with brain damage too; then, the patient could be mentally retarded. That work was done, when Betty Banker was in neuropathology with us.

RL: *You mentioned your report on toxoplasmic myositis and your book on polymyositis. Please elaborate on your contribution to the study of inflammatory myopathies.*

RA: Well, we showed very clearly with the use of steroids that the patients, who did not have cancer, showed improvement and loss of high muscle enzyme levels in blood. About a fourth of them became normal, but more often they would improve up to a certain point and then remain with some degree of weakness. We also realized that there were degrees of polymyositis that were often being overlooked. We had a Yale Professor, whose head flopped. He couldn't hold his head up. To lecture to his students—he had devised a little holter that he would fasten to his back with a headband to keep his head up. He also had slight weakness in his shoulder muscles and that's all. And they were going to do an ankylosing procedure. I looked at the pathology, and it was a polymyositis. We put him on steroids in a low dose, and he improved to the point where he was chopping wood; we increased the dose and he was cured.

We showed that there were tremendous variations in the intensity of these cases and most of them, with very severe generalized proximal muscle weakness, were being called dystrophy at a number of centers. So the concept of an idiopathic polymyositis, long since forgotten, was resurrected, to some extent, by our studies. Earlier, it had been recognized in Vienna and elsewhere in central Europe.

RL: *Are you saying that inflammatory myopathy in association with some other disease had not been forgotten, but the idiopathic type had been?*

RA: That's right and we had some striking examples. We began receiving cases from other places and had a chance to treat quite a number of them with Walter Bauer, who was a rheumatologist and chief of the medical service, Jackson Professor of Medicine.

RL: *Were you and your colleagues the first to use steroids for polymyositis?*

RA: I'm not sure about that. Soon after cortisone was discovered at the Mayo Clinic, almost within weeks, Walter Bauer started using it in rheumatoid arthritis. He had problems with it; some of the patients became psychotic. He invited Cobb to join him in the study of these cases. When I began seeing these cases of inflammatory muscle disease, we started using corticosteroid preparations in them. But I wouldn't be sure that we were the first to do that at Mass. General. Certainly, early on we were quite active in the field.

RL: *Did you attempt to produce an experimental myositis?*

RA: Waksman and I tried to produce polymyositis by injecting extracts of muscle and adjuvants. The animals, instead of developing a polymyositis, all came down with severe arthritis. (*laugh*) Finally we gave up on that approach. There are others who have taken it up since.

RL: *Was anybody ever successful in producing an experimental myositis?*

RA: Byron Kakulas and his group used better antigens, and they did produce a polymyositis in animals in their institute at Perth.

RL: *Could you comment on the sequence of events in human disease or in Kakulas' animals. Is there damage to the fibers before or after the inflammatory cells appear in the lesion?*

RA: In a report to the American Society of General Pathology, I pointed out that in these inflammatory diseases, whenever there was muscle fiber necrosis, there was an infiltrate of lymphocytes and mononuclear cells in or next to that fiber.

RL: *Are you implying that there are other places where you saw the lymphocytes without the muscle necroses?*

RA: Yes, that's right.

RL: *I gather that you were viewing this inflammatory myopathy as analogous to experimental allergic encephalomyelitis or neuritis?*

RA: Yes, I thought that was exactly the case, that it's non-infective inflammatory parenchymal process and that the lymphocyte and mononuclear cell are involved in the mechanism of the parenchymal lesion.

RL: *Did you remain active in the field of muscle disease?*

RA: I had lectured here and there on muscle. In 1973, I gave the Thayer lectures at Johns Hopkins . . . three of them on neuromuscular disease, summarizing our work and that of others.[4]

I realized that any further progress was really going to come from electron microscopy and genetics, and I was not versed in these techniques. I abandoned the field pretty much but kept an interest in it, made a good many visits to the muscle dystrophy center in Perth and also to the muscle dystrophy center in Newcastle, England.

Ray Adams cultivated the field of muscle diseases. The early fruits were the first book on muscle pathology in half a century, the description of two new forms of muscular dystrophy, the discovery of inclusion body myopathy, and the creation of a logical classification of polymyositis and dermatomyositis.

The seeds of these fruits have spread across continents, as indicated in the above interview.

Notes

1. Lorenz H. Die Muskelerkrankungen, Spec Pathologie und Theropie. XI Band, III Theil Edited by H. Nothnagel. Wien, Alfred Holder, 1904, 727 p.
2. Andrus S, Kan ES, Adams RD, et al. Toxoplasmosis in the adult. *Arch Int Med* V89, pp 759–782, 1952.
3. Adams RD, De Reuck J. *Metrics of Muscle International Congress Series* 294 (ISBN 9021901633). Basic Research in Myology Part I of the Proceedings of the Second International Congress on Muscle Diseases held in Perth, November 1971.
4. Adams RD. Thayer Lectures. I. Principles of Myopathology. II. Principles of Clinical Myology. *Johns Hopkins Med J* V131, pp 24–63, 1972.

Hydrocephalus

By mid-century the pathology of hydrocephalus had been analyzed by Dorothy Russell. Dandy had shown that ventriculography facilitated diagnosis and that ventricular drainage improved the neurological manifestations. Although there was good understanding of hydrocephalus, Raymond Adams was able to make important additions to our knowledge of the subject.

RL: *Your study of hydrocephalus spanned your career.*

RA: We had the first cases of hereditary aqueductal stenosis; it was sex linked. The acqueduct seemed to be congenitally narrowed, not because of chronic inflammatory change around it. It was only in males; it was present at birth; in fact our case had to be delivered by trephination of the ventricles.

RL: *Where did you encounter this patient?*

RA: This was at the Boston City Hospital. And that same family had had two other males die of hydrocephalus. And I discovered through the mail that the following generation had at least one case. So all the males of three generations had died of hydrocephalus. That was published under my name and that of Bickers, who was fellow in the neuropath lab at Boston City [see Chapter 5 and Figure 45]. And there have been other cases found in England like that.

RL: *Tell me about your investigation of normal pressure hydrocephalus.*

RA: A woman, the wife of a businessman in Columbia, South America, had become mentally "scatty," as her husband said, no longer able to thoughtfully discuss a topic, forgetful, unsteady afoot, and occasionally incontinent. She was sent to us by Solomon Hakim, who didn't know what was the matter with her. Nor did I when I first examined her. I verified the findings in general, mental status and unsteady gait. The spinal fluid pressure was normal to high normal, about 160–170 mm of water, and the total protein was normal as was the cell count. Since we had no CT or MRI scans at that time, I performed a pneumoencephalogram. The lateral and third ventricles were markedly enlarged. Afterwards she was virtually stuporous; she wouldn't speak, was inattentive to everything going on about her. We were appalled by what had happened, as was her husband. About three days later I obtained another X-ray of her skull and found the enlarged ventricles were still full of air.

Not knowing what to do, I asked William Sweet to drain the ventricular air and fluid through a catheter and later through a one-way valve, which was then available. To our astonishment, in the following week she was back to not only the state in which she entered the hospital, but, according to her husband, she had regained her normal level of mentation. She proved then to be an intelligent woman; her gait returned to normal. She was grateful to our staff, and she was buying cookies for our residents, knew them all by name and joked about their affairs. We were extremely pleased; we got another x-ray and the ventricles were smaller than they were in the pneumoencephalogram. The valve blocked two or three weeks later and she began to relapse but recovered when it was replaced. We thought about this case at some length, and I wrote Hakim about this and suggested that, for some reason or other, she had had a hydrocephalus with a high normal CSF pressure, which seemed related to her dementia. We didn't know the cause of the ventricular enlargement.

We had other cases coming along and were able to verify the original observation, that the ventricles could be greatly enlarged and the patient have difficulty in walking, impaired mentation, and incontinence. Miller Fisher noted that gait disorder was the most constant part of the syndrome. Their statutory base was widened, their legs were not rigid, and there was no real cerebellar type of ataxia. It seemed to be some type of frontal lobe gait disorder.

Miller Fisher was brought into the study of the syndrome early on. In fact, I told him about the first case and, if I remember correctly, he may have seen the first patient, the one from Columbia. He suggested the term "normal pressure hydrocephalus." That was the origin of the concept of normal pressure hydrocephalus as a type of dementia with a gait disorder and incontinence. [see Chapter 5 and Figure 46]

We were quite impressed with it. It was infrequent, of course. But the fact that some of these patients, treated by a shunt, could recover their mental function, meant that one had to look at the larger group of demented patients to make sure that such cases were not being inadvertently included in the syndrome of Alzheimer disease or senility. I thought we had made an interesting observation that might have value in clinical neurology. If you can find one treatable cause, even if it's a rare one, in an otherwise hopeless clinical state, it reorients the profession to a larger problem viz. the dementias. That's, I think, the significance of it.

Also it was quite evident that the hydrocephalus could have a good many different causes. One of my patients was a professor from Ithaca, who had declined to the point where he was sitting, idly and witless, having before been a highly successful author of textbooks. He had to be led into my office. It turned out that he had hydrocephalus due to Paget's disease of bone. Decompression of the lower part of the cerebellum and a shunt put him back on his feet, and he was reediting his textbook of geology and walking briskly, when I saw him six months later.

RL: *That must have been gratifying.*

RA: Yes. I think that was a highly instructive. Two physicians contacted me, telling of their dementia being diagnosed as Alzheimer disease, until they were treated successfully for NPH.

RL: *I was told that Houston Merritt was your patient.*

RA: They brought Merritt to me to see if he had normal pressure hydrocephalus, and I thought he didn't have it and sent him back. He had Babinski signs and he had had two instances of what sounded like brief strokes to me. And so we refused to shunt him. Then two or three years later he was getting to be quite helpless. Mabel was having a lot of trouble taking care of him. Bud Rowland brought him back up. Miller and I both saw him. I still felt that he didn't have that condition. Miller said, "Since he was so helpless it might be worth a trial." That was done. A day or two later he had an embolus to the leg and gangrene. It was down hill from there; he went back to New York and died. He had Alzheimer disease. I guess no harm was done.

RL: *You also wrote about focal neurologic disorder as a manifestation of hydrocephalus.*

RA: I lectured at the international neurology meeting in Budapest, and made the point that when there is a lesion in the brain and an associated tension hydrocephalus, there can be progressivity of the focal abnormalities. In other words, the hydrocephalus is expressed not just by the more general gait disturbance and mental abnormalities, as was described in normal pressure hydrocephalus, but at times by a progression of a focal abnormality. For example, a partial hemiparesis could become more severe as hydrocephalus develops. That part of the brain, wherein lay the lesion, would give way to pressure more than any other part of the brain and would allow the ventricle to deviate towards that defect. [see Chapter 5]

We had one patient, who was a very brilliant engineer. He had devised many of the lighting arrangements for American hospital operating rooms. A fairly heavy drinker, he had a head injury, quite a severe one, and was comatose for a time and then gradually recovered. He was back at work and years later had a focal seizure or two. He had a pneumoencephalogram about a year or so later, and his ventricles were slightly enlarged but the right frontal horn a little more so than other parts of the ventricular system. About five years later he became quite incompetent and seemed indifferent to his wife and family and neglected his work. He was reexamined and thought to exhibit frontal lobe symptoms. On CT scan, ventricles showed the right anterior horn of the lateral ventricle to be enormously dilated and extended as a diverticulum towards the frontal region. He was shunted and within a few weeks he was pretty well back to a normal level and returned to work. So it looked as though that enlarging ventricle, related to his marginally advancing hydrocephalus, was manifested by the frontal lobe signs.

Also we had a child, with a birth injury, who, when seen at several years of age, had very mild pyramidal signs on one side. The hemiparesis seemed to worsen in childhood. The slight hemiparesis had become a hemiplegia, and the lateral ventricle on the side opposite the hemiplegia had considerably enlarged in comparison to the other one. The hemiplegia lessened with a shunt of CSF. Dorothy Russell had reported a case in which there seemed to be worsening of symptoms on one side with hydrocephalus. And I thought we confirmed that principle, that hydrocephalus could be a responsible factor, even in unilateral cerebral lesions.

Dorothy Russell's classic work on the pathology of hydrocephalus appeared in 1949. In her discussion of congenital hydrocephalus with aqueductal stenosis, she hypothetically mentions several possible causes. In the same year, Ray Adams proved that some cases of congenital hydrocephalus with aqueductal stenosis are heredo-familial (see Chapter 5). Russell also mentions that in hydrocephalus a diverticulum of the lateral ventricle can push into the cerebral white matter and cause hemiplegia. Ray Adams added to the few such cases reported, analyzed the subject, and drew attention to it. (see Chapter 5)

Furthermore, Adams alerted the general medical community to the fact that hydrocephalus, under normal cerebrospinal fluid pressure, can cause progressive dementia, gait disorder, and urinary incontinence (see Chapter 5). Unlike Alzheimer disease, which can cause the same syndrome, hydrocephalus was treatable. Adams et al. thereby changed the approach to the demented patient. Instead of assuming that dementia was a manifestation of a hopeless degenerative disease, the neurologist began to look for evidence that the dementia might have a reversible cause, hydrocephalic or otherwise.

Pathologic and Clinicopathologic Concepts

RL: *Can we turn to the subject of selective vulnerability of particular territories of the brain in a given metabolic disease of the nervous system?*

RA: Those ideas, of course, go back to the nineteenth century. Always, when one is conceptualizing a nervous system disease, one should at least consider its location within the nervous system. Some diseases have a random distribution of lesions all through the brain and spinal cord. Others have a specific topography, and this was finally capitalized as a process by Oscar Vogt as "pathoclisis," just a fancy way of saying the same thing. I believe that all neurological clinicians recognize the topographic aspect of disease. We differentiate the diseases not only on the basis of topography but also by the nature of the lesion, their time course, and cause or causes.

RL: *At least at a couple of times during your career you sectioned a specimen in an unconventional plane. In pernicious anemia you made some longitudinal cuts in the cervical spinal cord. In studying midline cerebellar degeneration, you made a midline sagittal cut as opposed to a transverse section. You were able to make important observations by looking at the nervous system in a different plane.*

RA: There could be two reasons for that. In demonstrating brains to students and to residents, it was worthwhile to let them look at the brain in an unconventional way rather than the standard sections, coronal of brain, horizontal of brainstem and spinal cord. And the second reason was that, when you looked at a lesion always in one plane you couldn't really compare spinal, brainstem, cerebral, and cerebellar lesions effectively. There was advantage for getting a better idea of the topography of the lesion, if it was cut in different planes. You would perhaps see it in a different form. That was the reason I often did that.

RL: *Earlier you mentioned artifact. For example, the spongiform encephalopathies were not immediately recognized because the spongiform appearance was mistaken for artifact. Has there been the opposite difficulty, mistaking artifact for something real?*

RA: That continues to be the case. As you know from your own experience, when you use immersion fixation with formalin, sometimes the central parts are relatively unfixed. If stains are applied, you cannot see nuclear structure, and that often is misinterpreted. Granular degeneration of the cerebellum, where all of the small cells in the granular layer of the cerebellum look half stained, has been written about repeatedly as a form of cerebellar disease. I think, in large measure, it's a fixation artifact.

RL: *You make the distinction, between organ pathology and tissue pathology.*

RA: Well this was not an original concept with me. I got the general idea working with Paul Yakolev and seeing the material of Dejerine and his textbook. In order to get an idea about the totality of disease in the nervous system, you had to develop a way of sampling the whole brain. Much of our pathology (based on just taking random blocks from several places, which were thought to be representative) failed to provide an idea of the totality of a disease process. That was brought home very forcibly a number of times with a disease that I thought was localized to one part of the nervous system. In stained whole brain serial sections we found that the topography was widespread. Of course, this is a labor, exhaustive.

It's difficult to combine looking at the pathology of the brain as an organ and concentrating on the tissue changes in one or two places. Sometimes, in whole brain studies, the histopathology is not as clear as it would be if you had early fixation and a variety of stains; for the whole brain studies you're usually limited to Nissl, myelin, and celloidin material. There are very few places, where you can do whole brain serial sections. Something intermediate is done on paraffin, where you can get very large blocks of brain and cut them up serially. We did that in our studies of Wernicke–Korsakoff, where we knew that most of our interesting histopathology was in the diencephalon and brainstem. So we had those parts in serial section.

RL: *Did you learn anything by doing the serial sections on paraffin blocks that you might not have noticed, had you only taken sample sections?*

RA: Oh, I think so. When studying a single lesion, if one takes the trouble to see it from its beginning to its end in serial section, you'll get a different concept of the disease than you would from a single well stained section. These are techniques, of course, that are variably applicable. If there was a major frontal lesion you could trace the secondary effects in diencephalon. In fact, I thought that studying the diencephalon in serial sections would provide a better idea of cerebral disease than studying the cerebral cortex and white matter. Sometimes you don't know to what extent a disease process has affected large parts of the brain, and since the diencephalic-cortical neurons die when the diencephalic axon is degenerate, you could perhaps find, in the diencephalon, representative change for every cerebral disease.

I don't think that the secondary changes have been pursued properly, for example, in the dementing diseases. I'm sure all of them, if properly studied at a diencephalic level, would have a characteristic topography. It might be easier to study it there than by sampling all parts of the cerebrum. Furthermore, when you try to figure out the degree of cell loss in, say, the Broca area or areas, it's very hard to identify the beginning and ending of that inferior frontal convolution. You don't know where the cortical area lies exactly. Whereas, if you looked at it from the diencephalic effect, you could measure neuronal loss because the diencephalic nuclei, for the most part, have a measurable beginning and ending.

RL: *Are there other studies that you would have liked to have done?*

RA: Well, I hoped to have been able to follow up what Jan Cammermeyer was doing, to make more careful study of immersion versus injection fixation to see to what extent artifact could be reduced. In my time the literature was full of reports of subtle neuronal changes. I thought that some of these were probably artifactual. They were promoted by the German pathologists with excellent techniques but without very careful control.

RL: *How does morphologic change lead to ideas about pathogenesis?*

RA: The lack of a finding is just as important as the presence of one. For example, an explanation for episodic global amnesia must take into account the lack of morphologic change.

RL: *Is there still an important role for the single case report?*

RA: Yes. There has never been a serial section study of the arteries and veins to determine whether there is primary involvement of them in Binswanger's disease.

RL: *Can you comment on the idea of determining a "center" for one function or another?*

RA: We're inclined; I think to be too strict in our localization. I've commented on this before, that we're inclined to attribute a given function to a given place in the brain, to try to relate it to a fiber system or a set of connections in one place. I have the impression, and increasingly so now, that the brain isn't organized along those patterns. The functional MRI is showing us that. Some of our ideas about anatomy are correct, but a very high degree of precision in localization is probably fallacious in most instances.

RL: *Geschwind used the term conduction aphasia, which he considered a disconnection syndrome due to a lesion of the arcuate fasciculus.*

RA: Yes, in the external capsule, I know about that. I supplied Geschwind with a couple of brains for his study. He made some excellent observations, but I don't believe that the anatomy of that conduction aphasia has held up.

RL: *Is the arcuate fasciculus a substantial structure that could be a main conducting link between the receptive and expressive areas?*

RA: No question about it being there, but when there's a "conduction" aphasia, I believe there's usually been something in the angular gyrus or in that general region; the lesion hasn't been limited to that fasciculus. Geschwind has an article on this subject in the *Handbook of Neurology*, one of the late issues, in which he softened his view of disconnection.[1] Probably it was just before he died.

Moreover I didn't think there was anything terribly original in Geschwind's analyses. He tried to be a little more precise about the observations of Broca, Wernicke, Dejerine and others. Nevertheless, he was a major force in turning attention to the localization of phenomena in the brain.

RL: *Nielsen referred to expressive aphasia as an apraxia for speech and to receptive aphasia as an agnosia for language.*

RA: I think, as long as one defines the terms very carefully, that's all right. Obviously, when he refers to expressive aphasia, he is referring to a large sphere of motor difficulty, but probably most of those patients would show some difficulty in understanding what was said. In fact, Pierre Marie discussed whether the difficulty in speaking is really an aphasia or just an apraxic state. The only criticism I had with Nielsen, who wrote authoritatively on speech disorder and was a very talented clinician, is that he tended to be too strongly localizationist, more so than I would think is warranted by observed facts. I think that strict localization of function nearly always proves to be inconsistent.

I tried to analogize the function of language to voluntary movement of hand. As you know, the physiology of precentral and premotor cortex, that was so neatly divided by John Fulton and Marion Hines, has not held up at all well. The motor cortex is just a lot more complicated than they ever realized. In Macaque they had worked out area 4 and 6 of the cortex and the marginal area in between and they gave a specific function to each. Sir Charles Symonds and Denny-Brown thought that to be a specious form of localization, that the cortex was not organized that way.

RL: *Comment further on mental functions and their anatomic correlates.*

RA: I agree more with Luria than with Geschwind. I was very respectful of Luria's general approach to neuropsychiatric problems, his way of looking at memory and such. Geschwind, I thought, was very astute but was trying to overcommit himself to precise localization of cerebral functions.

Notes

1. Damasio AR, Geschwind N. Anatomical Localization in Clinical Neuropsychology. In Fredericks AM (ed.), *Handbook of Clinical Neurology, V1 (45). Clinical Neuropsychology.* Elsevier Science Publishers, Amsterdam, 1985, pp 7–20.

Writing

Adams' *Principles of Neurology* has been described as a "classic text...written with an enviable clarity and elegance of style."[1] Another Adams' book, *The Wenicke–Korsakoff Syndrome*, has been described as follows: "The writing style, as expected from these incredibly literate scholars, is crisp and direct."[2]

RL: *It has been said that your Principles of Neurology was the most lucid piece of medical writing since the time of Cushing.*

RA: That is a nice compliment.

RL: *How did you learn to write?*

RA: I learned to take care. At first I didn't write well.

RL: *How did you turn yourself into a good writer?*

RA: By writing. I didn't have a natural facility. Byron Waksman could just sweep through once, and it seemed to come out all right...very skillful.

RL: *And you would go through drafts.*

RA: Yes.

RL: *But you ended up able to write an entire neurology text book in a matter of months.*

RA: That was after I'd been writing for a medical textbook for years.

RL: *How did you decide to write your textbook* Principles of Neurology?

RA: I was being pushed very hard for space, by the other editors of Harrison's *Principles of Internal Medicine.* Thorn and Kurt Isselbacher, who had become the editor of gastrointestinal disease in the Harrison, came to me and they urged that I write a book on neurology and reduce the amount of material in Harrison. I wasn't very keen on that. I had had a policy, in writing for Harrison, of including in each chapter that I wrote, the name of one of the residents or assistants in the department, to help them in their careers. To reduce all of that, I thought, would hurt them. And, I think I can say fairly that the neurology part of the Harrison had become sort of the general physician's neurology book. It finally came to be about 500 pages out of a 2000-page book. This upset some of the other editors, especially when Resnik and Harrison retired and Petersdorf and Braunwald came in. They claimed that the Harrison had become *Principles of Internal Medicine with the Details of Neurology!*

RL: *Did any of your teachers survive to see your textbook published?*

RA: When I wrote the introduction to the psychiatry section in my book, I asked Cobb's opinion of it. He read it carefully, and he said that it was well written but that he disagreed with every word. And he was irritated that, after my exposure to psychiatry in his department, I would come up with such alien ideas.

RL: *How successful has* Principles of Neurology *been?*

RA: It is now going into the 8th edition in thirty-two years.

RL: *You mentioned that Kubik taught you about writing.*

RA: He would spend hours writing a few paragraphs, when we wrote a paper together. It was the first paper he had written since he had left Queen Square. He had written a paper when he was working with Greenfield. (He was Greenfield's first assistant.) F.M.R. Walsh looked over the paper Kubik had written and sent it back with a remark, "Please rewrite this in English." And Kubik was so hurt that he never published anything thereafter. Ayer tried to get him to report some of the wonderful material he had studied, but he refused. Finally, I spent so much time writing up our cases on subdural empyema that he was embarrassed to not to be involved. I would write something. He would take it and start analyzing it. We worked on that fifteen-page paper for one year. Sometimes, a whole evening we would spend on one or two paragraphs.

And then we wrote several more papers together, one on basilar artery occlusion and one on the brain lesions in pernicious anemia, and a very good paper on the pathology of meningitis. So I think that I learned how to write in large measure through my association with Kubik. Also clarity of thinking about pathologic changes came from him.

RL: *What were your experiences in dealing with publishers and their lay editors?*

RA: Well, I think that was a headache. I've been badly treated by them. For the neuropathology book, the publisher selected the editor, who never spoke to me, never came to Boston to find out what the purpose of the book was. I had assembled with Sidman, a wonderful set of illustrations, I thought. I spent a lot of money on these illustrations. When they printed the first draft, they reduced all the illustrations to half size. I had very carefully arranged them so they would show best when published just in the original size. The publisher was quite indifferent. They didn't care. And, finally, I told them they had ruined the illustrations. They said, if I didn't like it, I could pay for reproduction of them the way I wanted. And at that point I refused to do that or to have the book published. And finally the editor came to Boston and talked to me about it, and asked about the purpose of the book, and they agreed to publish it with the illustrations the way I wanted them. [see Chapter 6]

On several occasions they would select an editor, who knew nothing about the field and would make all kinds of outlandish suggestions. For each edition of Harrison they would have a different editor.

RL: *Was there a reason for the lack of continuity?*

RA: The main reason was that the previous editor would quit and go to another company or something like that. And they would just choose someone else and tell him to speak to the authors. That happened repeatedly. They think nothing of charging authors for all of the secretarial work that's done. They charged an outlandish price for doing an index poorly, unless we would protest. Tinsley Harrison, himself, would fight with them about the royalty that they would pay; he got them to agree to pay an 18% royalty on the Harrison medical textbook, which they thought was outlandish.

RL: *I have never heard of a royalty that high.*

RA: Yes. They usually will pay 10 or 12% and then try to charge you for the index out of the royalty . . . charge several thousand dollars. But Harrison not only would refuse to work with them, unless they would pay the royalty that he thought we deserved, but he insisted that each editor and his family (there were five of us) should be permitted to have meetings in New York every few months, putting the book together.

And once every four years the publisher would pay our way with our families for a two-week meeting in some part of the world, planning for the next edition. So we would have wonderful trips in various parts of the world, where we would get together and think, in Madeira, Sicily, Madrid, London, and Italy. I came to know the other editors very, very well. In fact, the international trips were so delightful that often, when we would have a meeting in New York, we'd spend most of our time trying to agree on the place where we wanted to go next. We'd spend more time arguing about that, than we did about the subject matter of the book. (. . .*chuckle*) [see Figure 48]

RL: *It sounds like Harrison was quite a businessman.*

RA: Yes. After he'd had a couple shots of whiskey, he could convince anyone that McGraw Hill was the luckiest company in the world to have such people as us as editors.

RL: *Once the book became so popular, he could negotiate from a position of strength.*

RA: Yes. I was able to get a good royalty on the *Principles of Neurology* because it was a successor book to the Harrison book. The royalties for Harrison enabled me to help with the education of my children and grandchildren.

Richard Sidman watched Adams edit his draft with "seemingly effortless writing." What seemed to come so easily was the result of much practice by Adams. Miller Fisher once bemoaned his own difficulty with writing to Elinor Adams, who tried to reassure him. Writing, she said, was not always so easy for Ray. When he first began writing papers, he had to go through fourteen drafts. Adams taught Allan Ropper that "clear writing is clear thinking."

Herb Schaumberg recalls his experience:

Well I have many memories of Ray as a teacher and a mentor and (*Ha*) I will tell you right now about one of the first big cases I had, as a neuropathology fellow. Someone, who died with what they thought was MS, turned out to have a reticulum cell sarcoma of the brainstem. Ray commented to me that somebody should look into this because he had a number of cases, over the years, that were thought to be microgliomas. So Charlie Plank and I got all the cases together and wrote a paper that Ray thought we should send to Brain. He didn't look at it. We finished, and he said, "Let me take it home and just look at it tonight." So we gave it to him. It was quite a long paper actually—and he brought it back. He had taken a regular pencil and rewritten every sentence above it. He handed it to me and said, "I made a few suggestions," a masterpiece of understatement! Every sentence in the paper! I would have been embarrassed, had it been anybody but Dr Adams. I mean he just tore my prose apart; that modified it into a very literate document. In the first sentence I had something about "the microglioma group of tumors was misunderstood." His first sentence was, "More than thirty years have elapsed since this tumor, first described as a microglioma but now recognized to be a reticulum cell sarcoma..." The man could write.

This striving for excellence in writing did not change. Very late in Ray's life, Bruce Price gave him a first draft. When Price received the manuscript back, he recalls, "I never saw so much red." This same experience was shared by many, perhaps most, of Adams' numerous co-authors.

In the basement of his Brookline home he had many tables, some actually doors supported by saw horses, upon which he spread the galley proofs of his books. When he would read an article, which he deemed worthy, he would go to the appropriate galley proof and add the information and reference. Thereby, when it was time to prepare a revised book, the next edition was practically ready for the secretary to type. This organized and disciplined method antedated the computer age but it was very effective, and it amazed those who witnessed it in action.

Notes

1. Aminoff MJ. Principles of Neurology. *J Am Med Assoc* V277, pp 1817–1818, 1997.
2. Daroff RB. The Wernicke–Korsakoff Syndrome. *Neurology* V39, p 1008, 1989.

Orienting Ideas in Neurology

RL: *You wanted to make some general comments.*
RA: I felt very strongly that in teaching neurology and in expository writing, e.g. in preparing a textbook of neurology, certain concepts should be respected.

One of primary importance is that all of neurology should be encompassed, not just the neurologic abnormalities of the adult but also neurologic disturbances of the maturing brain, those of the infant and child and of the aging brain as well. Stages of growth and maturation and of advanced age give completely different baselines for evaluation of neurological status. For example, in the study of epilepsy,[1] there are many forms, which, in part, vary with the age of the nervous system. Obviously, many parts of the brain, which can be altered in adult disease, are not functioning in the infant.

Another orienting principle is considering the time factor in evaluating the effects of a lesion. For example, a stroke, affecting a particular part of the brain initially, has a much wider effect than it will have later. Proper clinical-anatomical correlates of such a lesion become dependable only when viewed after six to twelve months or more, when all of the peripheral diaschisis effects, which are variable in each case, have resolved. This is a concept proposed by von Monikov, that these transient effects gradually disappear over time and that the residual lesion, by itself, does not explain these effects.

Clinical neurology textbooks and teachers of neurology should include references to the major neurophysiologic, neuropsychologic and neuropathologic data relevant to clinical phenomena. For example, one cannot discuss consciousness without reference to a specific afferent reticular cortical system in the subthalamus and thalamic region, separate from the afferents to the sensori-motor regions of cortex. Magoun and I believe, Morouzzi took great pains to identify this upper reticular–diffuse cortical system and showed that a lesion in the thalamic region could abolish consciousness. These neurophysiologic and neuroanatomic data, which relate to consciousness, are being neglected in most theoretical essays of consciousness. In our own material, those patients, who had survived for months or years in vegetative state, all had lesions in this region of the brain. Thus, even in the discussions of normal function, references to the deficits produced by disease are of value.

Another principle I thought to be important is the necessity of study of the whole brain and not just the most obvious lesion(s), in the study of the anatomy of disease. In the book that Sidman and I wrote on neuropathology, it was pointed out that many diseases of the CNS have a specific identifying general topography, viz. organ pathology.

I was quite careful to point out that our concept of neuropathology in the broadest sense includes the morbid changes and the functional deficits of all disorders of the nervous system. Reynolds, an earlier pathologist, defined pathology as all morbid processes that alter the structure and function of the body and all processes, that limit life, and its powers, enjoyment and duration. In the nervous system one must include not only those changes which are obvious by the present day methods of examination but those that are present but still not visible by present day methods. Neurology, in general, encompasses all diseases of the nervous system from the simplest disorder of muscle function to the most elaborate psychological derangement such as impaired memory, alertness and attention.

At a clinical level there are not one but two medical methods of collecting data. One approach utilizes the standard methods of medicine, such as history taking, use of treatment, physiologic and psychologic laboratory procedures, the pathology (where pathology can be defined), and, where one could envision, prevention and cure. I view this as the principal subject matter of neurology, neurosurgery, and psychiatry. Not only does it include all of the diseases that are commonly recognized in neurology but also diseases such as delirium, anxiety states and other neuroses, manic depressive disease, schizophrenia and persistent psychopathies, which are principal components of psychiatry.

There is a second method, a subjective, interpretive analysis of the patient's introspections about his past life, that is, his biography. The latter method is much utilized by contemporary psychiatrists, but the interpretation of behavior in terms of life experience has rather little value. Thus the Freudian approach to neurologic disease is believed to be invalid. Nevertheless, for understanding the patient and having a close and sympathetic relationship, this second type of information is essential.

Thus each approach, the neurological and the psychological, has its place in medicine. There's certainly a tremendous sphere of activity for psychiatrists in the study of a major category diseases of the brain, with which they have a large experience, including neuropharmacology. Also we depend on psychiatrists who can express the view of modern medicine towards all of these social phenomena that are so troublesome.

It's a little surprising to me that most of the older scholars of human behavior from Plato and St. Augustine, on through Descartes, always set aside higher mental function as being something not understandable in terms of brain anatomy and function. Even more modern scientists like Sherrington and Eccles, when confronted by disorders of the mind, always felt that these lay beyond their understanding. They had made their mark in the elucidation of single cell circuits. They concluded that mental function lay at a higher order of complexity. They ended up as dualists, separating physiological and psychic functions. I disagreed, being a monist. I felt very strongly that there was one clear proof that mind and brain function were equivalent: the loss of insight with cerebral lesions. In all types of widespread cerebral disease, the patient not only loses some aspect of behavior, but he also loses the capacity to introspect, to know that his mental function is deranged—that he is not functioning normally. In other words, there is a loss of insight in addition to the extrinsic expressions of the cerebral abnormality. Thus, neurology informs us that the only proper philosophic view of the brain and mind is one of psychophysical monism.

These are ideas that I thought were rather important in a modern neurologist's general orientation. And they place neurology and neurosurgery and psychiatry in proper relationship to one another.

Adams comments that two Nobel Prize winning neuroscientists could not free themselves from dualism, the notion that brain physiology could not explain the human mind. Into the second half of the twentieth century neuroscientists continued to try to find a way out of this difficulty. Penfield, having discussed monism and dualism, quoted a third view, that of Gilbert Ryle. "The umbrella titles of 'Mind' and 'Matter' obliterate the very differences that ought to interest us. Theorists should drop both of these words."[2] Thus he suggests that the terms themselves interfere with clear thinking about the subject. The foregoing interview includes Adams' own original thoughts about the relationship of mind and brain.

Notes

1. Salam MZ, Adams RD. L'epilesie processus physiopathologique on relation avec l'age. *Schweiz med Wchnschr* V97, pp 1707–1716, 1967.
2. Penfield W, Roberts L. *Speech and Brain Mechanisms*. Princeton University Press, Princeton, NJ, 1959.

4

FAMILY, RETIREMENT, AND OLD AGE

Family Life

In 1944 Ray and Elinor Adams bought a decrepit old New England farm house in Milton, Massachusetts. They borrowed the money from Ray's mother to make the purchase. He couldn't afford to have it painted. For a year before they moved in, Ray's father and Ray worked to repair the structure. Three years later he bought the adjacent field with a loan from his mother.

Eventually, their son recalls, they had 4 or 5 acres, 1½ acres of which was their vegetable garden. Everything that they ate was grown by Elinor who canned and froze the foods. The neighboring acres were vacant and provided more room for recreation including baseball games at neurology picnics.

The Adams grandparents, both of whom survived into their eighties, lived in the vast home. Ray's father was growing demented. Eventually his door was locked at night to avoid any incident. At mid-century there was no appropriate institution for patients with Alzheimer disease or other dementing illnesses. Ray did not want to send him to a mental hospital. Yet, his presence in the home was a strain. Ray's wife and mother, both strong personalities, did not mix well in the same household.

RA: My parents came to live with us. My father retired from the railroad. My sister, whose husband was in the army, came to live. My poor wife Elinor tried to put up with this household keeping. It was a large home… about twenty rooms. My father and I put the roof on the three-story house and barn and painted the whole thing on weekends and evenings.

RL: *Your purchasing the Milton property allowed your father to take up farming again.*

RA: Yes. He was helpful. And then there were incompatibilities between my parents and my wife, Elinor. Finally my sister—she was a social worker in Maine—and her husband, a pediatrician, took them in and they spent their remaining years with her.

    Elinor was at the time in graduate school at Harvard, making excellent marks; she was extremely bright. And was forced out of that by her last pregnancy. She went on and did her doctoral degree in Romance languages at Boston University. Later she taught at Boston State College, looking after this household and canning vegetables and so on at the same time. This was all going on during that period of the forties and early fifties, late fifties. So it obviously had a great deal of influence on my life.

RL: *Did your large family and the tensions in the house affect your professional work?*

RA: No, my wife was very protective and never interfered in any way. Elinor made it possible for us to live in a very lovely home—took the whole burden of the family on her shoulders and my parents for a short time. Did everything she could to be helpful to me.

RL: *Did your professional work affect your home life?*

RA: I am sure it did. But Elinor just devoted her entire energy to looking after that house and the family. The town of Milton had an elite society of older New England families. She tried to adjust to that, and they were rather rude to her, an uncouth westerner.

RL: *Why would they perceive of her as uncouth?*

RA: They were cliquish and rather haughty.

RL: *So it had nothing to do with her fluency or accent or intelligence.*

RA: No, she was brighter than they were.

RL: *It was just a matter of social snobbery.*

RA: Yes, but she was hurt by it.

RL: *I see.*

RA: And later, she got around some of them by joining the league of women voters and became an officer. That brought her in relation to a group of more intelligent women. And she got all of our children into the Milton Academy, which is a very fine private school, about a mile from the house. It was expensive but we managed to put them through.

    It was quite evident, when we moved to Milton, that the public school was very poor. There was a lot of politics in the town, and the wealthy people did not take any interest in the public schools. They all sent their children to the Milton Academy. So we had to turn to that school, if we wanted to stay in Milton. And I must say that it proved to be a very good school . . . excellent teachers . . . and they provided a good primary and secondary education.

RL: *How many children did you have?*

RA: Four.

RL: *Did they all go to Milton Academy?*

RA: All of them. And my son went to another preparatory school and then Harvard College. But the other three went south, one to Duke and two to the University of North Carolina. In the meantime I was traveling a lot, as a consultant to individual patients in Syria and Switzerland, France, England, and Algeria. I was away a great deal. So that finally it led to our separation. And I finally became involved with Maria Salam who was a pediatric neurologist in Lebanon. So, the family sort of broke up after that.

RL: *Tell me about Maria Zabnienska Salam.*

RA: I think we actually met, for the first time, when I was giving the Wilder Penfield Lecture at the American University in Beirut at the Mid-East Medical Assembly. And she came and visited Boston a number of times, and on one of these visits we developed a very close relationship. We began living together, but I couldn't get a divorce for years. Finally we married. Maria was extremely passionate, highly emotional woman, very sociable, very attractive and romantic, with a wide circle of friends, assistant professorship at Harvard for twenty-five years. Excellent pianist, entertainer, and her life was really very agreeable. She contracted in 1979, two years after I retired, multiple myeloma, and she bravely faced that. She kept on working at Mass. General, didn't let anyone know she was ill for twelve years, I think it was, and finally succumbed to it.

RL: *What became of Elinor?*

RA: She later retired and became a teacher in Mexico, later built a house in the mountains in eastern Oregon, finally died of carcinoma.

RL: *You remain close to Maria's daughter, Nina Salam.*

RA: Antonina has never married. I couldn't live here alone without her help. She's been devoted. I've known Nina since she was twelve years old and she's now fifty, I think. So I've known her very intimately for a great part of her life. She has been tremendously supportive.

All of the Adams children agree that their father's overwhelming devotion was to medicine. In their words: "For my father work came first," "his profession consumed him," "he loved neurology . . . it was his entire life," "he was 99% medicine and 1% biography."

Neurology permeated the Adams' household. "He always had brains in the refrigerator; there were slides everywhere" (Carol). He sometimes saw patients in the home (Mary). Every free minute he spent in his study. He was often not home for supper with the family. When he was home for dinner, he would nap in his easy chair in his library, eat dinner, and then work at his desk. His back was to the window as he wrote on yellow pads." [see Figure 49]

This work in the library went on until 1 a.m. according to Carol. There would be 4–5 hours of sleep. He would arise at 5 a.m. to exercise. Sometimes he would work the land. They had 4 or 5 acres of their own, which for many years he mowed with a push mower. Later he did the job with a power mower, which still required that he push it through the grass. Bill and Sarah remember watching their father from their bedroom windows; he would climb to the neighboring acres where he would run back and forth on a path along the wall of the property; he would then leave for work before the children would arise.

It was not only the unceasing work in the library which made the home a neurological outpost. The family constantly had foreign doctors, living with them. The visitors lived on the third floor, which was somewhat separate. Bill loved having these families from Norway, Sweden, and England in the home. There were times when there were twelve to fourteen people in the house. Often there were French-speaking people from whom the children would learn their language. With this ever-changing extended family, the children on one occasion would celebrate Bastille Day , on another Norwegian Christmas customs.

Family life was enriched by the flow of neurologists through the house. Interesting characters like Maurice Victor and Mandel Cohen often visited on Sundays. Bill and the others remember Phil Dodge, C. Miller Fisher, Justin Hope, and others as gracious and interesting and interested in the children.

The neurologic environment in the house directly affected the family in another way. Off at college, Mary began dating a man named Dudley. For holidays they would drive from North Carolina to see his family in Long Island. Then they would drive to Milton. On this leg of the trip, Mary would read to her boyfriend from her father's neurology section in Harrison's *Principles of Internal Medicine*. They hoped that the undergraduate might thereby be prepared to understand Ray Adams' comments, when Ray would take him on rounds at Massachusetts General Hospital. Eventually Dudley entered medical school and found that he understood neurology better than his classmates, at least in part due to his education by the Adams' family. He thus found himself drawn to the field and became a neuropathologist.

One of the most memorable days of family life in Milton related to a professional incident. Ray Adams had decided to leave Boston City Hospital to head neurology at Massachusetts General. Not long after he made his intention known, the finished manuscript of his book on muscle disease disappeared from Boston City Hospital. This disastrous loss meant that he would have to rewrite the book. Ray was so upset that the household was in an uproar. The emotion of the incident remains imprinted on the children over half a century later.

Although neurology was a main vein of the Adams' household and although their father was not home very much, Mary recalls that "we did not know anything else." At the time the children did not feel that career was interfering with family life. Ray never hit a child—he would wave his arms around instead. He did refuse to let them play cards on Sunday, although he resisted going to church himself. Carol recalls that the children did not suffer; "it was a wonderful life." There were always two or three dogs around. Great credit goes to Elinor Adams, who raised the children to a large extent by herself. To friends the Adams seemed a nice couple, but the marriage failed.

The neurologic connection to family life continued in his second marriage. Maria frequently entertained neurologists in the home. Maria and Ray saw patients together, and they wrote papers together. Outsiders found him to be happier in his second marriage. Perhaps, at a different stage of his career, he had more time for family life or, perhaps, the personality of his second wife, Maria, somehow suited him. "She got him up on the dance floor." They golfed together. This marital warmth was evident to Joseph Martin, who was struck by Ray's extraordinary affection for Maria. Ray was despondent on her death.

Retirement and Old Age

Retirement as chief of service was mandatory at age sixty-seven. For the occasion some 200 former residents, fellows, and colleagues assembled in the Ether Dome of Massachusetts General Hospital to honor Ray Adams in 1977. Over two days, eighty-nine papers were read by authors he had educated. At that time more than twenty-five headed major neurology departments in the United States and Western Europe. He continued at the hospital as a senior neurologist, and he remained director of the Shriver Center, where he worked three days a week. During these years he wrote the *Neurology of Hereditary Metabolic Disease* and he co-edited the 2,500-page *Histology and Histopathology of the Nervous System*. In the mid-1990s an annual Raymond Adams' Neurodevelopmental Disabilities Conference was initiated at the Shriver Center. As he reached the age of ninety, there was established a Raymond Adams lectureship, which is given at the annual meeting of the American Neurological Association.

RL: *What did you do after you retired as chairman?*
RA: Miller and I were kept on by Joe Martin as voluntary teachers. I was teaching the residents five times a week. To see patients one afternoon a week, I had to rent an office. So they got good work for their money. [see Figure 57]
RL: *You continued to work full time between Massachusetts General Hospital and the Shriver Center.*
RA: Yes, for about ten years.
RL: *During this time you wrote the book* Neurology of Hereditary Metabolic Diseases of Children.
RA: Well, that all came about through the Shriver Center. I had become involved in the pathology and clinical expressions of hereditary diseases that blighted the development of the brain at various epochs during infancy and childhood, and thought it worthwhile putting all these together. I thought there was a place for a small book

that would segregate the diseases according to the periods of time when they were most likely to be encountered by pediatricians. And Gilles Leon, who had been a research fellow in my department at Mass. General, was interested in the same thing. Gilles is French and didn't feel confident in writing things in English. So I composed most of the book, and he edited the content. It is a concise review of some of the main features, clinical and pathologic, of this whole category of diseases.

RL: *When did you give up your remaining responsibilities?*

RA: I turned the directorship of Shriver Center over to Hugo Moser, who moved there from the Kennedy Laboratories in the mid-1980s. I stopped teaching residents at MGH in the mid-1990s. Until the late 1990s I remained active each Friday, when I would see outpatients at McLean in the morning; then I would give a clinical conference at the Shriver Center in the afternoon.

RL: *Late in life you continue to be honored.*

RA: I received an invitation yesterday to become an honorary member of the American Academy of Neurology, and I've not been a member.

RL: *Never?*

RA: I don't think so. They rejected me at first because of that dispute that I'd had with Abe Baker.

RL: *I didn't know that you had had a dispute with Abe Baker.*

RA: Well, that one that I had over the protoplasmic astrocytes in the hepatic encephalopathies.

RL: *You must be referring to your response to his comments at the Association for Research in Nervous and Mental Diseases meeting, when you correlated hepatic encephalopathy with change in the protoplasmic astrocytes and he attributed it to myelin pallor.*

RA: Yes, I pointed out that he was describing a myelin artifact. He took it very seriously. And now someone has given money for an Adams fellowship. Since they wanted the fellowship in the American Academy of Neurology, they want me to become an honorary member.

RL: *Will you accept this honor?*

RA: Oh, yes.

RL: *Tell me about your stroke. You said you noticed it right after you got into bed one night.*

RA: Yes. My hand was totally paralyzed, and there was some altered feeling on the ulnar side of hand, but delicate sensory tests could not bring it out. It was not revealed by punctuate cutaneous testing. The recovery of motor function was remarkably rapid. The lesion, which was seen by MRI, was sharply localized in the upper part of the motor cortex, extending a little into the parietal lobe. I became quite conscious of the fact that, even though only my wrist and fingers were paralyzed, there were other more subtle distant effects in the motor system. For example, I thought that my speech was slightly dysarthric, when I was fatigued, even though the speech areas were distant from the lesion. And I thought that my shoulder and leg were slightly affected, even though it was only the hand that was paralyzed.

I mention this because it shows the inadequacy of our views of the very sharp localization of motor function to just areas 4, 6, and 8 in the motor cortex itself. It calls attention to the fact that we don't understand fully the physiology of the motor system.

RL: *Tell me about the temporal profile of your stroke.*

RA: Instantaneous. Instantaneous. I could date it almost to the minute it occurred.

I made the diagnosis, while I was still in bed. I thought it had to be an embolus. It had to be strictly localized to a part of the upper division of the left middle cerebral artery, what we call the Rolandic division. However, it included less than the full extent of that arterial territory—a branch occlusion.

RL: *How did you feel about it?*

RA: I wasn't very happy about it. I immediately called my daughter and went downstairs, and she drove me to the hospital. They didn't do an ordinary arteriogram. They did two CT scans about 12 hours apart and two MRIs, and only on the last MRI did they think they could see the lesion. I went quickly to the hospital, thinking that, with all the newer work on clot dissolution, they might want to try a drug on the lesion. They did an MRI arteriogram. In the left internal carotid artery, about a centimeter above the bifurcation, there was a kind of a shelf like lesion that narrowed the lumen about 50–60%. They conjectured that this might have been the source. The cardiac rhythm was normal, and an echocardiogram was normal. Since there was rapid spontaneous improvement, Miller Fisher, Walter Koroshetz, and Phil Kistler decided not to do anything except to put me on an aspirin-like compound. They added a cholesterol-lowering medication.

They didn't want to use anticoagulants because that would require that I come to the hospital to have my prothrombin time checked. It's almost impossible for me to do that. Moreover, Miller thought that some of his patients had had a single embolus and had gone for a long time without anticoagulant and without recurrence.

RL: *Do you have problems residual from the stroke?*

RA: My hand is a bit awkward and my speech is not easily fluent as in the past. After about a year I was able to write more legibly by writing slowly and intentionally large.

RL: *Could you share your observations on the effects of aging?*

RA: In a sense, the life span and the duration of adequate function is ended by a combined declination of multiple organ systems that are of vital importance.[1] That includes the brain, the heart, the endocrine glands, the kidneys, and the bone marrow. All of these organs do fail gradually, and they begin to fail conspicuously in the senium. These gradual declines, including those in the nervous system, represent the aging process per se and are not easily differentiated from diseases. And, of course, there can be disease in one organ system that interferes slightly with life span and still there will be the aging processes in other organs. That's why a student, looking at the post-mortem findings in an old person, is surprised not to see serious disease that could possibly account for death. I think death is a combination of these gradual declines in all these various organs. I remark on this because I think, in neuropathology, one of the biggest problems right now ,with all the emphasis on dementias, is a failure to differentiate age-linked disease from the aging process, which has been going on for about fifty years already. This process needs to be more fully studied.

RL: *So, how does this apply to you? You don't seem to be suffering multiple organ failure, from what you've told me.*

RA: Oh, yes I think I am. I don't have the cardiac reserve that I did. I have to go up the stairs holding on to a bannister, a step at a time. And I puff three or four times when I reach the top. I have developed a little anemia. My hematocrit has fallen off about three or four points. They are watching that. My blood urea nitrogen has gone up to about thirty or forty and they are watching that. So I can see that there are multiple organ failures. Of course you have no way of proving it. The doctors who look after me find excuses for it, which I don't agree with.

RL: *Tell me about your visits to the doctor.*

RA: He did that (*gesture: hitting the side of his hand against the palm of his other hand*). I said, "What are you doing?" "Testing your knee jerk." (*Laughter*). I said, "Why don't you get a reflex hammer?" He said he didn't have one.

RL: *There was a time when skills in physical diagnosis were highly developed.*

RA: I was taught how to percuss a chest and listen to breath sounds. There is a real art to examining a chest. I remember Ayer's brother-in-law, Palfrey, who had written several books on clinical examination. He was a master clinician. He looked after the nurses at the Boston City Hospital. Whenever the Thorndike staff had a clinical problem that they couldn't solve, they'd call the old man, and he would come and tap and tap and tap. He'd spend a half hour going over a chest; "Well the fever's due to a little something in the pleural cavity here... put a needle there, even though the X-ray doesn't show anything; there's some pus there." They aspirated pus from the chest!

I had a friend who had a gastrointestinal problem that no one could solve. He'd had many X-rays and all, and I asked Palfrey to see him. One Saturday afternoon he went over to the hotel with his little paper for testing hemoglobin, and he went to work on his abdomen. He must have spent 45 minutes palpating, localizing his stomach and duodenum, and he found a spot in his duodenum. He thought he had an ulcer on the back side of his duodenum, prescribed three or four medicines, charged him $25, and sent him home. He never had any more symptoms! But that's the art of medicine. He could locate every organ in the abdomen, unless the person was enormously fat. Now, that level of clinical skill is nonexistent.

RL: *What other changes have you noticed with aging?*

RA: Quite apart from my auditory threshold being slightly elevated, auditory perception is a little impaired. I don't assimilate a spoken command or remark as readily as before. Also, I'm conscious of an increase in tearfulness. Of course, this is a well-known phenomenon in the aged. I don't like to hear the Battle Hymn of the Republic or something like that for it brings an embarrassing tear.

RL: *What other observations have you made about aging?*

RA: Sleep is troublesome. I think I have sleep apnea to some degree. So I try to prevent it by lying on my side and arranging pillows. Usually I have a book in bed, but I don't read more than three or four pages before becoming noticeably drowsy. I fall asleep and I will stay asleep for 3 hours, maybe, and then I awaken. From there on I sleep intermittently; I doze and have curious mixtures of reminiscences and dreams that are almost indistinguishable. So I probably only have 4, 4½, 5 hours of solid sleep. And, of course, I make up for that by dozing, when I sit in my chair during the day. I'll be reading a book or an article in a journal, and it will fall out of my hands, and I pick it up and drop it again in another 2 or 3 minutes. These are microsleep periods that probably don't last more than a very few minutes.

The other day, for some reason or other, I had a momentary visual memory of riding in a railroad car through the Sierra Nevada mountains in Western Oregon on the way to the beach. My mother and sister were there. I don't know what aroused that memory. I suppose I would have been seven or eight.

RL: *You lead a life of hard work. In retrospect how do you feel about it?*

RA: I don't think I've ever worked very hard. I've always found time to do other things. Throughout my life I played tennis three times a week. Maria persuaded me to return to golf, when I was around fifty. I always had time for leisure. I never felt like I was working hard. I've never been conscious of the sensation of fatigue particularly. It's a sensation I'm not familiar with, mentally or physically. Some people experience that very much and give an account of bodily sensations.

"One of the great tragedies of urban civilization that hamper the treatment of elderly people slipping into second childhood, is the inadequacy of institutions for medical care and for independent living; one treats old people as if they were insane. In rural and primitive cultures, such individuals are cared for by their relatives in the familiar environment of their homes."[1]

Ray Adams, age ninety-seven, lives in a stately home in Chestnut Hill, Massachusetts. He spends most of his day in his study, on the second floor adjacent to his bedroom. He is surrounded by walls of books. He sits at the desk where he did his important writing. There he reads mysteries and medical journals.

His four children, growing old, are scattered from Oregon to Virginia. The loving care of Nina Salam makes it possible for him to remain in his home, where she also resides. She or his sister-in-law, Iga, brings him lunch in his study, usually peanut butter on a hamburger bun or American cheese on white bread. Lumbar stenosis is a source of chronic pain. Trips for doctor's appointments are an ordeal. His hearing is failing. He is accepting of but frustrated by a slowly increasing difficulty remembering names. With the emergence of West

Nile virus in North America he is afraid to sit in the garden; he knows that the elderly are particularly vulnerable to this encephalitis.

Three decades earlier he had written:

"Atherosclerosis and neoplasm are now the chief factors in preventing our decline into second childhood and overstaying our biologically allotted span of life too long. As O.W. Holmes observed:

'Little of all we value here
Wakes on the morn of its hundredth year
Without both feeling and looking queer.
In fact there's nothing that keeps its youth,
So far as I know, except trees and truth.'"[1]

Note

1. Adams RD. Ageing, Involution and Senescence. *SA Med J* V43, pp 1239–1244, 1969.

5

MAJOR ORIGINAL CONTRIBUTIONS

Neoplastic Diseases

1) *Reticulum cell sarcoma of brain.* First series of cases reported. Adams pointed out that this tumor was mistakenly viewed as microglioma and that it did not arise from cells resident in the brain. Instead, he argued, it was a hematologic type malignancy. Dorothy Russell, the great English neuropathologist, did not agree with Adams. (See: Russell DS et al. Microgliomatosis: A Form of Reticulosis Affecting the Brain. *Brain* V71, part (1), pp 1–15, 1948.) Adams' analysis has prevailed. By the terminology of that day Adams called it reticulum cell sarcoma. Today this tumor is classified as a high-grade form of primary brain lymphoma, non-Hodgkin's in type.

Kinney TD, Adams RD. Reticulum Cell Sarcoma of the Brain. *Arch Neurol Psychiatry (Chicago)* V50, pp 552–564, 1943.
Schaumberg HH, Plank CR, Adams RD. The Reticulum Cell Sarcoma Group of Brain Tumors. *Brain* V95, pp 199–212, 1972.

2) *Lymphoma of brain.* Survey of cases, at the Mallory Institute of Pathology, comparing and contrasting the clinical and pathological effects of different types of central nervous system lymphoma, including the first reported cases of primary Hodgkin's disease of brain. There were nineteen clinicopathologic cases from the Mallory Institute of Pathology. Also included were two cases from other hospitals and seven cases biopsied at the spinal level. A classification of malignant lymphoma of the nervous system was offered.

Sparling HJ, Adams RD. Primary Hodgkin's Sarcoma of Brain. *Arch Pathol* V42, pp 338–344, 1946.

Sparling HJ, Adams RD, Parker F. Involvement of the Nervous System by Malignant Lymphoma. *Medicine* V26, pp 285–332, 1947.

3) *Pituitary apoplexy.* First thorough description of necrosis of and/or hemorrhage into a previously unknown pituitary tumor and its clinical manifestations. Four of these five autopsied cases were given to Adams by Timothy Leary, the coroner of Suffolk County. Adams wrote the article and asked colleagues from the neurosurgery service to contribute. [see Figure 64]

Brougham M, Heusner AP, Adams RD. Acute Degenerative Changes in Adenomas of the Pituitary Body—With Special Reference to Pituitary Apoplexy. *J Neurosurg* V7, pp 421–439, 1950.

See also multiple myeloma under Nerve Disease and polymyositis/dermatomyositis under Muscle Diseases.

Cerebrovascular Diseases

4) *Occlusion of the anterior inferior cerebellar artery.* First definition of the clinicopathologic syndrome when no other vessels are occluded. This was a single case report with a systematic discussion of the main cerebellar arteries and the lesions and syndromes which occur consequent to their occlusions.

Adams RD. Occlusion of the Anterior Inferior Cerebellar Artery. *Arch Neurol Psychiatry* V49, pp 765–770, 1943.

5) *Aortic dissection.* First clear presentation of the patterns of nervous involvement. Series of eleven autopsied cases, all with clear neurologic findings definitely related to the dissection. All were cases of ischemic injury including extension of dissection along a carotid artery (cerebral lesion), thoracic artery (myelopathy), and brachial artery (multiple mononeuropathies of the arm).

Weisman AD, Adams RD. The Neurological Complication of Dissecting Aortic Aneurysm. *Brain* V67, part 2, pp 6–92, 1944.

6) *Syndrome of basilar artery occlusion.* First detailed series delineating the clinical and pathologic features of embolic and thrombotic occlusion of the basilar artery, a previously neglected entity. Eighteen autopsied cases and four cases with survival were reported.

Kubik CS, Adams RD. Occlusion of the Basilar Artery. *Brain* V69, part 2, pp 73–121, 1946.

7) *TTP (Thrombotic thrombocytopenia purpura).* First complete study of the neurological manifestations and neuropathology of TTP (then known as Moschowitz syndrome of platelet thromboses). Four patients with autopsies were studied.

> Adams RD, Cammermeyer J, Fitzgerald P. The Neuropathological Aspects of Thrombocytic Acroangiothrombosis: A Clinico-anatomical Study of Generalized Platelet Thrombosis. *J Neurol Neurosurg Psychiatry* V11, p 27, 1948.

8) *Embolism as a common cause of stroke.* Clinicopathologic data established embolism or probable embolism as the most frequent type of stroke.

> Fisher CM, Adams RD. Observations on Brain Embolism with Special Reference to the Mechanism of Hemorrhagic Infarction. *J Neuropathol Exp Neurol* V10, p 92, 1951.
> Fisher CM, Adams RD. Observations on Brain Embolism with Special Reference to Hemorrhagic Infarction. In Furlan AH (ed), *The Heart and Stroke Exploring Mutual Cerebrovascular and Cardiovascular Issues.* Berlin, Springer-Verlag, pp 17–36, 1987.

9) *Distal migratory embolism as the pathogenesis of hemorrhagic infarction.* First clinicopathologic data to establish the concept that distal migration of a fragmenting embolus was an explanation, alternative to vascular spasm, for the failure of the pathologist to find occlusion of a vessel in many autopsied cases of cerebral infarction. Reperfusion of the proximal portion of the infarction, after distal migration of the embolus, explained the association of brain embolism with hemorrhagic transformation of the infarction.

> Fisher CM, Adams RD. Observations on Brain Embolism with Special Reference to the Mechanism of Hemorrhagic Infarction. *J Neuropathol Exp Neurol* V10, p 92, 1951.
> Fisher CM, Adams RD. Observations on Brain Embolism with Special Reference to Hemorrhagic Infarction. In Furlan AH (ed), *The Heart and Stroke: Exploring Mutual Cerebrovascular and Cardiovascular Issues.* Berlin, Springer-Verlag, pp 17–36, 1987.

10) *Complete classification of stroke for the second Princeton Conference on cerebrovascular disease.* Authorship attributed to an ad hoc committee established by the National Institutes of Neurological Diseases and Blindness. Miller Fisher states that the document was written almost in toto by Raymond Adams and himself. Basis of all modern classifications of stroke.

A Classification and Outline of Cerebrovascular Diseases. In Millikan CH (ed.), *Cerebral Vascular Diseases Grune and Stratton*. New York, 1958, pp 185–216.

11) *Meningeal cerebrovascular anastomoses.* Noticed by early anatomists, these connections had been neglected. This was a study of twenty-five normal brains and ten brains with infarctions due to major vessel occlusion, showing that there are end-to-end anastomoses of the three major cerebral arteries and also of the three major cerebellar arteries. Demonstration that the final form of an infarct depends on the residual circulation from such anastomoses, thereby explaining the variable and unpredictable effects of obstruction of a particular blood vessel. In a given individual the anastomoses may be large and numerous and in another small and poorly developed.

Vander Eecken HM, Adams RD. The Anatomy and Functional Significance of the Meningeal Arterial Anastomoses of the Human Brain. *J Neuropathol Exp Neurol* V12, pp 132–157, 1953.

12) *Operations on the neck.* Exposition of the neurological disorders consequent to surgery on the neck and thorax. This clinicopathologic study of ten autopsied patients included various ischemic strokes and anoxic encephalopathies. These disorders remain common complications of chest and neck surgery to this day.

Cammermeyer J, Adams RD. An Analysis of the Mechanism and a Study of the Morbid Anatomy of Neurological Disorders Incident to Operations on the Neck and Thorax. *Acta Psychiatr Neurol Scand* (Suppl 96) Munkgaard-Copenhagen, pp 1–61, 1954.

Demyelinative Diseases

13) *Multiple sclerosis.* Comprehensive review of the neuropathologic cases on file at Massachusetts General Hospital with analysis of the different features including demyelination, axon injury, cavitation, and the inflammation. This paper explained that the difficulty in defining demyelinative disease stems from the entire concept being an abstraction. In other words, the pathology is not simply demyelination; the axis cylinders and even interstitial tissue and blood vessels can be affected. There was also comment that there are other demyelinative diseases that are not included under the term multiple sclerosis. This paper showed that these diseases

are by and large perivenous in location. A classification of these diseases was presented.

Adams RD, Kubik CS. The Morbid Anatomy of the Demyelinative Diseases. *Am J Med* V12, pp 510–546, 1952.

14) *Experimental allergic encephalomyelitis.* Confirmation in a series of papers that injection of small quantities of proteolipid extracts of myelin with adjuvants could produce this disease just as injection of extracts of myelin, itself, had been previously shown to do. Demonstration that the microscopic findings evolve in a characteristic sequence from venous endothelial change to lymphocytic-monocytic infiltration and paravenous demyelination.

Demonstration of the basic similarity of the elementary lesions of acute multiple sclerosis, acute post-infectious encephalomyelitis, and the lesions of experimental allergic encephalomyelitis.

Waksman BH, Adams RD. A Histological Study of the Early Lesion in Experimental Allergic Encephalomyelitis in the Guinea Pig and Rabbit. *Am J Pathol* V41, pp 135–162, 1962.

Waksman BH, Adams RD. *Tubercle Bacillus* Lipopolysaccharide as Adjuvant in the Production of Experimental Allergic Encephalomyelitis in Rabbits. *J Infect Dis* V93, pp 21–27, 1953.

Waksman BH, Porter H, Lees MD, Adams RD, Folch J. A Study of the Chemical Nature of Components of Bovine White Matter Effective in Producing Allergic Encephalomyelitis in the Rabbit. *J Exp Med* V100, pp 451–471, 1954.

15) *Experimental hemorrhagic allergic encephalomyelitis (Hurst type).* Addition of meningococcal toxin to the experimental allergic encephalomyelitis model resulted in a Schwartzman reaction. In addition to the demyelinative lesions, there were deposits of fibrin and injured vessels and necrotizing and hemorrhagic changes, more than those seen in usual EAE and similar to those seen in the Hurst variant of hemorrhagic encephalomyelitis in humans. This experimental model strengthened the concept that the acute necrotizing hemorrhagic encephalopathy of Hurst was related to other "demyelinative" disorders.

Waksman BH, Adams RD. Studies of the Effect of the Generalized Schwartzman Reaction on the Lesions of Experimental Allergic Encephalomyelitis. *Am J Pathol* V33, pp 131–153, 1957.

16) *Progressive multifocal leukoencephalopathy*. From clinical analysis, Ray Adams recognized that the patient had a unique disease and not a direct effect on the central nervous system of his chronic lymphocyte leukemia. He was not an author of the pathologic article on this disorder, but his contribution was acknowledged by the authors both in the paper and especially in a later article of reminiscence.

See Aström KE. Under the Ether Dome. *Brain Pathol* V4, pp 189–195, 1994.

Muscle Diseases

17) *Pretibial compartment syndrome*. Description of central traumatic necrosis of the pretibial muscles due to repetitive overuse and its association with myoglobinuria in soldiers on forced marches.

Pearson C, Adams RD, Denny-Brown D. Traumatic Necrosis of Pretibial Muscles. *N. Engl J Med* V239, pp 213–217, 1948.

18) *Pathology of muscle disease*. First book on the subject in half a century. The first edition with Carl Pearson and Denny-Brown was published in 1953. The second edition was under the names of the same three authors.

Adams RD, Denny-Brown D, Pearson C. (eds). *Diseases of Muscle: A Study in Pathology* (2nd edition in 1962). Paul Hoeber, Inc., New York, 1953.
Adams RD. (ed.). *Diseases of Muscle: A Study in Pathology*, 3rd edition, Harper and Row, Hagestown, MD, p 569, 1975.

19) *Polymyositis and dematomyositis*. Monograph based on study of forty (thirty-five pathologically proven) cases on file at Massachusetts General Hospital with clarification of the classification of this condition, some with malignancy, some with connective tissue disease, and some with neither. This modification of the classification of Lee Eaton put more emphasis on the association of polymyositis with cancer. It was important that the book was published in Great Britain, where polymyositis was being overlooked or misdiagnosed. This book was comprehensive in its clinical detail, pathologic detail, illustrations, historical perspective, and discussion of nosology.

Walton JN, Adams RD. *Polymyositis*. E & S Livingstone Ltd., Edinburgh and London, 1958.

20) *Congenital muscular dystrophy*. First careful description of this entity with thorough pathologic study in two autopsied male siblings. First clear

exposition of the spectrum of pathologies underlying arthrogryposis multiplex.

Banker BQ, Victor M, Adams RD. Arthrogryposis Multiplex Due to Congenital Muscular Dystrophy. *Brain* V80, pp 319–334, 1957.

21) *Acute inclusion body myopathy*. First description of the clinical features and its distinctive pathologic features, the introcytoplasmic and intranuclear inclusions.

Adams RD, Kakulas BA, Samaha FA. A Myopathy with Cellular Inclusions. *Trans Am Neurol Assoc* V90, p 213, 1965.

22) *Myopathy in the quokka, an Australian marsupial experimental animal*. Recognition that the pathology was that of vitamin E deficiency. As a result of the appropriate modification of their diet, the laboratory animals were protected from this muscle disease. Kangaroos in zoos were likewise protected.

Kakulas B, Adams RD. Principles of Myopathology as Illustrated in the Nutritional Myopathy of the Rottnest Quokka. *Ann NY Acad Sci* V138, pp 90–101, 1966.

23) *Regenerative ability of muscle in muscular dystrophy patients*. Experimental trauma to muscle, by alcohol injection in seven human dystrophy patients, resulted in good regeneration. Even in the nondystrophic muscle. Important in disproving Denny-Brown's idea that inability to regenerate was the fundamental defect in the muscles of patients with muscular dystrophy.

Walton JN, Adams RD. The Response of the Normal, the Denervated and the Dystrophic Muscle-Cell to Injury. *J Pathol Bacteriol* V72, pp 273–298, 1956.

24) *Oculopharyngeal muscular dystrophy*. First demonstration that this known familial disease of late life was a genetic disease of muscle, dystrophic in type, disproving the then prevailing concept that this was a disease of brainstem nuclei. The disease was traced through three generations. Pathologic study was made of a biopsy of the temporalis muscle in one patient in the original article. A later article detailed an autopsied case. (One of Adam's predecessors, E.W. Taylor, thought that the dysphagia was due to degeneration of the vagus and glossopharyngeal nuclei. He had no pathology to support his speculation.)

Victor M, Hayes R, Adams RD. Oculopharyngeal Muscular Dystrophy. *N Engl J Med* V267, pp 1267–1272, 1962.

Rebeiz JB, Caulfied JB, Adams RD. Oculopharyngeal Dystrophy—A Presenescent Myopathy in Progress in NeuroOphthalmology. *Proc Int Congr Neurogenet Neuro-Ophthalmol* V8, pp 12–31, 1967.

Nerve Diseases

25) *Experimental allergic neuritis.* First demonstration that injection of peripheral myelin can induce peripheral neuritis, sparing the central nervous system.

Waksman BH, Adams RD. Allergic Neuritis: An Experimental Disease Induced by the Injection of Peripheral Nervous Tissue and Adjuvants. *J Exp Med* V102, p 213, 1955.
Waksman BH, Adams RD. A Comparative Study of Experimental Allergic Neuritis in the Rabbit, Guinea Pig and Mouse. *J Neueropathol Exp Neurol* V15, p 293, 1955.

26) *Human dipththeritic polyneuritis.* First comprehensive clinical and pathologic study of this disease. Clinical information was correlated with the necropsy findings in six cases, in which brain spinal cord, spinal root ganglia, plexi, peripheral nerves, and muscle were studied. The paper provided clear demonstration that the characteristic pathology was an intense noninflammatory demyelinative process of nerve fibers in the dorsal root ganglia; there was variable involvement of paraganglionic anterior and posterior nerve roots and spinal nerves.

Fisher CM, Adams RD. Diptheritic Polyneuritis. *J Neuropathol Exp Neurol* V15, p 243, 1956.

27) *Experimental diphtheritic polyneuropathy.* Duplication of the neurologic, temporal, and pathologic features of the human disease by subcutaneous injection of diphtheria toxin (with a slight amount of antitoxin). In rabbits the characteristic lesion was purely demyelinative, noninflammatory damage in the posterior spinal roots and ganglia.

Waksman BH, Adams RD. Mansmann: Experimental Study of Diptheritic Polyneurirtis in the Rabbit and Guinea Pig. *J Exp Med* V105, p 591, 1957.

28) *Experimental allergic autonomic polyneuropathy.* Original experimental model of this disease produced by injection of sympathetic ganglia and Freund's adjuvants. Inflammatory changes were found in sympathetic ganglia; antibodies to sympathetic ganglia were detected. Altered vasomotor reflexes were the clinical correlates.

Comment: A human disease of this type was not documented until a later date. See below.

Appenzeller O, Arnason BG, Adams RD. Experimental Autonomic Neuropathy: An Immunologically Induced Disorder of Reflex Vasomotor Function. *J Neurol Neurosurg Psychiatry* V28, p 510, 1965.

29) *Acute pure-autonomic polyneuritis.* First clinicopathologic demonstration of this human disease of sympathetic and parasympathetic ganglia. This was a detailed report with long-term follow-up of a case, which had been briefly reported by the authors six years earlier. There was a comprehensive review of relevant interim literature.

Young R, Asbury A, Corbett J, Adams RD. Pure Pan-dysautonomia with Recovery, Description and Discussion of Diagnostic Criteria. *Brain* V98, pp 613–636, 1975.

30) *Uremic polyneuropathy.* First clinicopathologic description. The four patients described had various causes of chronic uremia, only one due to hereditary renal disease. One patient had uncertain evidence for diabetes. All had burning feet and symmetrical distal motor-sensory polyneuropathy on examination. There was distal destruction of myelin and axons. Prior to this article there had been scant mention of polyneuropathy in uremia. There had been an article about hereditary nephritis with the incorrect implication that the neuropathy was also hereditary. Adams' article was the first report of cases in which the nervous system was studied fairly completely.

Asbury AK, Victor M, Adams RD. Uremic Polyneuropathy. *Arch Neurol* V8, pp 413–428, 1963.

31) *Polyneuropathy of multiple myeloma.* This paper was the first clear clinical and pathological description of the subacute to chronic, progressive sensorimotor, distal, noninflammatory polyneuropathy associated with multiple myeloma. Four of the five patients had autopsy or biopsy of nerve. The absence of compression, tumor invasion or amyloid involvement of the nerves was emphasized. The authors pointed out a "striking lack of parallelism between the symptoms of neuropathy and those of myeloma," that the neuropathy could dominate the clinical picture long before there was any other manifestation of myeloma. Furthermore they clearly documented that the neuropathy could improve with the treatment of myeloma.

Comment: Interestingly, Dr Waldenstrom called the authors to inform them that one of their carefully described patients actually had Waldenstrom's macroglobulinemia rather than multiple myeloma. This correction the authors came to accept. (Maurice Victor, personal communication).

Victor M, Banker BQ, Adams RD. The Neuropathy of Multiple Myeloma. *J Neurol Neurosurg Psychiatry* V21, p 73, 1958.

32) *Guillain–Barré syndrome.* Monographic article. First detailed study of neuropathology of demyelinative form. Prior study of Guillain–Barré syndrome from the Armed Forces Institute of Pathology material (Kernohan and Haymaker) had included only the nerve roots; peripheral nerve specimens were not available to those authors. It was by the systemic investigation of the entire peripheral nervous system in nineteen autopsied cases that Adams and colleagues delineated the inflammatory lesion. A neurologist had examined each patient. It was largely by analogy with the microscopic pathology of experimental allergic neuritis that they inferred an autoimmune mechanism.

Asbury AK, Arnason G, Adams RD. The Inflammatory Lesion in Idiopathic Polyneuritis. *Medicine* V48, pp 173–215, 1969.

33) *Pseudo-hypertrophy of cervical nerves due to mononeuritis multiplex of nerves and roots.* First description of the clinical and pathologic features. This localized, steroid responsive inflammatory condition caused masses in the neck. The enlargement of nerves was due to endoneurial collagen deposition and to onion bulb formation.

Comment: Dr Arthur Asbury, Adams' coauthor, states that one of these cases later evolved into a motor sensory familial neuropathy. He adds that Charcot Marie Tooth disease can sometimes present with patchy involvement including lumps in the brachial plexus. In other words, one of these cases, in retrospect, was an atypical presentation of a generalized Charcot Marie Tooth type neuropathy.

Adams RD, Asbury AK, Michelsen JJ. Multifocal Pseudohypertrophic Neuropathy. *Trans Am Neurol Assoc* V90, pp 30–33, 1965.

See also tremor in pure polyneuropathy under Movement Disorders, experimental B vitamin deficiency polyneuropathy under Nutritional Diseases, diabetic ophthalmoplegia under Neuro-opthalmic Disorders, and herpes zoster under Infectious Diseases.

Infectious Diseases

34) *Subdural empyema.* First clear detailed differentiation of the clinical and pathological features of this disease from brain abscess and from subdural hematoma. Emphasized the importance of early drainage.

Kubik C, Adams RD. Subdural Empyema. *Brain* V66, p 18, 1943.

35) *Ramsay Hunt syndrome*. First pathological study of the peripheral nervous system after herpes zoster with facial paralysis. There was seventh nerve inflammation with only slight change in the geniculate ganglion. Ramsay Hunt had inferred, from the clinical features, that geniculate ganglionitis was the correlate of the facial palsy, but he had no pathology.

> Comment: The coauthors, Ray Adams and Denny-Brown, disagreed about the interpretation of the autopsy result. Denny-Brown felt that the minimal ganglion involvement confirmed the Ramsay Hunt hypothesis. Ray Adams felt that the prominent seventh nerve inflammation offered an alternative explanation for the facial weakness. Adams' analysis prevailed in the paper, which emphasized the idea that a motor neuritis, independent of any ganglion involvement, could cause facial weakness.
>
> Denny-Brown D, Adams RD, Fitzgerald PJ. Pathologic Features of Herpes Zoster: A Note on "Geniculate Herpes". *Arch Neurol Psychiatry* V51, p 216, 1944.

36) *Bacterial meningitis*. Classic study of the neuropathology of acute and subacute bacterial meningitis, exemplified by *Hemophilus influenza* meningitis. There were analyses of its chronology, distribution, and effects on meninges, brain, and nerve.

> Adams RD, Kubik C, Bonner F. The Clinical and Pathological Aspects of Influenzal Meningitis. *Arch Pediatr* V65, pp 354–376, 408–441, 1948.

37) *Neurosyphilis*. Monographic book, which was a complete statement of modern concepts and exposition of the spectrum of the disease. Based on the clinical material from the neurosyphilis clinic of Boston City Hospital and the pathologic material at the Mallory Institute of Pathology.

> Merritt HH, Adams RD, Solomon H. *Neurosyphilis*, Oxford University Press, New York, 1946.

38) *Experimental measles encephalitis*. First demonstration that the pathology was not related to vessels, i.e. that its pathology was different from that of allergic encephalomyelitis.

> Waksman B, Bernstein T, Adams RD. Histologic Study of the Encephalomyelitis Produced in Hamsters by a Neurotropic Strain of Measles. *J Neuropathol Exp Neurol* V21, pp 25–49, 1962.

39) *Herpes simplex (inclusion body) encephalitis*. Demonstration, in a series of cases, of the special topography in the temporal lobes, cingulate gyri, and

orbital frontal regions. Original in providing pathological support for the association of temporal lobe involvement with the memory disorder in survivors.

Drachman DA, Adams RD. Herpes Simplex and Acute Inclusion Body Encephalitis. *Arch Neurol* V7, pp 61–79, 1962.

See also human diphtheretic neuropathy and experimental diphtheritic neuropathy under Nerve Diseases.

Hydrocephalus

40) *Familial aqueductal stenosis.* First pathologic description of this sex linked, often fatal, form of obstructive hydrocephalus in a family with multiple affected males in each of two successive generations. There was detailed clinicopathologic description of one case with a comprehensive review of relevant literature.

Bickers DS, Adams RD. Hereditary Stenosis of the Aqueduct of Sylvius as a Cause of Congenital Hydrocephalus. *Brain* V72, part 2, p 246, 1949.

41) *Hydrocephalus with focal signs.* When progressing, it can cause a focal lesion in the cerebrum to become clinically manifest. First complete description.

Adams RD. Diverticulation of the Cerebral Ventricles—A Cause of Progressive Focal Encephalopathy. *Dev Med Child Neurol* V17 (Suppl 35), pp 135–137, 1975.

42) *Normal pressure hydrocephalus.* First comprehensive description of a previously unemphasized syndrome. Mental impairment, gait unsteadiness, and urinary incontinence were the clinical manifestations. Demonstrated reversibility of the clinical syndrome by a shunt in properly selected patients.

Adams RD, Fisher CM, et al. Symptomatic Occult Hydrocephalus with "Normal" Cerebrospinal-fluid Pressure. A Treatable Syndrome. *N Engl J Med* V273, pp 117–126, 1965.

Liver Diseases

43) *Gray matter changes of hepatic coma.* Confirmation that there is hyperplasia of protoplasmic astrocytes (Alzheimer type II) without nerve cell changes

in severe liver failure. This liver–brain relationship was strengthened by grading of astrocytic change; brains of cirrhotic patients who had not experienced hepatic coma were compared to those of patients who had experienced hepatic coma.

Adams RD, Foley JM. *IV Congres Internationale. Vol. II: Communications.* Masson et Cie, Paris, 1949b, p 62.

Adams RD, Foley JM. The Neurological Disorder Associated with Liver Disease. *Res Proc Assoc Nerv Ment Dis* V32, pp 198–237, 1953.

44) *Asterixis.* Although there had been mention of abnormal movements in patients with hepatic coma, this unique movement disorder had never been characterized before the work of Ray Adams. The discovery of asterixis as a manifestation of hepatic encephalopathy, preceding hepatic coma, gave hepatologists a tool to study which factors precipitated precoma (See Davidson CS. Liver Diseases and Nutrition in the Harvard Medical Unit, at Boston City Hospital by Maxwell Finland. VI. Frances A. Countway Library of Medicine, Boston, 1982, p 536).

In their initial description of what they later called asterixis, Adams and Foley used the term "tremor" for this phenomenon. They soon recognized the distinctive lapses of sustained contraction of groups of muscles were arrhythmic, irregular, and worthy of a specific term. Foley, over a bottle of Metaxa at the Athens Olympia Cafe, consulted a classics scholar from Boston College. A word was needed to denote the lack of steadiness, the characteristic inability to maintain a fixed posture such as dorsiflexion of the wrists and fingers. Eventually selected was the term "asterixis" (a— privative, sterixis—maintenance of posture).

Adams RD, Foley JM. The Neurological Disorder Associated With Liver Disease. *Res Proc Assoc Nerv Ment Dis* V32, pp 198–237, 1953.

Adams RD, Foley JM. The Disorder of Movement in the More Common Varieties of Liver Disease. *Electroencephalogr Clin Neurophysiol J* (Suppl), V3, p 51, 1953.

45) *EEG in hepatic coma.* First description of the increasing amount and distribution of bilateral slow activity in the electroencephalogram with worsening hepatic encephalopathy. This paper also included the first description of "blunt spike and wave" activity in hepatic coma. The latter feature was later named "triphasic wave" by Bickerstaff. His term, triphasic wave, has become widely accepted to denote this characteristic, but not specific, feature of the EEG in hepatic coma.

Foley JM, Watson CW, Adams RD. Significance of the electroencephalo-
graphic changes in hepatic coma. *Trans Am Neurol Assoc* V75, pp 161–165,
1950.
Adams RD, Foley JM. The Neurological Disorder Associated With Liver
Disease. *Res Proc Assoc Nerv Ment Dis* V32, pp 198–237, 1953.

46) *Neuropathology of hepatic coma in hemochromatosis.* Of eighteen autopsied
patients, nine had died in liver coma. Two categories of change were noted:
direct deposition of characteristic pigments in certain specific structures;
indirect alterations in brain parenchyma including pronounced hyperplasia
of protoplasmic astocytes in those cases dying with liver failure.

McDougal DB, Adams RD. The Neuropathological Changes in Hemochromatosis. *J Neuropathol Exp Neurol* V9, pp 117–124, 1950.

47) *Human pure Eck fistulas.* First neurologic study showing that "liver coma"
could be replicated in the presence of a normal liver in humans. As a treatment for cancer of the head of the pancreas, the portal vein was removed
and a surgical anastomosis was made between the superior mesenteric
vein and the inferior vena cava. (Earlier cases of portal-caval shunts had
been performed in humans to treat esophageal varices. In these patients
there was portal hypertension with extensive collateral venous circulation, through which some blood may have reached the liver.) In Adams'
report there was no collateral circulation; the liver was totally excluded
from receiving blood from the intestine. Thereby the first human pure
Eck fistula was created. In this human, episodic stupor, indistinguishable
from hepatic encephalopathy, was induced by the oral administration of
excess protein, urea, ammonium chloride, or an ammonia and potassium
cation exchange resin. Concomitant with stupor there was elevation of
blood ammonia.

McDermott WF, Jr, Adams RD. Episodic Stupor Associated with An Eck
Fistula in the Human with Particular Reference to the Metabolism of
Ammonia. *J Clin Inv* V33, pp 1–9, 1954.
Adams RD. The Encephalopathy of Porta Caval Shunt (Eck Fistula). In Pop-
per H, Schaffiner F. (eds), *Progress in Liver Disease*. Grane Stratton, New
York, 1965, pp 442–455.

48) *Chronic hepatocerebral disease.* First detailed study of the clinicopathologic
features. The monographic article of fifty pages was based on observations
on twenty-seven cases, seventeen of which had been studied at autopsy.
Tremor, dementia, dysarthria, gait ataxia, and choreoathetosis were common features. In no case were there Kayser-Fleischer rings or familial

incidence of the disease. Brains showed a diffuse increase in size and number of protoplasmic astrocytes, diffuse but patchy pseudolaminar necrosis of the cerebral cortex, and polymicrocavitation in the striatum and at the corticomedullary junction. There was no abnormality of brain copper, serum ceruloplasmin, or other measurements indicative of Wilson disease.

Victor M, Adams RD, Cole M. The Acquired (non-Wilsonian) Type of Chronic Hepatocerebral Degeneration. *Medicine (Baltimore)* V44, pp 345–396, 1965.

49) *Wilson disease.* The paper with Porter showed that the non-Wilsonian cases of chronic hepatic encephalopathy exhibited no increase in copper in the brain or liver. Adams argued that this fact and the similarity of the neuropathology of the acquired hepatocerebral disease to that of Wilson disease excluded simple copper neurotoxicity as an adequate explanation for the brain lesions of Wilson disease.

Porter H, Adams RD. The Copper Content of Brain and Liver in Hepatic Encephalopathy. *J Neuropath Exp Neurol* V15, pp 61–64, 1956.
Victor M, Adams RD, Cole M. The Acquired (Non-Wilsonian) Type of Chronic Hepatocerebral Degeneration. *Medicine (Baltimore)* V44, pp 345–396, 1965.

Alcohol Withdrawal

50) *Delirium tremens.* First rigorous study of the relation of delirium tremens to abstinence in the chronic alcoholic. This detailed experimental human study of 101 patients resolved the controversy as to whether alcohol intoxication or alcohol withdrawal is the cause.

Victor M, Adams RD. The Effect of Alcohol on the Nervous System. *Res Publ Assoc Res Nerv Ment Dis* V46, p 431, 1968.

51) *Alcohol withdrawal syndromes.* Description of the timing of appearance of various manifestations of withdrawal and the relationships between them. Included were eighty-eight cases with seizures.

Victor M, Adams RD. The Effect of Alcohol on the Nervous System. *Res Publ Assoc Res Nerv Ment Dis* V46, p 431, 1968.

52) *Auditory hallucinosis.* Demonstration (in a study of seventy to eighty cases) that this condition is also due to abstinence and that some patients

can be left with chronic auditory hallucinosis, reminiscent of paranoid schizophrenia.

Victor M, Hope J. The Phenomenon of Auditory Hallucinations in Chronic Alcoholism. *J Nerv Ment Dis* V126, p 451, 1958.

Nutritional Diseases

53) *Pernicious anemia*. Demonstration that central nervous system involvement shows a distribution of lesions depending on the intensity and duration of the disease. Lesions appear sequentially in the posterior columns, lateral columns, then anterior columns, and finally in the cerebral white matter. In the spinal cord and in the brain the lesions were in multiple, contiguous foci. Two autopsied cases were described.

Adams RD, Kubik CS. Subacute Degeneration of the Brain in Pernicious Anemia. *N Engl J Med* V231, p 2, 1944.

54) *Experimental B vitamin deficiency polyneuropathy*. Controlled pathologic study, in thirty swine, of the peripheral nerve lesions of pyridoxine and pantothenic acid deficiency. A confirmation of the findings of Wintrobe in a different species. Although Wintrobe had reported that the pathology of the neuropathies of these two deficiency diseases differed, Adams and Swank showed that they were identical.

Swank RL, Adams RD. Pyridoxine and Pantothenic Acid Deficiency in Swine. *J Neuropathol Exp Neurol* V7, p 274, 1948.

55) *Wernicke disease*. Detailed study describing a neuropathologic series with clinicopathologic correlation and analysis. Original observations were made on 245 patients, 82 with autopsies.

Victor M, Adams RD, Collins GH. *The Wernicke–Korsakoff Syndrome and Other Disorders Due to Alcoholism and Malnutrition* (1st edition in 1971). Davis, Philadelphia, 1989.

56) *Midline cerebellar degeneration in the alcoholic*. The most comprehensive description of this disease in a monographic article, original in its clinico-pathologic analysis, in its localization of the lesion to the superior vermis and anterior lobe of cerebellum, and in propounding its nutritional basis. Half a century later the tenets of this classic article remain unchallenged. (See Laureno R. Nutritional Cerebellar Degeneration with Comments

on its Relationship to Wernicke Disease and Alcoholism. In Subramony and Durr (eds), *Handbook of Clinical Neurology, Ataxic Disorders*. Elsevier, Amsterdam, 2010).

Victor M, Adams RD, Mancall EL. A Restricted Form of Cerebellar Degeneration Occurring in Alcoholic Patients. *Arch Neurol* V1, p 577, 1959.

See also alcoholic dementia under Memory.

Other Metabolic Disorders

57) *Central pontine myelinolysis*. First description of this disease and its clinical manifestations. A clinicopathologic study of four cases. Large lesions caused tetraplegia, pseudobulbar palsy, and death. Small lesions were asymptomatic. The unique histology was analyzed. The symmetry and stereotyped location of the lesion was taken to imply a metabolic or chemical cause. Possible etiologies were discussed.

Adams RD, Victor M, Mancall EL. Central Pontine Myelinolysis. *Arch Neurol Psychiatry* V81, p 154, 1959.

58) *Lance–Adams syndrome*. Original study of four cases of action polymyoclonus/cerebellar ataxia as a sequela of anoxic brain injury.

Lance JW, Adams RD. The Syndrome of Intention or Action Myoclonus as a Sequel to Hypoxic Encephalopathy. *Brain* V87, p 111, 1963.

59) *Increased intracranial pressure with encephalopathy in respiratory failure with hypercapnia*. First complete report of the reversible neurologic disorder, headache, papilledema, impairment of consciousness, and asterixis.

Austen FK, Carmichael MW, Adams RD. Neurologic Manifestations of Chronic Pulmonary Insufficiency. *N Engl J Med* V257, pp 579–590, 1957. *See uremic neuropathy under Nerve Disease.*

Memory Disorders

60) *Korsakoff psychosis*. Detailed studies of the amnesic state and its thalamic origin (medial dorsal nucleus) in Wernicke disease. This study included detailed observation on eighty-two autopsies.

Victor M, Adams RD, Collins GH. *The Wernické Korsakoff Syndrome: A Clinical and Pathologic Study of 245 Patients, 82 with Postmortem Examination*. Davis, Philadelphia, 1971.

61) *Alcoholic dementia*. Demonstration that most patients so labeled had Korsakoff psychosis as a chronic manifestation of Wernicke disease.

Victor M, Adams RD, Collins GH. *The Wernické Korsakoff Syndrome: A Clinical and Pathologic Study of 245 Patients, 82 with Postmortem Examination.* Davis, Philadelphia, 1971.
Victor M, Adams RD. The Alcoholic Dementias. In Vinkn PJ, Bryn GW, et al. (eds), *Neurobehavioral Disorders, Handbook of Clinical Neurology,* V2 (46). Elsevier, Amsterdam, pp 335–352.

62) *Episodic global amnesia.* A monographic article, comprehensively delineating the clinical syndrome and establishing it as a clinical entity.

Fisher CM, Adams RD. Transient Global Amnesia. *Acta Neurol Scand* V40 (Suppl 19), p 1, 1964.

See also herpes simplex encephalitis under Infectious Diseases.

Movement Disorders

63) *Striatonigral degeneration.* First description of the disease with clinical detail and autopsy study of three patients. The spinal cords were not available for study. In today's terminology this disease is classified by many as a form of "multiple system atrophy."

Adams RD, Van Bogaert L, Van Der Eecken H. Degenerescences nigro-striees et cerebello-nigro-striees. *Psychiatr Neurol Basel* V142, pp 219–259, 1961.
Adams RD, Van Bogaert L, Vander Eecken H. Striatonigral Degeneration. *J Neuropathol Exp Neurol* V23, pp 584–608, 1964.

64) *Tremor in pure polyneuropathy.* First description of the occurrence of fast-frequency postural tremor in polyneuropathy.

Shahani BT, Young RR, Adams RD. Neuropathic Tremor: Evidence on the Site of the Lesion. *Electroencephalogr Clin Neurophysiol* V34, p 800, 1973.

65) *Post-hemiplegic athetosis.* Complete study of its pathology in serial section of whole brain. Four autopsied patients for whom there was long-term clinical information. Extensive damage to the putamen was present in all cases.

Dooling EC, Adams RD. The Pathological Anatomy of Post Hemiplegic Athetosis. *Brain,* V98, pp 29–48, 1975.

66) *Corticobasalganglionic degeneration.* First recognition, from the apraxia and extrapyramidal rigidity of limbs, that this was a clinically unique syndrome. Adams followed the patients long term with Miller-Fisher, but Adams did not participate as an author of the pathology paper on his patients.

> Rebeiz JJ, Kolodny EH, Richardson EP. Corticodentatonigral Degeneration with Neuronal Achromasia. *Arch Neurol* V18, p 20, 1968.

> *See also asterixis under Liver Disease and Lance–Adams syndrome under Other Metabolic Disorders.*

Neuro-ophthalmic Disorders

67) *Apraxia of gaze in bifrontal lesions.* First adequate clinicopathologic report of patients, who could not move their eyes on command as a result of acquired lesions.

> Cogan DG, Adams RD. A Type of Paralysis of Conjugate Gaze (Ocular Motor Apraxia). *Arch Ophthalmol* V50, pp 434–442, 1953.

68) *Diabetic ophthalmoplegia.* First description of the neuropathology with serial sections of entire third nerve and midbrain. Unfortunately, portions of the other third nerve were lost and control tissue was thus lacking. Over a decade later one of Adams' ex-residents studied another case and demonstrated more clearly a demyelinative lesion in the intracavernous portion of the third cranial nerve. (See Asbury et al. Oculomotor Palsy in Diabetes Mellitus: A Clinicopathologic Study. *Brain* V93, pp 505–556, 1970.)

> Dreyfus PM, Hakim S, Adams RD. Diabetic Opthalmoplegia. *Arch Neurol Psychiatry* V77, pp 332–349, 1957.

Miscellaneous Contributions

69) *Bedside observation.* Essay on bedside observation of clinical phenomena as sources of new leads to scientific study of the human nervous system.

> Adams RD. Important Contributions to an Understanding of the Mind and Nervous Function, Which Have Emanated from the Clinic. In Beecher HK (ed.), *Disease and the Advancement of Basic Science.* Harvard University Press, Cambridge, 1960, pp 265–314.

70) *Horizons*. Essay on the horizons of clinical neurology stressing the importance of including developmental and congenital attributes of the nervous system when analyzing the pathogenesis of diseases.

Salam MZ, Adams RD. New Horizons in the Neurology of Childhood. *Perspect Biol Med* V9, pp 384–419, 1966.

71) *Brain death syndrome*. Original definition of neurologic criteria for the diagnosis of brain death (Harvard criteria). Raymond Adams wrote the neurological portions of the report. According to Wjdicks this report "defined totally destroyed unsalvageable brain for the first time." (See *Neurology* V61, pp 1920–1976, 2003.)

Report of the Ad Hoc Committee of the Harvard Medical School to Examine the Definition of Brain Death. A Definition of Irreversible Coma. *J Am Med Assoc* V205, pp 337–340, 1968.

72) *Maturation and seizures*. Discussion of the effect of the level of maturation of the nervous system on the pattern of seizure disorder.

Adams RD, Salam MZ. Lepilepsie processes pathophysiologique in relation avec l'age. *Schweiz Med Schr* V97 (Nr 51), pp 1707–1716, 1967.

73) *Neurology and the skin*. Classification and description of neurocutaneous diseases in many editions of the Fitzpatrick textbook of dermatology. A grand synthesis of information about diseases that "implicate the skin and nervous system either simultaneously or successively."

Adams RD. Neurocutaneous Disease. In Fitzpatrick TB, Eisen AZ, Wolf K, et al. (eds), *Dermatology in General Medicine* (3rd edition). McGraw Hill, New York, pp 2022–2062, 1987.

6

MAJOR BOOKS OF RAYMOND D. ADAMS

1. Merritt HH, Adams RD, Solomon HC. *Neurosyphilis*. Oxford University Press, New York, 1946, 443 p.
2. Adams RD, et al. *Diseases of Muscle: A Study in Pathology*. Hoeber, New York, 1953, 556 p.
   (*Note*: The fourth edition of this book was published in 1985 under the authorship of Adams RD and Kakulas B.)
3. Walton JN, Adams RD. *Polymyositis*. Livingston, Edinburgh, 1958, p 269.
4. Adams RD, Sidman RL. *Introduction to Neuropathology*. Blakiston Div., McGraw-Hill, New York, 1968, 629 p.
5. Victor M, Adams RD, Collins GH. *The Wernicke–Korsakoff Syndrome: A Clinical and Pathological Study of 245 patients, 82 with Post-Mortem Examinations*. F.A. Davis, Philadelphia, 1971, 206 p.
   (*Note*: In 1989 the same authors published a second edition under the title "The Wernicke–Korsakoff syndrome and related neurologic disorders due to alcoholism and malnutrition.")
6. Adams RD, Victor M. *Principles of Neurology*. McGraw-Hill, New York, 1977, 1041 p.
   (*Note*: This book is in recent editions entitled Adams and Victor's *Principles of Neurology*. Edition 8 was by Ropper A and Brown R; Edition 9 by Ropper A and Samuels M is expected in 2009).
7. Haymaker W, Adams RD. *Histology and Histopathology of the Nervous System*. Thomas, Springfield, IL, 1982, 2597 p.
8. Adams RD, Lyon G. *Neurology of Hereditary Metabolic Disease of Children*. Hemisphere Pub. Corp, Washington, DC; McGraw-Hill, New York, 1982, 442 p.

(*Note*: Under the authorship of Lyon G, Kolodony EH, and Pastores GM, the third edition was published in 2006.)

9. Harrison TR, Adams RD, et al. *Principles of Internal Medicine*. McGraw Hill, New York. Adams was an editor for nine editions beginning with the second edition in 1954 and concluding with the tenth edition in 1983. The core group of editors, with whom he had continuity in the early editions, were WR Resnick, MM Wintrobe, GW Thorn, IL Bennett, and TR Harrison. This book has been translated into sixteen foreign languages.

(Note: To this day, a neurologist, SL Hauser, formerly Adams' resident, is an editor of this textbook.)

7

ACCOMPLISHMENT AND LEGACY OF RAYMOND ADAMS

Rᴀʏᴍᴏɴᴅ Aᴅᴀᴍs ʙᴜɪʟᴛ ɪɴsᴛɪᴛᴜᴛɪᴏɴs, discovered new diseases and phenomena, and made classic descriptions of previously known diseases. His systematic studies contributed to our knowledge of most of the categories of neurologic disease. He transformed internal medicine by his writings about alcoholism, the commonly seen metabolic encephalopathies and the nutritional and infectious disease of the nervous system. As much as any other individual, he expanded the frontiers of neurology to include muscle disease, stroke, pediatric neurology, and mental retardation. He educated innumerable leaders in neurology. Through his neurology sections of *Principles of Internal Medicine* and *Principles of Neurology*, he educated doctors of internal medicine and neurology around the world. Through his psychiatry sections in *Principles of Internal Medicine*, he defended the medical approach to psychiatry during decades, when the psychoanalytic approach was dominant at American medical colleges.

The very vocabulary of modern neurology shows the impact of Raymond Adams. Nonexistent before his contributions were the terms, asterixis, transient global amnesia, striatonigral degeneration, corticobasal degeneration, normal pressure hydrocephalus, oculopharyngeal dystrophy, inclusion body myositis, central pontine myelinolysis, and pituitary apoplexy. Although he and those whom he educated have provided us much of our basic terminology, he is remembered by only one eponym, Lance–Adams syndrome.

Muscle Diseases

Raymond Adams introduced the field of muscle pathology. According to Andrew Engel, the first edition of Adams' 1953 book on pathology of muscle was a "classic work . . . a great contribution." He considers it "the first contemporary book on muscle pathology," a book which was a "great influence on Greenfield, Shy, Walton, Kakulas, Mastaglia and myself." In fact Adams' text was the first book on pathology of muscle since that of Lorenz half a century earlier.

Often overlooked is Walton and Adams' book on polymyositis, a detailed clinicopathologic study with abundant illustrations and a beautiful synthesis on this disease. It is also neglected that Adams was the first to describe inclusion body myopathy. Engel considers Adams' paper on oculopharyngeal dystrophy a "classic" article. With Betty Banker, he wrote a standard description of congenital muscular dystrophy. Adams not only advanced the field of dystrophies and inflammatory myopathies but also added to knowledge of myopathy due to vitamin E deficiency.

The most important books on muscle disease, to appear in the half century since Adams' first edition, were those of his fellows: John Walton[1] and Betty Banker.[2]

Cerebrovascular Diseases

C. Miller Fisher reports that he and Raymond Adams authored virtually the entire classification of cerebrovascular disease distributed nationally and internationally by the National Institute of Neurological Diseases and Blindness. This classification and outline became the "lingua franca of the international stroke community."[3] The concepts underlying this document were publicized to the general medical community by the Fisher–Adams' chapter on stroke in the leading medical text, *Principles of Internal Medicine*.

In the early 1950s, 70% of strokes were attributed to vasospasm; there was a major German textbook on this subject. Adams made the vasospasm hypothesis unnecessary. Infarctions, for which the pathologist found no corresponding vessel occlusion, could be explained in another way, fragmentation of an embolus and distal migration of the fragments, sometime after embolic occlusion of a vessel. Adams, having abandoned vasospasm as an important cause of stroke, propounded the idea that cerebral embolism is a common cause of stroke. Furthermore, it was he and Fisher who associated hemorrhagic infarction with cerebral embolism and proffered the idea that distal migratory embolism is the basis of hemorrhagic transformation. Adams also explained why occlusion of a given artery gave rise to infarctions of variable size and symptoms in different patients: there were variations in cortical arterial anastomoses from one person to another.

With Kubik, Adams wrote "one of the most important and influential reports in the field of cerebrovascular disease,"[4] a paper on basilar artery occlusion. This article included discussion of the pathologic distinction between embolism and thrombosis in situ.

Peripheral Neuropathies

According to Arthur Asbury, Ray Adams brought the method of clinicopathologic correlation to the study of peripheral neuropathy. He carefully studied the spinal cord, posterior roots, anterior roots, spinal ganglia, spinal nerves, and peripheral nerves. Adams determined the location of the lesions and the type of microscopic change, and he correlated the clinical features with the pathology. In this way he was able to recognize the distinctive patterns of peripheral pathology underlying diseases such as shingles, diptheritic polyneuropathy, and tabes dorsalis. More than his predecessors he included examination of both proximal and distal nervous elements as well as the autonomic nervous system in his study. He brought this same thoroughness to the study of cranial nerves. Waksman and Adams' study of experimental allergic neuritis was listed as one of the major accomplishments in the study of peripheral nerve in the years after World War II. This work was important enough to be listed with the discovery of the mechanism of action potential transmission, the discovery of the axonal flow, and the advent of nerve conduction studies in clinical medicine.[5] Adams and colleagues' study of the clinical and autopsy features of Guillain–Barré syndrome established the inflammatory nature of the lesion, and, by analogy with experimental allergic neuritis, its immunologic nature.

Demyelinative Diseases and Neuroimmunology

Adams and colleagues contributed to landmark studies on allergic diseases of humans and experimental animals.

In humans he clarified the spectrum and classification of demyelinative diseases. According to Byron Waksman, Adams' paper with Kubik on the neuropathology of multiple sclerosis was responsible for a paradigm shift from theories of vascular or infectious cause to one of immune mechanism.[6] It illustrated the perivenular nature of the disease and the involvement of gray matter more clearly than the classic study of Dawson at the beginning of the century.

Waksman and Adams showed that in experimental allergic encephalomyelitis the histopathology was different from that of the viral encephalitides. They also demonstrated that a fraction of the myelin antigen could successfully elicit the experimental disease.

The experimental studies on demyelinative disease were so important that they opened an entirely new view of immunologic disease. They showed that during the first few hours, in the presymptomatic phase of disease, there was the appearance of lymphocytes and monocytes. Only later did demyelination and macrophages appear. Waksman: "We initiated a whole field in the area of inflammatory autoimmunity by realizing that this was mediated by live mononuclear cells, not by antibody. Most neuropathologists knew nothing about immunological cells. They thought only in terms of antibody and complement at the time." Without Adams, Waksman went on to show that there was a very large class of similar experimental inflammatory, autoimmune diseases affecting a large variety of organs and that these diseases were all, fundamentally, the same as contact allergy, tuberculin sensitivity, and allograft rejection.

Metabolic Diseases

All modern concepts of the hepatic encephalopathy originate with Raymond Adams. The histopathology, the characteristic clinical syndrome, and the EEG findings were described by him and his colleagues. He added considerably to the idea that blood ammonia was related to the encephalopathy. The recognition that asterixis was the harbinger of coma gave liver researchers a tool to study the cause of hepatic coma.

Furthermore, he and colleagues fully characterized the chronic neurological disease, which follows repeated bouts of acute encephalopathy. His analogy of the neuropathology of Wilson disease to this chronic hepatocerebral disease has never been adequately noticed and pursued.

Adams clarified the neurology of alcoholism. For once and for all he and colleagues settled an old issue by showing that delirium tremens was a withdrawal phenomenon and not a problem of intoxication. They fully described the spectrum of withdrawal syndromes. They showed that polyneuropathy was nutritional in origin, they wrote the classic work that fully characterized Wernicke disease, and they defined the nature of cerebellar degeneration in the alcoholic.

Ray Adams' contributions to metabolic brain disorders were not limited to his studies of alcoholism, liver disease, and malnutrition. Adams and colleagues discovered and described central pontine myelinolysis. Furthermore, he made important contributions to the neurology of anoxia, uremia, and hypercapnia.

Dementia and Memory Disorders

Adams and colleagues were the first to emphasize the reversibility of the clinical syndrome of normal pressure hydrocephalus. His demonstrating a reversible dementia reoriented neurologists and internists toward the demented patient. Much more attention was paid to searching for treatable causes of dementia in the wake of this article.

Adams and colleagues fully described transient global amnesia, offered evidence that bilateral temporal damage was the basis of amnesia in herpes simplex encephalitis, and showed that the amnesia of Korsakoff was due to bilateral medial thalamic lesions of Wernicke disease.

Anatomy

The demonstration that Korsakoff psychosis was due to bilateral medial thalamic, not mamillary body lesions, was an important contribution to understanding normal brain anatomy and physiology. From Adams analysis we learned that the medial thalamus plays an important role in memory. Similarly Adams' clinicopathologic analysis in midline cerebellar degeneration has provided the best evidence that the anterior superior vermis plays an important role in the gait of humans.

Clinical Teaching

It is instructive to compare Adams to other great clinical teachers, whose careers overlapped his. Adams' systematic method of diagnosis was teachable in a way that the approach of Sir Charles Symonds or Houston Merritt was not.

RICHARD JOHNSON:

"One of the most interesting comments I ever heard was from Henry Miller from New Castle. Henry Miller was one of the showiest neurologists I've ever known. He could entertain crowds, tailor his comments, a real performer, in the nicest sense—he was a great performer. He said to me that there were only two people in all of neurology who he really felt intimidated by, by their breadth and depth of knowledge, two neurologists that he respected that way. One was Sir Charles Symonds and the other was Ray Adams. And he never worked with Ray. I think that's probably true. They were the two most impressive clinical neurologists I've ever seen.

Sir Charles Symonds, people said, read very little. He kept enormously detailed notes on every patient he saw, and he saw enormous numbers of patients. His wife was a librarian, who cross-indexed. The story goes that he used to study his own records every night, his own records. It was a librarian type of approach to neurology, unlike the analytical approach that Ray used."

In the decades that spanned mid-century, Houston Merritt was another great American clinical neurologist.

HERBERT SCHAUMBURG:

"Houston Merritt was a very different man than Ray. Actually it's quite a contrast because I knew Merritt and presented patients to him on several occasions. Houston Merritt was somebody, who did not discuss a patient. You gave him this very complicated patient, and he would say that it's probably herpes simplex—next case. So when he came as a visit, you are prepared to show him five or six difficult cases, which, with his computer-like mind, he would analyze and give the answer, and that was it. Houston was very intuitive. He could not expound in any depth on the pathophysiology of most conditions. Ray, you would show him one case, and he would discuss every aspect of it. That was the difference. He had this deep understanding of the pathogenesis." Elliott Mancall was in a good position to know both men because he was first a resident with Merritt at Columbia and then a fellow with Adams in Boston. Mancall agrees with Schaumburg's description of these two leading neurologists.

Herbert Schaumburg: "Nobody was in Ray's league as far as integrating all these different aspects of a disease. Nobody could do what Ray did. I presented cases to Sir Charles Symonds, McDonald Critchley of Queen Square, and John Walton, who were all very good, but Ray could discuss a twitch for an hour and leave you taking pages of notes. He would go into every aspect of it."

Principles of Neurology

As always, Adams had a sense for what person was suited for what enterprise in neurology. When it came time for him to write his magnum opus, *Principles of Neurology*, he recruited Maurice Victor to be his co-author. He recognized Victor's literary bent, his "nice way with the English language." They made beautiful music together, but it is clear that the score was fundamentally that of Adams. Herbert Schaumburg compares Adams' book to Merritt's *Textbook of Neurology*: "Houston wrote a wonderful book" but "Victor and Adams' book— you read it and it's like listening to him talk." It is unique as a textbook in that "you can read it from beginning to end," according to Richard Johnson. "It is not written like an encyclopedia."

Other great English language syntheses of neurology are those of Wilson and Gowers. Like Wilson, Adams made a nice historical summary of a topic early in a chapter. This author views Adams' grasp of the history more complete and his writing of it more elegant. Like Gowers, Adams' book frequently refers on his own experience, published and unpublished. Adams had not only deep clinical experience but also the vast experience as a neuropathologist who had studied thousands of brains. Hence he was able to classify neurologic diseases and understand them anew. *Principles of Neurology* is one of the best neurology books ever written in English or perhaps any language. Having been translated into at least six languages over its first forty years, this one volume text is a guide for students and doctors all over the world.

Builder of Institutions

C. Miller Fisher:

"Before Raymond Adams came to Massachusetts General Hospital, residents were leaving before finishing. His first group of four residents all became national figures." When Adams arrived, there was one full-time neurologist. Ten years later there were 150 full-time members of the department. At about this time C. Miller Fisher was at a meeting in Europe, when a prominent figure commented to him that there were three principal neurological institutions in the world. In the same breath he mentioned Massachusetts General Hospital with the venerable and long-established neurology programs at La Salpêtrière and the National Hospital at Queen Square. It was an extraordinary achievement to have transformed a small neurology service into one so highly regarded in such a short time. This large research department had eight floors of laboratories by the time of Adams' retirement as chairman in 1977. Under his successors there has been continued development of the department, which remains one of the world's great programs in neurology.

Expansion of Neurology

When Ray Adams entered neurology:

1. Neurologists knew little about children, and pediatricians knew little about neurology.
2. Orthopedists and internists took care of patients with muscle disease.
3. Neurology departments did not want to admit stroke patients and foisted many of them onto the medicine service.
4. Mental retardation was a neglected area of study.

Ray Adams contributed greatly to changing this state of affairs. He developed the first division for cerebrovascular disease in a neurology department. He revived interest in muscle disease and stimulated the next generation of neurologists to pursue this field of study. In his department he developed the first sizable division of child neurology with both clinical affairs and extensive research laboratories. Furthermore he developed the Shriver Institute, where scores of scientists applied themselves to research on various problems related to mental retardation.

In a sense an empire builder, Ray Adams expanded the role of neurology at his hospital and thereby set an example for neurologists elsewhere to do the same. He also tried to expand neurology's role in the medical school. In fact, he envisioned a major department of neuropathology at the medical school campus. Foiled in this plan, he, nevertheless, developed an outpost—an experimental neuropathology laboratory in the Warren Museum on the medical school campus. Today, at Harvard Medical School, there is no anatomy department, but there is a department of neurosciences. In a sense, what Adams proposed, decades ahead of the trends, eventually came to be. On the other hand, some of what he built has faded. Adams, late in life, is disappointed that the Shriver Center is no longer affiliated with Harvard and is no longer a thriving facility for scientific and medical research on mental retardation.

Psychiatry

Raymond Adams was, perhaps, the most prominent figure in American medicine to fight against the psychoanalytic approach to psychiatry, which was pervasive in the United States. He brought into his neurology department a psychiatrist, one of his own teachers, Mandel Cohen. Cohen advocated rigorous, scientific research in psychiatry and boldly confronted psychoanalysts. Ray Adams' department tirelessly argued that psychiatry should find its way back to brain function.

The importance of Adams' strong stance must be understood in the context of the era. At Harvard Medical School, psychoanalysis had been accepted in the mid-1950s, not only by the psychiatrists but also by leading internists and surgeons such as Oliver Cope. Robert DeLong, who attended in the 1960s, remembers that over 25% of his Harvard class became psychiatrists. Adams was one of few in the United States trying to inform medical students that psychoanalysis was not the only kind of psychiatry. Through his chapters on psychiatry in *Principles of Internal Medicine*, Adams influenced doctors all over the world. He had no effect at all on the national psychiatry organizations. Dismissed by many as a Freud basher, Adams was not daunted.

No career better exemplifies Adams' enduring concern about psychiatry and his positive impact on it than that of Paul McHugh. George Thorn, the great endocrinologist, was disappointed to hear that McHugh wanted to enter into psychiatry. He urged the student to study neurology first. McHugh's application to Denny-Brown was promptly rejected. Denny-Brown informed him that he did not want residents who were interested in psychiatry. However, Raymond Adams received McHugh's application differently. "This is just what we want," he told McHugh. "The brain is central to anybody interested in psychiatry." After a few weeks of neurology residency, McHugh recalls, "The scales fell from my eyes." He realized that an inductive approach was needed in psychiatry. As a Harvard medical student, he had been taught a deductive approach to psychiatric diagnosis based on the idea that "mental disorders were invariably the consequence mishandled early life conflicts of a sexual nature."[7]

McHugh sought guidance from Adams about where to study psychiatry after his neurologic education; he followed Adams' advice and went to the Maudsley Institute in London. McHugh states that Adams "rescued me from Harvard psychiatry...he helped me in career management, always wonderfully kind to me in the process." This combined education in psychiatry and neurology put McHugh on a path to becoming the chairman of psychiatry at Johns Hopkins, where for three decades he educated residents and students in medical psychiatry. His residents have gone elsewhere and done likewise. McHugh: "If it hadn't been for Ray Adams, I would have been a psychoanalyst in Marblehead."

Pediatric Neurology

Perhaps because of his prominence as a neuropathologist and neurologist, Adams' enormous contribution to child neurology is sometimes overlooked. As early as anyone he saw the need for educating pediatric neurologists, and he arranged for those interested to spend one year of the three-year residency in child neurology. This opportunity drew Guy McKhann, for example, to the MGH program.

Adams fostered not only the educational program of Phil Dodge but also the development of the very productive Kennedy Laboratories at Massachusetts General Hospital. This lab, directed at problems of children, was the world's premiere research group for examining newborn screening results and for developing new tests for the screening of newborns for metabolic diseases. This lab identified the enzyme defects in metabolic diseases such as hydroxyprolinemia. His researchers identified variants of phenylketonuria. Mary Efron and Hugo Moser developed a method for chromatographic analysis of blood or urine dried on filter paper. This method was widely adopted for a time. Vivian Shih and Harry Levy carried on at the Kennedy Laboratories, after the death of Efron and the departure of Moser for the Shriver Center at Fernald School.

Moser: "It was Ray Adams' weekly rounds at Fernald State School that established the field of mental retardation as a meaningful activity for neurologists." Adams made clear to me his pride that Moser and others published the *Atlas of Mental Retardation*. It was Moser, however, who revealed to the author the extent to which Adams facilitated the whole project by his taking up different topics at the weekly rounds at Fernald, by providing staff support and so on. Moser: "Whatever neurology did in the field of mental retardation...is all due to Ray Adams." One senses Adams' deep knowledge of the subject in his book, *Neurology of Hereditary Metabolic Diseases of Children*.

Adams' advancement of child neurology was not limited to the chronic diseases. With Phil Dodge he wrote an important article on acute

encephalopathies in children. It is not included on the list of his major contributions because, in retrospect, it is clear that the cases in this paper did not
constitute a homogenous entity. Several, however, had acute brain swelling
attributable to aggressive fluid administration on the pediatrics floor. The
impact of the study was great at Massachusetts General Hospital, where Dodge
proselytized the pediatricians and to a large extent eliminated such cases. This
realization, that one could prevent iatrogenic brain swelling in the young,
affected pediatric practice nationally.

The literature on adrenoleukodystrophy, once encompassed by the rubric
of Schilder's disease, shows the mark of Raymond Adams. Two men whom
Adams educated are responsible for much of the progress in this field. There is
the series of papers, by Schaumburg and colleagues at Albert Einstein medical
school, and there is the later work of Moser at Johns Hopkins medical school.

What does not appear in the literature is explained by Schaumburg himself:
"Actually, the best memory I have of him is one that was a real career maker for
me in a crazy way. We had a neurology clinic on Friday mornings, and if you
picked up an interesting piece of phenomenology, we would try to bring the
patient into the amphitheater (there were no video tapes in the 1970s). Ray had
a phenomenology round. We'd show the patient-unequal pupils, nystagmus,
a movement disorder, numb feet . . . and Ray would just discuss it with all the
residents, grouped around him. I had this patient who had a severe case of
spasmodic torticollis. She told me that she had a tough life, that she had a child
who just died of Schilder's disease, and she thought her older child had it as well.
So I was curious if the torticollis could be psychogenic in this poor woman.
So I brought her in and I presented her to Ray. Ray talked to her and the
patient left. Ray asked me if I thought it was psychogenic, and I said 'I just don't
know, I don't understand this.' He said, 'it's not'; he was convinced that this
was a fragmentary dystonia. A more interesting aspect to this case, he thought,
was that she allegedly has two children with Schilder's disease. 'I have never
been comfortable with the concept of Schilder's disease. The neuropathology is
always strange.' He knew there had been some hereditary cases, which made no
sense for an inflammatory demyelinating disorder. He suggested that I should
look into the family.

Well, his suggestion was my command. The next weekend I went down to
Foxborough, the state hospital, with her permission, and hauled out the records
on this child. And then I got the names of some male cousins who had also died.
I called the families, and, for a number of weekends, my wife and I drove all over
Massachusetts, looking at family bibles, and uncovered this huge kinship.

It turned out that one of them had died years before at Massachusetts
General. Luckily they had saved all the organs. They hauled out the brain,
the adrenals, and the liver. I looked at the pathology with Dr. Castleman; he
commented that there is something funny about adrenals with this case, but
the kid had no adrenal failure. He said, 'Go over to Richard Cohen who is in

charge of pathology at Beth Israel. He is an adrenal pathologist.' So I took the slides over to Richard Cohen, and I just showed them to him blindly, and he said, 'Is this a kid with Schilder's?' I said, 'Yeah.' He said that adrenal autoyzes very quickly; the only way to find out is to get a biopsy, and you can't justify that. Well we wrote a paper on x-linked Schilder's and talked about the adrenal a little bit.

About two years later I went back to Albert Einstein, and one of my colleagues there was an adrenal pathologist, who was fascinated with these slides and urged me to get a biopsy on one of these kids. We biopsied the adrenal of one of these children we thought had Schilder's with normal adrenal function, and the biopsy turned up these inclusions, which were then characterized as C26. That's the whole story. But it was Ray who had the idea. That's the sort of thing he did. His breadth of interest and knowledge was just astonishing."

Perhaps Adams' greatest contribution to pediatric neurology was the number of early leaders in the field, whom he and Phil Dodge educated: Huttenlocher, DeLong, Rosman, Volpe, McKhann, DeVivo, Kolodny and others.

Greatness

In adult neurology the list of leaders educated by Adams is vast. Joseph Foley cannot think of another person who has made such important contributions and brought along other people to make similar contributions. Adams "trained some of the greatest leaders of modern American neurology." Suffice it to say that simultaneously at Johns Hopkins the neurology chairman, another neurologist in an endowed chair, the psychiatry chairman, and the director of neuropathology were all Adams' trainees. In New York, Adams' trainees chaired the neurology departments at Albert Einstein NYU and Cornell medical schools, all at the same time. His residents and fellows held professorships in Europe, Australia, Canada, South America, and elsewhere. There is a neuropathology laboratory named for him in Brussels and a library named for him and Maria in Beirut.

Some great medical men or women do not make headlines by winning famous prizes. They are great by virtue of a large body of very important works, which make a permanent impact on the profession. This is not the greatness of a single twist but a greatness of decades of systematic work of observation, discovery, classification, and exposition. Raymond Adams is such a figure. His expansion and transformation of neurology are unprecedented.

Notes

1. Walton J. *Disorders of Voluntary Muscle* (3rd edition). Churchill Livingstone, London, 1974.
2. Engel A, Banker B. *Myology Basic and Clinical*. McGraw Hill, New York, 1986.

3. Goldstein M. Remembrance of Things Past: A Summary of the Development of Cerebrovascular Terminology in Modern Times. *Journal of Stroke and Cerebrovascular Diseases* V17, pp 47–48, 2008.

4. Caplan LR, Manning WJ. *Brain Embolism.* Informa, New York, 2006, p 9.

5. Dyck PJ. PK Thomas MD (1926–2008). *Neurology* V70, p 2196, 2008.

6. Murray T. *Multiple Sclerosis: The History of a Disease.* Demos, New York, 2005, p 268.

7. McHugh P. *The Mind Has Mountains.* The Johns Hopkins University Press, Baltimore 2006, p 120.

8

EPILOGUE

Raymond Adams' health progressively declined during the months after his ninety-seventh birthday. Worsened anemia required transfusion. Eventually, he spent most of his days bedridden. Finally, a hospital bed was needed. He spent his last night in his home. On October 18, 2008 he was in duress. The ambulance attendants would not take him to the distant Massachusetts General Hospital. He died with congestive heart failure not long after arriving at Brigham and Women's Hospital. He was buried next to the grave of his wife, Maria.

9

APPENDICES

Appendix A: Interview with Maurice Victor, Boston, Massachusetts, 2000

RL: *You first encountered Raymond Adams in Denny-Brown's department at Boston City Hospital.*

MV: Ray Adams was a tremendously stabilizing force. He would not permit Denny any flights of imagination. He would always bring him back to earth, based on what he had seen in the pathology laboratory. So he created a fine sense of balance in the department. Ray Adams' official duty at the Boston City Hospital was to run the neuropathology laboratory in the Mallory Institute of Pathology. In addition, be visited a few months out of the year and, most importantly, he was available to the resident for opinions about an individual patient or about the career of an individual resident, something for which Denny had very little patience. In my own case, after several years at the neurology service and faced with a need to move on in my career, Denny-Brown did not even ask me on a single occasion what my plans were, what I intended to do. He had nothing against me; it was just his way. He didn't consider that part of his job.

Ray Adams was quite the opposite. With Ray Adams, one could sit down for 10 minutes and he could straighten out your life and set appropriate goals much better than you could yourself. I know that, as far as I personally am concerned, he was the one that put me on the track. He was the only one who took any interest in my future and how it should be shaped and what I should do about my advancement as a neurologist. And this was just one of his extraordinary qualities.

Now Ray Adams is still with us. Ray Adams, in February of 2001, will celebrate his ninetieth birthday. I had a chance to speak with him yesterday. And there, sitting in his chair, because he has a lot of difficulty with his walking, he looked at least twenty years younger than ninety, and his ability to express himself, which always was superb, seemed totally unaffected or undamaged. It could take a long time, really, to enumerate the tremendous influences that he exerted on American neurology.

I would say that, firstly, he created at the Mass. General Hospital the proto-type of what should be a neurology teaching service in a major medical school. He created a huge department from a neurology department that was really run by one person. For the first time, Ray Adams created divisions within the neu-rology department, pediatric neurology, vascular disease neurology, immunology within neurology, and developmental neurology. And all of these were firsts. When it came time to build up vascular neurology . . . Ray Adams immediately went to Miller Fisher and got him to come down to the Mass. General. (Miller had been a fellow with Ray Adams from July 1949 to July 1950, and that is when Miller developed his interest in vascular disease of the nervous system.) And he got Phil Dodge to develop a division of pediatric neurology. (There were very, very few pediatric neurologists in the United States then; they were functioning, of course, as individuals. There was Buchanan in Chicago, and there was Ford at Hopkins. And Sidney Carter was seeing pediatric patients at Columbia but that was about it.) There were no real formal divisions of pediatric neurology within a department of neurology. Byron Waksman, a very good immunologist, was invited to the depart-ment to develop neuro-immunology. At the medical school, Ray developed the section on developmental anatomy of the nervous system. For this purpose, he brought in Paul Yakovlev, who made sections of the entire brain, traced pathways and their development from birth until old age. Ray started a unit at the Shriver Institute, in which he developed a large cadre of people to study the chemistry as well as the clinical aspects of developmental disease and inherited metabolic dis-ease, including Ed Kolodny and Hugo Moser, both of whom are now occupying positions of great prominence in that field. So it was his remarkable capacity to embrace many disciplines under the umbrella of neurology; to get the very best people out of his own program and others to come and develop those aspects of neurology and to sort of capture them for neurology.

It was his characteristic, literally in regard to every neurologic problem that came by, not only to teach residents who were on the service at that time how to go at a case and work it out, but always it would end with a question of what do we know about this condition, how can we find out more about it?

Now he has trained generations of neurologists. I know no one who comes close to him in the number of neurologists that have been trained by that department. Several years ago, there was an alumni meeting of all these people, and hundreds and hundreds of them turned up. It really was a sight to see.

Now Ray Adams had a number of other attributes that absolutely set him apart from the rest of the crowd. He was a great bedside teacher not only because he was knowledgeable but also because he understood neuropathology. This was a man that personally had supervised between 800 and 1,000 post-mortems per year for ten years at the Boston City Hospital, and he had digested all of that material and had written it up. So that his neurological teaching was grounded in a profound understanding of neuropathology. And he passed that along to a few people, to Betty Banker, and to EP Richardson, who then followed in his footsteps.

RL: *Where did he acquire this approach of combining neuropathology and clinical neurology?*

MV: Now this is an interesting question. He invented it! His brain cuttings were the first of their kind, in which a resident would present a very, very detailed clinical history of a patient who had come to autopsy, and then Ray Adams presented the autopsy findings, which were discussed by the staff. The method of clinical pathologic correlation as we know was invented by him.

RL: *Did the famous German neuropathologists do nothing like this?*

MV: Not that I am aware of. They did fine neuropathology in its own right, and, of course, some of them even were psychiatrists and neurologists. It was strictly solo work; it wasn't part of the academic program. Ray's clinical-pathologic conferences were legendary, attended by huge numbers of people, very disciplined. Always the discussion would begin with asking the resident what he thought of the case and then the chief resident and then the junior staff person and then (during my residency years), Denny-Brown. And then he would cut the brain in front of everybody and show them how short they had fallen of the tree. In my estimation, it was the single finest form of clinical teaching that I have ever experienced. It just increases your understanding of neurological disease no end, and it gives you a respect for how the nervous system reacts to disease so that you don't make all kind of foolish conjectures, that can't exist neuropathologically. I think that is one of his very great contributions.

On the ward he was absolutely superb, and in this way he differed from or I think superseded many of the best neurologists in the country. Not only could he make a correct diagnosis, prognosis, and so forth but he could teach the residents how to do it. And once again, I think he developed a systematic, logical approach to a clinical problem that was quite unique. In this way he differs from most of his contemporaries. If you listened and kept your eyes open, you could learn how to do it. His method was eminently teachable. I think that's a very, very important contribution that he made, because we had all kinds of fine diagnosticians who could come to the right conclusions and give the patients the right management and treatment. But it didn't help the residents much if their mentor could not transmit to them how to come to that conclusion in a very methodical way. So I think, as a teacher of clinical neurology, he occupies a position of his own, and I think that, as a neuropathologist, he, for many years, stood alone in terms of clinical–pathological correlations and the teaching of that subject.

In addition to all these things, I think it's worthwhile reviewing what the man has written to see how many concepts, that we now accept as in our field, really sprung from his observations. For example, he made excellent observations on the neurology, of platybasia and basilar invagmation of the brain. He made early observations of subdural abscess. His early observations on the natural history of bacterial meningeal infections are still a standard in the field. If you want to know what a meningeal exudate looks like five days after the onset of the infection, you have to turn to that article that he wrote with Kubik and Bonner. On neurosyphilis, he wrote a book with Houston, Merrit, in 1944, I believe, in which for really the first time, they documented how all of the neurologic and neuropathologic complications of neurosyphilis came from chronic syphilitic meningitis. Take the entire concept of acute hemorrhagic necrotizing encephalitis. Although he didn't describe the first cases, the first comprehensive description of that disease he did author.

And he got just countless people working on certain aspects of disease (and he participated in all these things). For example, he got Bill Mc Dermont working on the pathophysiology of ammonium intoxication of hepatic encephalopathy. He first adequately described the neuropathology of hepatic encephalopathy. He got me working on all the neurologic aspects of alcoholism. And, when he did something like this, he made certain by his own attendance and his own interest that you were working along proper lines.

Here was a man who's dreadfully busy. He ran the neuropath lab at the Boston City, which paid very little. He had to make a living with four children to bring up. He did that by going over to what was called the Pratt, now called the New England Center Hospital, where he worked three afternoons a week, seeing patients, doing lumbar punctures and air studies, simply because he had to make a living. At 6 o'clock in the afternoon, after a heavy day at the New England center, he would come back to the City Hospital, where he would make rounds with me on the complications of alcoholism that I had seen in the last few days. He taught me how to think about these things and how to begin to classify them. He would do that for example with Byron Waksman. And he would see pediatric neurology cases with Phil Dodge. He got Miller Fisher started on vascular disease, which then Miller developed to a tremendous degree. He had this remarkable ability to conceptualize the problems that we were seeing at the bedside and how to go about working them out, until we reached a stage where we could carry on by ourselves.

RL: *Did he sleep? . . . You make it sound like he worked all day long!*

MV: He didn't . . . he had a tremendous energy and a tremendous capacity for sustained effort, high-class mental activity.

RL: *Was he not distractible?*

MV: He went right to the point. He didn't make small talk. He was all business when it comes to professional undertakings, looking at slides and things like that. And you're quite right; he had tremendous ability to work late hours, day after day after day. He had a remarkable ability to get people to work along those lines. He trusted people too. If he saw they had any ability he'd get them going and then let them continue on their own. I can't think of any other person, in the time that I have been associated with neurology, that's over fifty years now, that has had that combination of capacities, of a tremendous intellectual endowment, a tremendous energy, the ability to stay focused on a subject, and the ability to perceive the needs of particular aspects of neurology, and to get people to work on them.

He had a great ability to write. He could write under all circumstances, and it would come out almost ready for publication. This was a man who would drive back home to Milton in an old beat up Plymouth that used to stall intermittently. When he had to wait until it was possible to get it going again or even to stop at a red light, he would have a pad next to him, and he would get down a sentence or two at that time. When he saw patients, between the time he took the history and the time that he examined the patient, he'd get a few lines written while the patient was getting into a dressing gown. He never wasted a minute. In an airport, he would sit there and write. On an airplane, he would sit there and write. And it wasn't just scribbling. He had trained himself in such a way to think logically, sequentially, and then to get the thing down on paper. He had a knack for doing that. Again, that I have never seen duplicated by anybody.

And if you just pick up his articles, the introductions are absolutely dazzling. He had the ability to conceptualize the subject for the reader. Take an individual chapter of our book for example. There's chapter on degenerative disease; you get an introduction on what is a degenerative disease, what is the source of the word, how it is used in neurology, what is the excuse for having the category of degenerative disease, what are the general characteristics of degenerative disease, what are the shortcomings of those generalizations and so on . . . and then, on to the individual degenerative diseases. He had the ability to do this.

I looked to the other day, for instance, at the chapter in our text on the complications of alcohol and nutritional disease on the nervous system. He and I first presented that subject at the ARNMD in the 1951 meeting, but the book was not published until 1953. He wrote the introduction for purposes of publication, and to this day, we've kept that introduction as the introduction to our chapter on alcoholism. And it's still the best conceptualization of the subject that I've ever read from anybody, from all the great experts on alcoholism.

He had that ability (and I don't think that's noticed by many people), this remarkable ability to conceptualize a subject. I think he does that better than anybody I've ever known. He used to like to do that very much because that was the real test of his understanding of the subject that we were dealing with, without getting into the details. And I think he found a certain excitement in that.

For instance, central pontine myelinolysis which you are very interested in. The original cases had come to his laboratory. I had done most of the work, getting them organized, making sure slides were made, going back to the families for the histories, and all those sorts of thing. But when it came to writing up the subject, Elliot Mancall and I, who were working on it, decided that it was only proper that Ray be the first author on the paper. We knew that it had never been described before and we felt that he had recognized it at post and knew what he was dealing with; he deserved primacy in description. Of course, he looked at all the slides and made sure the pathological reports were correct and all that but he took it on himself, as his contribution, to write the introduction to the article on central pontine disease. He did that with all the things we did together. And I remember he called me late at night. He had been working on the introduction to the article, and he read it to me on the telephone. I was thrilled. I thought it was sheer poetry when I read it. He had the ability to put things together and use the English neurological language, I think, with the greater facility and experience.

Then, of course, I have to personalize things, in relation to Ray Adams because I think, next to my father, he's the most wonderful man I have ever met in my life. He had the ability to be responsive to individuals, to have a feel for their problems, these various people who had been trying to make it in the profession. He always could get them in the track, to give them the ideas, as to how to develop their work and their work habits.

If he saw me wandering around at the Boston City Hospital on Christmas day, he'd put me in the car and take me home to dinner. At the Boston State Hospital, we had to round out our work on the Korsakoff amnesic state, which meant that we had to examine all the patients there with Korsakoff psychosis. He would come one afternoon and work with me until we got it going. Finally he'd take me home and feed me, so to speak. He had an innate understanding of how to deal with people. And none of this is sentimental in any way. (In fact he's the opposite of sentimental; he used to hold people at the arm's length.) He was never maudlin about any subject, he just did it in a very natural way. And he wasn't a man to pay compliments unnecessarily; he never buttered anybody up. You could always get a very straightforward answer from him about any subject, a critical judgment on any person or idea.

RL: *As I recall, you took him to see the first patient you found to have central pontine myelinolysis.*

MV: Yes. The first case, that we reported, I saw, when I was a resident in consultation on the alcoholic ward, so-called. There was a man with delirium tremens...who had recovered from delirium tremens, only to find that he was anarthric. He couldn't chew, couldn't swallow, and couldn't move his limbs. I remember Ray Adams seeing him; I can reconstruct the scene. He placed the lesion in the central part of the basis pontis. He didn't know what to call it, but that's where he placed the lesion. The patient did us the courtesy of dying, and it was a rather large lesion that occupied most of the basis pontis. In all his neuropathology Ray Adams was fully cognizant about what the patient showed clinically. That was the great strength of his writings on a neuropathologic subject.

I think that, when the history of neurology is written in this country, he will occupy a position in neurology, comparable to what Osler occupied in general medicine a half century earlier. He is, in a sense, the Osler of neurology.

RL: *You say this, despite his many distinguished predecessors?*

MV: No, I wouldn't say despite them. I would say he, certainly in terms of accomplishment, is in the same class as Gowers, Kinnier Wilson, and Gordon Holmes. I would single those people out as the giants at Queen Square. I think he occupies the same position in the hierarchy of teachers as Charcot. I would say that, in second half of the twentieth century, he was the leading neurological figure, just as Harvey Cushing was in neurosurgery and just as Holmes and Kinnier Wilson were in England during the first half of the century. I think he stands in that particular firmament.

Appendix B: Department of Psychology, University of Oregon

Small but strong, the psychology department at the University of Oregon had well-developed experimental laboratories. The department offered an eclectic approach to psychology with considerable emphasis on instruments, measurement, and numerical analysis.[1] Its chairman, Harold R. Crosland, gave a course on general psychology, which was greatly admired by the undergraduates. On the Oregon faculty were two other professors who would later chair departments. Edmund S. Conklin became chairman of the psychology department at the University of Indiana, and he held offices in national scientific and psychological organizations. He authored books about abnormal psychology, psychology and religion, and genetics in psychology. Robert H. Seashore was a junior faculty member who had come from the illustrious psychology training programs at Iowa and Stanford. He advocated careful laboratory research on the biological basis of human behavior. His publications appeared in journals such as *Science* and *Annual Reviews in Physiology*. Seashore went on to chair the department at Northwestern University.

This constellation of professors provided the rich environment, in which Ray Adams, previously unfocused, blossomed into a superior student. In this department Raymond Adams first became interested in the nervous system, where he learned general psychology from Crosland, abnormal psychology from Conklin, and research methods from Seashore. Adams' master's thesis project with Seashore resulted in a publication in *Science* within months of his receiving the degree.[2] In addition to his publication on the thesis work, he and a technician in the lab wrote an article on motor skills and typewriting proficiency.[3] Furthermore, Adams wrote a book review in the *American Journal of Psychology*.[4]

Psychology was an enduring interest. Decades after Adams left Oregon, he became president of the American Neurological Association. One of his responsibilities was to select the guest speaker for the annual meeting. He chose Harry Harlow, the famous experimental psychologist.

Notes

1. Crosland HR. Certain Points Concerning the Reliabilities of Experiments in Psychology. *Am J Psychol* V40, pp 331–337, 1928.
2. Seashore R, Adams R. The Measurement of Steadiness: A New Apparatus and Results in Marksmanship. *Science* V29, pp 285–287, 1933.
3. Walker RY, Adams RD. Motor Skills: The Validity of Serial Typewriting Proficiency. *J Gen Psychol* V11, pp 173–186, 1934.
4. Adams RD. The Free Association Method and the Measurement of Adult Intelligence. *Am J Psychol* V46, p 174, 1934.

Appendix C: Correspondence of Frederic W. Hanes, MD, Chairman, Department of Medicine, Duke University, related to Raymond Adams*

March 12, 1937

Dr. J. B. Ayer
319 Longwood Avenue,
Boston, Massachusetts.

Dear Dr. Ayer:-

On my staff at present is one of the soundest men I have ever had. He has just about everything that one hopes for from a house officer, above all, he has a brain. His name is Dr. Raymond Adams. He would like to work with you in neuro-psychiatry, and I am writing you much in advance of the usual time for such letters since he would like to know whether you think it would be possible to consider him. He will be available for work in December 1938. It is possible that this time could be shifted a little to fit any requirements which you may make.

I realize that it may be impossible for you to give me a definite answer, however, I promised Adams I would write at once so as to get his name on record. Any thing you can tell me in regard to what he should do further will be greatly appreciated.

Sincerely yours,

Frederic M. Hanes
Professor of Medicine

May 21, 1937

Dr. J. B. Ayers,
Massachusetts General Hospital,
Boston, Massachusetts.

Dear Dr. Ayers:-

This note is being written at the request of Dr. Raymond Adams, whom I wrote you about some time ago. You will recall that Adams was very keen to work with you beginning some time after July 1938. He came to me today to know whether he should make application to some other clinic besides

---

*Reference is made to Dr Lyman, the newly appointed chair of the Department of Psychiatry at Duke.

yours in case you did not decide to take him. I told him that it might be impossible for you, at this time, to say anything definite, but that I would drop you a line in regard to the appointment. Adams is such a splendid fellow that I really feel safe in advising you to take him if you feel that you can do so. If you find that you can give a definite answer it would relieve his mind and prevent him from making applications elsewhere. I dislike troubling you about this matter further, but I know you will appreciate the circumstances.

With kind regards,

Sincerely yours,

Frederic M. Hanes

January 13, 1938

Dr. J. B. Ayer,
Massachusetts General Hospital
Boston, Massachusetts.

Dear Dr. Ayer:

You were good enough to take Dr. Raymond D. Adams, who is at present on my staff here at Duke, as a house officer for a year. Recently, Dr. Robert Lambert, of the Rockefeller Foundation, has suggested that Adams take a fellowship, since he is preparing himself as a teacher of psychiatry. I told Dr. Lambert of your kindness in taking Adams and that I wanted to write to ask if it would incommode you in any way if Adams should come to work with you under a Rockefeller fellowship instead of accepting a house officer appointment.

We are helping Adams with his education with the prospect of his returning here as a teacher of psychiatry, and Dr. Lambert thinks that he might under a fellowship be able to work with both you and Dr. Stanley Cobb. Adams is very keen to do some neuro-pathology while in Boston. I think it probable that he will be on this fellowship for three years, or as much of three years as is required. Will you be kind enough to write me at your convenience telling me whether Adams has your permission to accept this fellowship? I do hope that this will not put you to any trouble, for I more than appreciate your kindness in taking Adams on my recommendation.

With best wishes,

Sincerely yours,

Frederic M. Hanes

November 15, 1938

Dear Adams:

Not having heard from you, I do not know whether you are still alive or dead. In any case, the enclosed notice is to cover your life insurance, and I don't know whether you are able to take care of this from your own funds or not. Please write me in regard to this and if you wish to take care of it in whole or in part.

With kindest regards,

Sincerely yours,

Frederic M. Hanes
Dr. Raymond D. Adams
Massachusetts General Hospital,
Boston, Massachusetts

February 16, 1940

Dear Dr. Hanes,

I don't know if you received the letter that I wrote about a month ago. The matter which needs to be settled soon is my plan for next years work. Dr. Lambert suggested that you and Dr. Lyman should decide on where I should spend next year.

So far this year has been very profitable to me in that I have been able to continue my work in clinical neurology and neuropathology as well as to see a great deal of the type of psychiatry that comes to a large general hospital. In addition to that I am working on several different research problems in neuropathology, pharmacology, and neurophysiology. Before I leave here I hope to spend about two months with Fuller Allbright in endocrinology and one month with Paul White in cardiology. My interests remain about the same, that in internal medicine and the psychiatry and neurology that is related to medical problems in general. So far I have had an excellent chance to see a great variety of neurological diseases and psychoneuroses.

Next fall I should like to go to a regular psychiatric Institution and get some experience with the major psychoses. I should prefer to have a house appointment if possible because the clinical opportunities are so much greater. The best places seem to be Yale, U. of Penn. c̄ Strecker or Phipps at Baltimore. I have no preference, really, and will do whatever you think best about next year.

Since hearing of Dr. Lyman's appointment I have been very anxious to meet him. Dr. Cobb & Lambert think so highly of him that he must be an excellent choice. Also I am anxious to know what place I shall have in the scheme of things. Recently I have had several offers for positions in neurology but of course have no idea of considering such in view of my obligation to you.

Mrs. Adams and I are now enjoying Boston much more than we did at first. It is really a grand place to study and I am sure Spike Harvey is wise in coming here.

Sincerely yours,

Ray Adams

March 29, 1940

Dear Adams:

Dr. Lambert gets pretty irritated with you because you do not write him from time to time telling him of your plans. When I saw him in New York last week he asked me if you had seen Dr. Lyman at Johns Hopkins and I could not tell him. It is very essential that you do see Dr. Lyman and talk over your next year's work. Dr. Lambert says that he will pay your expenses down to Baltimore and I hope you will make arrangement at once to get down to see Dr. Lyman. Please write Lambert from time to time.

All goes well here and we hope you have had a better winter than we have.

Sincerely yours,

Frederic M. Hanes

February 11, 1941

Dr. Robert A. Lambert,
The Rockefeller Foundation,
49 West 49th Street,
New York City.

Dear Count:

The enclosed letter will explain itself. Lyman has not got a place in his budget for Adams at present, but did intend to make a place for him beginning in September. Lyman says that it will be all right with him if he can have the option on Adams' services for September 1942. I have asked Lyman to drop you a word in regard to all of this, since your advice in the matter has always been helpful. I think myself that Adams would do well to stay on with Merritt for another eighteen months.

Sincerely yours,

Frederic M. Hanes

February 11, 1941

Dear Dr. Hanes,

By now you have probably received a letter from Houston Merritt telling of the temporary vacancy in neurology at Harvard & Boston City Hospital. I am writing to acquaint you with some of the details of this matter.

During past two years in Boston I proved to be a better than average neurologist but a rather poor psychiatrist, whether from lack of interest or aptitude I don't know. The men with whom I have worked urge me to continue to work in neurology rather than psychiatry. When this vacancy at Harvard occurred Stanley Cobb recommended two people for the job—Charles Aring of Cincinnati and myself. Since Aring could not leave he recommended that I take the position. His argument was that in another 18 mo.—which is the duration of the appointment—I could become a first class neurologist, begin several research problems which could be continued in subsequent years, and be more valuable to Duke as a result of this.

You are probably thinking what an ungrateful whelp I am and that I merely want an excuse to break my agreement with you. That is not entirely so. I shall be delighted to return to Duke but dread the thought of doing formal psychiatry, psychotherapy etc. at which I am no good. My real interest is internal medicine, neurology and in the type of psychiatry that is encountered on medical wards. With all the people who are working there in neurology I wonder if there will be a place for me. If there is a chance for me in neurology at Duke I should like to have the privilege of working at Harvard for another 1½–2 yrs. If there is no place and you insist that I just do psychiatry of course I shall do it as by agreement.

So far I haven't written to Dr. Lambert about this but shall do so as soon as I hear from you. Please let me know if there is any chance for me to continue to work in neurology and whether I may take this appointment at Harvard before returning to Duke. The salary they offerred was $3500 or more depending on my needs—which I might say are growing since we are soon to have the 3rd child.

I trust you are well and happy.

Sincerely yours,

Ray Adams

February 17, 1941

Dr. Raymond Adams,
Boston City Hospital,
Boston, Massachusetts.

Dear Ray:

I think that all concerned are willing for you to stay on at Harvard. Just what the future will bring forth I can't say, but we can leave that alone for the present.

Sincerely yours,

Frederic M. Hanes

Appendix D: Rockefeller Foundation Correspondence Related to Raymond Adams

THE ROCKEFELLER FOUNDATION

February 10, 1938

Dear Dr. Ayer:

Regarding Dr. R.D. Adams of Duke—I thought best to defer writing you until you and Dr. Hanes had exchanged views on the practicability of the suggested fellowship.

I have read carefully your letter of February 4th to Dr. Hanes and I see no real difficulty in our granting Adams a modified training fellowship such as we occasionally give younger candidates. (Our regular grants, as you know, are intended primarily for research and therefore go to individuals who have had basic training in their special fields.) Under the arrangement to which I refer Dr. Adams could accept the residency with the duties you describe. While the stipend could be substantially lower than that given our more advanced research fellows, who of course receive nothing from the institutions where they work, the allowance would help take care of the family. We would anticipate a second year's grant for clinical psychiatry probably on the regular basis. This might be either for work with Dr. Cobb at the Massachusetts General and at McLean, or in some other center, as circumstances indicated.

I think you understand that our interest in Adams derives largely from his assured future at Duke. I have no doubt that he is an exceptional young man—otherwise he would not have been selected for the place there. Though action on his appointment to a fellowship may have to wait a few weeks, as I would like to talk with him first, the question of his reporting to you for duty on July 1st(?) may be considered settled. There is just one bit of information I should like to have in advance of our action—it is the amount of remuneration, if any, Adams would receive from the hospital in addition to meals and optional use of room.

Sincerely,

ROBERT A. LAMBERT

Dr. James B. Ayer
Massachusetts General Hospital
Boston, Massachusetts.

RAL: GC

THE ROCKEFELLER FOUNDATION

The Medical Sciences
Alan Gregg, M.D., Director
Robert A. Lambert, M.D., Associate Director

December 16, 1938

Dear Doctor Adams:

After talking with Doctor Hanes a few days ago, I presented to our officers a recommendation for a renewal of your fellowship and I wish to report that the grant was made. The appointment is for twelve months beginning August 1, 1939, with stipend at the rate of $200 a month. The rate would be modified in case you were given a residency in a hospital such as you hold now. I doubt if such an arrangement would be indicated.

The place of study may be left for decision until you have looked into several possibilities. We discussed last year the advisability of your continuing at the Massachusetts General in the service of Doctor Cobb. But as Doctor Cobb's department will be crowded until the new building is completed I suggest visits to the psychiatry departments of Yale, the Institute of the Pennsylvania Hospital (Philadelphia), the Phipps Clinic at Johns Hopkins, and the Payne Whitney Clinic at Cornell (New York). For such a trip the Foundation would make a travel allowance if you will let me know in advance when you might get leave to go.

It is my feeling that you should study preferably in some institution where there is a close relation between the psychiatry department and other clinical departments, such as obtains at the Massachusetts General and at the New Haven Hospital.

You understand, of course, that no definite arrangements for next year's study should be made until we have cleared the matter again with Doctor Hanes.

Yours sincerely,

Robert A. Lambert

Doctor Raymond D. Adams
Massachusetts General Hospital
Boston, Massachusetts.

RAL: K

THE ROCKEFELLER FOUNDATION

The Medical Sciences
Alan Gregg, M.D., Director
Robert A. Lambert, M.D., Associate Director

March 3, 1939

Dear Doctor Adams:

I was disappointed not to see you when you were here. We are so accustomed to have our fellows call whenever they are in the city that it never occurred to me that you would pass through New York twice without dropping in, particularly since the question of your plans for next year were under discussion. On receipt of a note from Doctor Diethelm on the 23rd that you had visited the Payne Whitney Clinic two days before I tried in vain to locate you. From the New York Psychiatric Institute I learned that you called there on the 22nd but that in the absence of Doctor Nolan Lewis you went away without meeting any one else. May I suggest in this connection that you should never hesitate, in the absence of the chief, to ask some one else to show you over an institution. There is a lot of good work going on at the Institute which I am sure you would have been interested to see, though I do not think at this stage of your training it is the place you would choose to spend a year.

Since you were in Durham last Friday and presumably back in Boston on Monday, I am wondering if you stopped in Philadelphia and Baltimore. Certainly you did not have time to see much of the activities in either place. You will doubtless have another opportunity to visit the clinics there, as well as those in New York which you did not see, but the purpose of this trip was to look into the various possibilities that you might decide where you could most profitably spend the second year of your fellowship. It is obvious that you really did not do this thoroughly.

There are certain advantages, of course, in your remaining at the Massachusetts General, as you wish to do. You have come to know and to be known by the people there and you have established a home in Boston. Furthermore, I am sure you can get with Doctor Cobb and his associates an excellent training in neuropathology, along with an introduction to psychiatry. We may therefore consider it settled that you will work there next year.

I hope you will write me promptly and frankly if you have anything on your mind, and that you will not fail to call the next time you are in New York.

Yours sincerely,

Robert A. Lambert

Doctor Raymond D. Adams,
Care of Doctor James B. Ayer,
Massachusetts General Hospital,
Boston, Massachusetts.

RAL: BR Copy to Dr. F.M. Hanes.

Appendix E: Nomination for the Bullard Professorship

CONFIDENTIAL

Report of the Joint *ad hoc* committee Appointed to Nominate
a Candidate for the Bullard
Professorship of Neuropathology
Recommendation of Dr. Raymond DeLacy Adams

In the selection of a candidate to be recommended for the position of Bullard Professor of Neuropathology, the joint *ad hoc* Committee gave consideration to the place of neuropathology in the Harvard Medical School and its associated institutions. It is the opinion of the Committee that neuropathology should properly form the center of an orbit around which neurology, neurosurgery and psychiatry revolve, as well as function as a subject in its own right. It has special responsibilities to these divisions of neuropsychiatry, as well as broad responsibilities to general pathology, medicine and surgery. While psychiatry tends to emphasize certain psychodynamic principles, while neurology emphasizes tissue changes of the nervous system and neurosurgery the surgical intervention, there is no sharp line of demarcation separating patients who have disorders in this general territory. Neuropathology has the opportunity to aid in distinguishing cases of anatomical lesions from those in which disturbance seems to be more definitely on a functional level. It would seem that it can afford equal service to all divisions of neuro psychiatry. It becomes evident, therefore, that an individual to be recommended for the Chair of Neuropathology should not only be aware of his responsibilities to these divisions, but should also have a background of training and experience such as to give him the competence needed to meet these responsibilities. He should accordingly be expected to be acceptable to the faculty members of these divisions. Needless to say, he should also be an individual having marked ability in the field of neuropathology. He should have investigative imagination and proven ability in research. He should be a good expositor and teacher in order to be able to inspire the student body, the young graduate and his associates.

A further opinion of the *ad hoc* Committee is that, for the continued development of neuropsychiatry at Harvard, the Massachusetts General Hospital is now the proper locus for the Bullard Professor of Neuropathology, for this arrangement would permit taking advantage of the extensive facilities of this large institution in an effort to achieve a balance with the Neurological Unit at the Boston City Hospital operating so effectively under the direction of Dr. Derek Denny-Brown.

With these various considerations in mind, the name of Dr. Raymond D. Adams emerges from a careful survey of his peers in the fields of neuropathology and neurology as the person above all others who is best qualified. His career began with specialized training in psychology under Dr. Robert Seashore at the University of Oregon. His master's thesis concerned techniques for recording motor skills. This experience has provided him with more than the usual insight in the value of psychological method in the study of diseases of the nervous system. Dr. Adams has also had good preliminary training in psychiatry. He has worked successfully for a number of years in collaboration with neurosurgical associates, and he has made a distinguished name for himself in the field of neurology and in neuropathology. He is most highly regarded and respected by his confreres in the associated fields already mentioned, and equally so by his peers in medicine, surgery, physiology and biochemistry. His bibliography will indicate that his interests have cut across many lines of specialization. It appears in each instance that the collaborations have been happy ones.

Dr. Adams' capacities were closely scrutinized three years ago when he was made Associate Clinical Professor of Neurology and Chief of the Neurological Service and Neuropathologist at the Massachusetts General Hospital. A distinguished committee made him its first choice for the directorship of the Neurological Institute at McGill University, Montreal, to succeed Dr. Wilder Penfield. This attractive opportunity he turned down.

In seeking a candidate for nomination as the next Bullard professor of Neuropathology, two fields of competence were carefully considered because of their essentiality, namely, ability in teaching and research. An appraisal of the status of Dr. Adams as a teacher brings out the following characteristics:

(1) His scholarship is distinctly of a high order, his knowledge of the literature is especially striking as is often shown in his ability to present extemporaneously the pertinent literature of a subject under discussion. Obviously this can be the case only when an individual has devoted himself to continual review of the literature. His papers indicate clearly that he is an excellent student of the subject matter presented. The chairman of the present *ad hoc* Committee, who is a co-author with Dr. Adams of a volume on Neurosyphilis, can attest to his scholarly processes. His literary style is clear, concise, and very readable.

(2) Clinical ability is an essential for a teacher who is to win the respect of the sophisticated medical student, intern and resident of today. All the evidence indicates that Dr. Adams has their complete respect and that of his colleagues too. His clinics, especially as developed on Thursday mornings at the MGH, are widely regarded as models of clinical presentation. His examination of the patient is a masterly demonstration of methodology. His erudition as aforementioned in referring to pertinent literature on the subject and his logical deductions and able diagnostic interpretations make these sessions attractive and stimulating. Similarly, his knowledge of gross and microscopic anatomical pathology of the nervous system is widely recognized. Over a period of years his brain-cutting sessions have been attended by large numbers of neurologists, psychiatrists, residents and interns. They are generally considered a high spot in our medical community.

(3) On the lecture platform Dr. Adams has the ability to hold his audience because of the clarity of his exposition, the orderliness of the approach to the subject at hand and the pertinence of the material presented.

(4) The capacity to inspire and to evoke interest is another important characteristic of the great teacher. Dr. Adams has shown this ability most adequately. Younger men in the field and, indeed, peers in associated fields of medical science have found working with him a valuable and satisfying experience.

(5) Administrative ability, by which is meant the capacity to think through an educational program and to accumulate able associates and assistants for the orderly development of the subject, is an important asset in a department head. Dr. Adams has given the matter of the philosophy and logic of the subject matter a great deal of thought and has been able to find able people to surround him in his present capacity as Chief of the Neurological Service at the MGH. His point of view on the teaching of neuropathology is concisely stated by him as follows:

"We envision a neuropathology course as being a joint enterprise, having three focal points:

(1) neuroanatomy in relation to neuropathology under Dr. Yakovlev;
(2) basic neurohistology in relation to neuropathology, which should be under the direction of Dr. Pope;
(3) the morbid anatomy of the more common disease of the nervous system."

Statements of Dr. Adams' colleagues corroborate our high evaluation of him.

Quotation from Dr. Cobb: "I think Dr. Raymond D. Adams is the ideal man for the Bullard Professorship. He is taking a marked interest in the advancing frontier of chemical pathology. He is to a marked degree able to integrate special laboratory work with clinical neurology. He does not narrowly limit himself to neurology, but has an unusual interest in, and knowledge of, special psychiatric syndromes as dementia, delirium and toxic states."

Quotation from Dr. Walter Bauer: "Dr. Adams' mastery of his chosen field of interest has gained him national recognition. His ability to impart his knowledge of the nervous system and its diseases in a well-ordered, systematic, interesting manner stamps him as one of the outstanding teachers of neurology in this country. In his bedside teaching he demonstrates in exemplary fashion the importance of history-taking, accurate observation and precise examination. In translating clinical findings in terms of disease he makes evident the many factors, which contribute to maintaining the integrity of the nervous system and its normal functions. His emphasis on interdependence of systems and organs orients the student more fully to the true meaning of comprehensive medicine and the need for investigation. This approach invites a maximum of student participation and mutual exchange of knowledge, so important to good teaching."

Quotation from Dr. Derek Denny-Brown: "Dr. Adams' clinical ability has enabled him to make outstanding contributions in the field of clinico-pathological correlation, which is the most important need in neurology and psychiatry. It is hard to find anyone up to him in all-round ability, stimulation of young men, original viewpoint and experience."

A review of Dr. Adams' publications from 1941 to 1954 (January)—61 articles, indicating great industry and productivity—shows a wide range of subject matter. The titles also indicate that he has knowledge of a variety of techniques, which include not only the conventional neurological and neuropathological methods but also those of internal medicine, biochemistry and general pathology. His collaborators outside of his special field throw some light on the breadth of interests and his ability to associate himself with men of real ability in a number of fields. Among his collaborators may be mentioned Denny-Brown in neurology, Schatzki in roentgenology, Scoville and Munro in neurosurgery, Parker in pathology, Weinstein in infectious diseases, Ham in internal medicine—to mention but a few.

The field which he has perhaps investigated most intensively is that of vascular disease, in which he has made a real contribution. He has brought orderliness into this subject. By exploitation of a combination of chemical and pathological methods, he has attempted to determine some of the mechanisms of apoplexy. This grew out of a series of studies of hemorrhagic infarction of the brain that not only brought order into a previously confused subject but put the histology of cerebrovascular disease on a dynamic basis.

His work on liver disease in relation to its effects on the nervous system is of great significance. It combines clinical acumen and originality in the use of histological, biochemical and physiological techniques.

Finally, it should be mentioned that Dr. Adams has been able to direct younger man in valuable investigative enterprises and, at the same time, he has been able to work fruitfully with his seniors such as Dr. Denny-Brown and Dr. Charles S. Kubik.

In summary it may be stated that Dr. Adams has proven his mettle at the Harvard Medical School and in the Boston community, where he is recognized as a man of outstanding ability in neuropathology, both nationally and internationally. As a teacher he has won the admiration of students, interns and residents; as a leader he has gathered about him men of distinction. There is no question that he has been found to be most acceptable at both the Boston City Hospital and the Massachusetts General Hospital. Furthermore, there is no question that he can work effectively with others in a wide variety of fields. The joint *ad hoc* Committee, therefore, recommends Dr. Raymond D. Adams unanimously as its one and only nominee for appointment as the next Bullard Professor of Neuropathology.

Respectfully submitted,

Walter Bauer, M.D.[1]
Allan M. Butler, M.D.[2]
George P. Berry, M.D.[3]
Dean A. Clark, M.D.[4]
Derek E. Denny-Brown, M.D.[5]
Arthur T. Hertig, M.D.[6]
Francis D. Moore, M.D.[7]
Harry C. Solomon, M.D.,[8] Chairman

Notes

1. Jackson, Professor of Clinical Medicine, Harvard Medical School, Chief of Medical Services, Massachusetts General Hospital.
2. Professor of Pediatrics, Harvard Medical School, Chief, Children's Medical Services, Massachusetts General Hospital.

3. Dean of the Faculty of Medicine, Harvard Medical School.

4. General Director, Massachusetts General Hospital.

5. James Jackson, Putnam Professor of Neurology, Harvard Medical School, Director Neurological Unit, Boston City Hospital.

6. Shattuck Professor in Pathology, Harvard Medical School, Chief Obstetrician, Boston Lying In Hospital.

7. Moseley Professor of Surgery, Harvard Medical School, Surgeon in Chief, Peter Bent Brigham Hospital.

8. Bullard Professor of Psychiatry, Harvard Medical School, Superintendent, Boston Psychopathic Hospital.

Appendix F: Announcement for Neurology Residency Applicants to Massachusetts General Hospital, 1962

THE NEUROLOGY SERVICE ******** MASSACHUSETTS GENERAL HOSPITAL
Raymond D. Adams, M.D.—Chief of Service

The Neurology Training Program at the Massachusetts General Hospital consists usually of three years of training (two in clinical neurology and one in neuropathology and basic neurological sciences).

There are six openings for the post of assistant resident, and these are awarded to men who have had a sound training in internal medicine—at least two years. One or two of these openings are awarded each year to men who come here for training in pediatric neurology and who have already completed their training in pediatrics. They spend this year in adult neurology in order to become acquainted with special neurological problems and techniques. Stipends vary from $4200 to $4500 during the first year (based on previous training and whether the candidate is married or not), and there is an increase in stipend during the second and third year. The Hospital contributes in part towards the salary of one resident and three assistant residents, with board, and the rest is supplemented from a Training Grant from the National Institute of Neurological Diseases and Blindness. The other assistant residents are paid entirely from the Training Grant—at the same rate.

First Year Residents

The Assistant Residents rotate for periods of two months each on the following services:

Neurology Ward
Neurosurgery Service

Private Neurology Service
Emergency Ward and Overnight Ward
Out-patient Service
Shuttuck Hospital

Neurology Ward: During this time he has charge of the neurological patients on the ward under the supervision of the Senior Resident. He supervises the work-ups of the medical house officer and assistant resident, in rotation, from the Medical Service, instructs and assists fourth year Harvard Medical students who come for a month's elective clinical work in neurology. He performs lumbar punctures, myelograms, and other neurological techniques, makes rounds and presents patients to the Visit, discusses problems with the Senior Resident in daily morning and late afternoon rounds, and takes responsibility for patient care.

Neurosurgery: During this time he performs the duties of an assistant resident in neurosurgery, works up patients, presents them to the Visit, assists at operations, does minor neurosurgical procedures, and attends the neurosurgical rounds and conferences.

Private Service: During this time he sees all patients admitted to the private service to members of the Neurological Staff and follows them with the Senior Staff member. He may help the Senior Staff member with certain procedures.

Emergency and Overnight Ward: During this time he sees acutely ill neurological patients at the time of their admission and requests consultations as needed and follows the patients in the overnight ward as necessary.

Out-patient Service: On this Service he sees patients in the Nerve Clinic and works in the special clinics and may do special work in the EEG and EMG laboratories.

Shattuck Hospital: This is a hospital for chronic neurological patients and it has an active neurological service under Dr W. H. Timberlake of our Staff.

All assistant residents go to the Nerve Clinic one half-day a week and attend conferences as time permits.

Second Year Residents

If resident is in the Pediatric Neurology Training Program, he works as assistant resident in pediatric neurology under the supervision of Dr P. R. Dodge and follows and works up patients there.

If resident is in the adult neurology training program and is doing neuropathology, he performs autopsies, works up cases, prepares for clinico-pathological conferences, attends microscopical-neuropathological sessions twice a week in the evenings, (two-hour sessions each), has opportunity to spend some time with Dr Yakovlev in the Neuropathology-Neuroanatomy Laboratory at the Warren Museum at the Harvard Medical School. He also has opportunity to have individual sessions with Dr E. P. Richardson, Jr regarding difficult cases and also to consult with Dr R. D. Adams, Dr C. S. Kubick and Dr C. M. Fisher on particular problems. There is some opportunity to do research work.

During this year also, he participates as assistant to senior members of the Staff in laboratory teaching of neuropathology, a course which is given to second year students of the Harvard Medical School. He also attends all the lectures in this course. Sometimes, he may assist in the course of neuroanatomy for the first year medical students.

All of the men go to the Nerve Clinic out-patient one half-day a week.

Third Year Residents

If resident is in Pediatric Neurology, he does neuropathology this year.

The senior residents in clinical neurology rotate through the Neurology Ward, Consultation Service and the Pediatric Neurology Service.

On the Ward, he has general supervision and teaching of assistant resident, the house officer and assistant resident in rotation from Medical Service, teaching of all neurological procedures, arranging for neuroradiological conferences, etc.

Consultation Service—during this time he sees all consultations from all the other Services in the Hospital and from the Massachusetts Eye and Ear and in the Overnight Ward, arranges for neurological grand rounds, and with assistant resident makes rounds of patients in Emergency Ward, and instructs assistant resident in care of patients, as necessary.

Pediatric Neurology—makes rounds with Visit and examines and treats pediatric neurology patients under the supervision of the Pediatric Neurology Visit and the pediatric neurology resident.

All residents go to the Nerve Clinic one half-day a week and attend all conferences, as time permits. Some years the Residents go to the Shattuck Hospital one afternoon a week for follow-up study of patients with cerebrovascular disease.

List of Conferences for Residents and Fellows on the Neurology Service

Weekly conferences in neuroradiology with Dr New about patients on the Ward Service

> One weekly clinico-neuropathological conference—Dr R.D. Adams or Dr E. P. Richardson, Jr
> Neurological Grand Rounds—one morning a week—Dr R.D. Adams.

Neurological out-patient conference—once a week—Dr M. Victor

Two evening sessions—microscopic neuropathology—Dr Adams and Dr Richardson

Journal club meetings—once a week and once a month combined with Neurosurgery

Weekly conference with Social Service about problem on ward patients

October–April Seminars in Neurological Sciences in the Department of Neuropathology, Warren Museum, Harvard Medical School—various members of the Senior Staff (These are evening sessions, held twice a week).

Special Clinics—Neurology Service

Pediatric Neurology—Dr P. R. Dodge

Seizure Clinic—Dr R. S. Schwab and Dr M. L. Scholl

Myasthenia Gravis Clinic—Dr Schwab and Dr V. P. Perlo

Parkinson Clinic—Dr Schwab and Dr England

Multiple Sclerosis Clinic—Dr P.M. Dreyfus

Stroke Clinic—Dr C. M. Fisher

Language Clinic—Dr E. M. Cole and Dr Perlo

The Senior Residents may take part in some research projects in the Department, and opportunities are available to them in the following laboratories:

EEG and EMG laboratories—Dr R. S. Schwab, Dr M. L. Scholl

Neurophysiology Laboratory—Dr J. S. Barlow

Laboratories for Immunology—Dr Byron H. Waksman

Laboratory of Experimental Tissue Neuropathology—Dr R. D. Adams

Electron Microscopy—Dr H. deF. Webster

The Charles S. Kubik Laboratory for Neuropathology—Dr E. P. Richardson, Jr

Laboratory for Lipid Chemistry—Dr Hugo Moser

Laboratory for the study of Nutritional Diseases—Dr M. Victor and Dr P. M. Dreyfus

Cerebrovascular Diseases—Dr C. M. Fisher

Laboratory for Chemistry of Muscle Disease—Dr J. Gergely

Tissue Culture Laboratory—Dr R.L. Sidman

Laboratory for Children's Psychology—Dr M. Sidman and Dr L. T. Stoddard

Kennedy Laboratories for the study of Children's Neurological
Diseases—Dr P.R. Dodge
Cortical Testing Laboratory
Laboratories of Neuropathology—Warren Museum, Harvard Medical
School—Dr P. I. Yakovlev

Appointments for residencies are made about October 10, 1962—Applications
and letters of recommendation should be sent by October 1, 1962.

Applications for posts as Research Fellows may be made at any time during
the year, and appointments are made if openings are available.

July, 1962
G

Appendix G

This 1962 report to the director of the Massachusetts General Hospital documents Raymond Adams' first decade as neurology chair. By building research,
clinical, and educational programs, he had created the first modern, large,
multi-divisional academic neurology program.

Report on the Neurology Service of the Massachusetts General Hospital

During the past decade, through the generous support of the administration
and Trustees of the Massachusetts General Hospital and of Dean Barry of the
Harvard Medical School, it has been possible for the Staff of the Neurology
Service to expand the sphere of its activities. By way of general remark, it should
be said that this has been relatively easy to accomplish for the Massachusetts
General Hospital has proved to be an ideal place for a medical or surgical
specialty to develop. There are powerful forces here which keep medical and
surgical groups in balance; they continuously thwart excessive specialism and
encourage the closest relationship between any particular field and the main
stream of medicine and surgery. It is our opinion that the isolation of any medical or surgical specialty, as in the establishment of an institute, deprives it of the
stimulus afforded by free competition, closes it off from the sources of many
fresh ideas so that its research program is always in danger of sterility, and may
interfere with the quick application of new techniques in the diagnosis and care
of the patients.

Expansion of the Neurological Staff to Meet Clinical Needs

Our first recognized need was to enlarge the Staff so that the Service would
at all times be capable of rendering expert service in the care of the neurologically sick. A number of new clinical workers were brought into the

Service. These were Dr C. Miller Fisher, whose special interest had been cerebrovascular disease, Dr Maurice Victor, who had been studying alcoholic and
nutritional problems, and Dr Philip R. Dodge, who had devoted himself to
pediatric neurology, Dr Mandel Cohen, the neurology of cerebral diseases and
Dr David Poskanzer, preventive neurology. We were fortunate in already having Dr Edwin Cole, whose competence in the field of language training and
speech therapy was well established, and Dr Robert Schwab, who for many
years has been active in studying myasthenia gravis, Parkinson's disease, and
epilepsy. Also he had established one of the first EEG labs in the United States,
and shortly afterwards Dr Cole had opened a laboratory for the psychological
testing of patients with disordered brain findings in the cortical testing laboratory of which Miss Elizabeth White has been in charge. Dr William Timberlake
and Dr Vincent Perlo had already had an association with the hospital, but their
role was strengthened by making Dr Timberlake the Chief of the Neurology
Service at the Shattuck Hospital (1954) where there are now 190 beds available
for neurological patients, and by having Dr Perlo take over the active direction
of the Neurology Clinic. Invaluable assistance has been given to Dr Schwab in
the EEG laboratory by Dr John Abbott, and in recent years by Dr Mary Louise
Scholl and Dr Albert England. Dr Ruth Stauffer and Dr Karol Toll have helped
Dr Perlo in the out-patient department.

As a result of this expanded clinical staff, a larger clinical material of
difficult neurological diseases has been attracted to the hospital, being sent
specifically for examination by some of these people who had an authoritative
knowledge of a given category of disease. In addition, both the ward and out-
patient service have strengthened and in the Shattuck Hospital a neurological
ward for chronic diseases became accessible to our resident staff.

Despite the increasing strength of the clinical service, there are some
obvious difficulties which must be corrected if possible:

A. The Neurology Ward is inadequate. Neurology and Neurosurgery share
   a 31-bed ward, at the moment reduced to 27 beds, which is hardly over
   large enough to take care of the number of patients. This requires that the
   patients be boarded around the hospital, often in places where the nursing
   personnel is without special training. Neurological nursing is difficult and
   time consuming and often the limited number of nurses has been inadequate for the task at hand. This has caused our most dedicated nurses to
   become discouraged.
B. There is great need of a special care unit for the neurologically and neu-
   rosurgically sick. Some of the most difficult problems in the hospital are
   on these two services. Ideally, it should be possible to put any stuporous
   or comatose patient into a unit where all the available facilities for management of temperature, blood pressure, respiration, etc., are available and
   where specialized nursing personnel can be concentrated.

C. It is not possible at the present time to fully integrate the private patient activities of the Staff with those of the resident staff. It is to be hoped that in a new out-patient building, it will be possible for all out-patients, whether private or clinic, to be seen in one area. This would tend also to bring the Senior Staff more constantly into proper relationship to the out-patient clinic.

D. It is our impression on the Neurology Service that all patients with a disease of the nervous system should be seen by a neurological physician. Ideally, if time permits, it would be best to admit these patients on a medical service such as ours, and as the work-up proceeds to have the neurosurgeon on call in constant contact with the problem from the time of admission, providing, of course, there is a neurological aspect to the case. This would free the neurosurgeon of some of the tedium of history taking and running down non-surgical problems and would also encourage a better medical follow-up on the cases after operation. The training of young neurosurgeons in these aspects of diagnosis could easily be managed by rotating an assistant in neurosurgery through the Neurology Service for a period of training. In fact such a rotation has been approved by the Neurosurgical service and will begin shortly. It will parallel a rotation of the assistant residents in neurology through neurosurgery, an arrangement which has proved to be extremely valuable over the past several years.

An Educational Program in Neurological Medicine

A great deal of thought and attention has been given to the instruction of medical students in neurology and the training of young physicians in neurological medicine. We have been fortunate in obtaining an excellent resident staff which appears to be constantly improving. Our policy of accepting men on the Neurology Service only after they have had at least two years of internal medicine has proved to be generally sound. We believe that a man should not be permitted to specialize until he is already well on his way to becoming a broadly experienced physician, and capable of handling almost any problem in general medicine. In the training of these men we have learned, more or less by trial and error, that the insertion in the period of training of a full year of laboratory work in neuropathology and anatomy has been of value. The majority of our past residents consider this training period in neuropathology to be, perhaps, the most fruitful since the beginning of their post-graduate education. It seems to us that this program keeps the man from becoming stale from an overdose of heavy clinical responsibility, and it allows time in which to mature and gain perspective. Men coming back to the ward after a year spent in this way, or in some other laboratory activity, seem to have a greater poise and a sounder sense of values. After completing two clinical years and one in neuropathology, most of our residents in recent years have sought further training in the laboratory. This varied according to their background and interests and includes such fields as neurophysiology, biochemistry, biophysics, immunology and neuropathology. Here they learn the methodology of one of these fields and its application to specific research problems, and most important, they acquire a way of thinking and a number of new approaches to unsolved medical problems.

In order to give some type of coordinated instruction to all residents and fellows, not only for those on our Service but also for those in neurosurgery and psychiatry at the Massachusetts General Hospital and at other Harvard hospitals in the area, we have instituted a seminar program at the Harvard Medical School. Lectures or seminars are given in neuroanatomy, cellular pathology, chemical pathology, neuroradiology and neurophysiology, two evenings a week. During the course of the year, nearly all the leading figures in neurology and related fields in Boston are seen and heard. With a minimum of effort it has permitted us to provide a high level of general instruction to all of the residents and clinical and research fellows in Boston and it has saved a great deal of duplication of effort in all the teaching programs.

A special plan for the development of pediatric neurologists has been instituted and there is now a Pediatric Neurology training program in effect. This is under the direction of Dr Philip Dodge. Well trained pediatricians spend a year on the Adult Neurology service; a second year with Dr Dodge in Child Neurology, and a third year in neuropathology. As with residents on the adult service, these young people are encouraged to enter a period of laboratory training after completion of their clinical work.

In neuropathology we have arrangement, through the generous cooperation of Dr Castleman, for bringing men from either neurology or pathology into the neuropathology laboratory for a year; and then, depending on their background, they spend a year in neurology or a year in general pathology, and will have a second year as Dr Richardson's assistant. Afterwards they can turn to the laboratories of cellular neuropathology here and at the Harvard Medical School under Dr Richard Sidman, or to the biochemical pathology laboratories directed by Dr Alfred Pope at McLean Hospital.

The attractiveness of this teaching program is perhaps indicated by the quality of men applying to our service for training. At the moment we do not see any serious flaws in it, though we would be quick to admit that there is a danger of unnecessary rigidity. As the laboratory facilities of our Service expand, we hope that some of these young people will do as one or two of the residents have done in the past few years, drop out of the program for one or two years and work in some special laboratory field.

The success of the medical student teaching program depends to a very considerable extent on having a large number of excellent instructors who are able to take a group of four students and put them through their paces at the bedside. For such instruction we rely heavily on the more senior Neurological Residents; they have, in general, proved capable of providing excellent instruction to our students. This experience provides another dimension in the training of neurological residents, most of whom are destined for careers in academic medicine. In the elective fourth year clerkship the student depends to a considerable extent upon the resident staff.

Expansion of Laboratory Facilities

The third and last area of expansion has been in relation to the laboratory facilities. At the outset we purposely made this secondary to the establishment and maintenance of a strong clinical unit. Originally we were much handicapped by lack of space and, of course, had no personnel for anything except clinical and pathological studies. Through the help of Dr Dean Clark, Dean Berry, Mr. David Crockett and Mr. Henry Meadow, we were able to obtain enough space for both service and research laboratories. The first of these laboratories was consigned to the improvement of the diagnostic facilities of the service. Thus, a new EEG laboratory was established on Warren 3 under Dr Schwab's direction and a temporary laboratory for neuromuscular physiology, including electromyography was built on Baker 12. Further expansion of service laboratories which will include a biochemical screening laboratory, a laboratory for children's EEG and a laboratory for behavioral assessment in children will be possible on the completion of the Joseph P. Kennedy, Jr. Laboratories in the Burnham Building. In addition, neuropathology has been expanded to provide adequate space for the study of approximately a thousand brains a year under the direction of Dr Peirson Richardson, Dr Charles S. Kubik, Dr Raymond D. Adams and resident staff. Some of these specimens are coming to us from the Dever and Wrentham State Schools whose neuropathology we are doing under a contract with the State of Massachusetts.

Dr Byron Waksman's laboratories in immunology have been provided more space on Warren 3 and for the past 10 years he had devoted himself to the study of the immunological basis of neurological, ophthalmological and other medical diseases. These laboratories and their work have provided a strong link to Dr Jordi Folch's research laboratories at the McLean Hospital and the Departments of Bacteriology and Pathology at Harvard Medical School.

New research laboratories have been or are being developed for the biochemical studies of lipid and for intermediary carbohydrate metabolism in diseases of the nervous system and for chemical pathology of muscle and nutritional diseases. In addition there is a neurophysiology unit which includes an area for instruments of communication and data analysis under Dr John Barlow, and a general department laboratory for neurophysiological studies. A new laboratory unit is being formed for experimental psychological studies of the behavior of infants and children with brain disease under Drs. Murray Sidman and John Stoddard. Animal quarters will be provided on the eighth floor of the Children's Unit. In connection with the expansion of the Kennedy Laboratory, some of the present space in Warren 3 will be used for an Electron Microscopic Unit to be under the direction of Dr Henry Webster, and Dr George Collins who has been assisting him in this.

Dr David Poskanzer has joined the service and is presently engaged in the study of neurological diseases by epidemiological methods. We hope that he will form a link between neurology and the School of Public Health where he is now finishing his graduate studies. Dr Alfred Weiss will soon return to an earlier research program in auditory perception and effects of age on CNS, a study to be done in conjunction with the Otology Department and the age center. Dr P. M. Dreyfus is in charge of a Special Multiple Sclerosis Clinic.

Aside from the development of laboratory space for the study of the nervous system of infants and children with brain disease, made possible through a gift by the Kennedy Foundation, probably the most important development in our research unit has been the establishment of two groups of laboratories for neuropathology on the quadrangle of Harvard Medical School. These are under the direction of Dr Paul Yakovlev and Dr Richard Sidman, both members of the Neuropathology Staff. It has been our belief that neuropathology is one of the fundamental medical science disciplines for neurology, neurosurgery and psychiatry, and that many of its teaching and research activities should be carried out in the Medical School itself. Dr George Packer Berry and Mr. Henry Meadow have permitted us to have space within the Warren Museum and these rooms have been assigned to the study of pathological anatomy which is done under the direction of Dr Paul Yakovlev, Dr J. Angevine and their assistants. The other laboratory area is in Cellular Neuropathology, most of which is under the direction of Dr Richard Sidman. Here there are laboratories for use of autoradiographic techniques, biochemical methods as applied to cells, tissue culture and organ culture. All of these are being applied to the investigation of inherited diseases in animals and certain disease processes which can be set up within the experimental neuropathology laboratory. These, in addition to our teaching efforts in neurology and neuropathology, represent our principal university activities.

The following is a list of the Research Laboratories in the Massachusetts General Hospital-Harvard Neurology-Neuropathology Department:

Massachusetts General Hospital

1. Physiology and EEG laboratories under Dr Robert Schwab with the assistance of Dr John Abbott, Dr Mary Louise Scholl and several Research Fellows. Technical staff of 16.

2. Electromyography Laboratory under Dr A. Salama formerly under Dr Ingrid Gamstorp.

3. Neurophysiology Laboratories for the investigation of the significance of EEG patterns and other brain rhythms, using computer techniques, under Dr John Barlow working in collaboration with Dr Rosenblith and Dr Norbert Wiener of M.I.T.

4. Laboratories for Immunology under Dr Byron H. Waksman with the assistance of Dr Barry Arnason, Dr B. Jankovic of Yugoslavia, Dr T. Kosunen of Finland. Technical assistants 12.

5. Laboratory for Experimental Tissue Neuropathology. Dr R. D. Adams, Dr Stanley Cobb. Technical assistant, Miss Carroll.

6. Electron Microscopic Lab. Dr Henry deF. Webster.

7. The Charles S. Kubik Laboratory for Neuropathology under Dr E. P. Richardson, Jr, with assistance of Dr George Collins. Technical staff 6.

8. Laboratory for Lipid chemistry. Dr Hugo Moser. Technical staff 1.

9. Laboratory for the study of Nutritional Diseases. Dr M. Victor and Dr Pierre Dreyfus. Technical assistants 2.

10. Laboratory for Chemistry of Muscle Disease. Dr John Gergely.

11. Tissue Culture laboratory. Dr Richard Sidman.

12. Laboratory for Children's Psychology under Dr Murray Sidman and Dr Stoddard.

13. Laboratory for Study of Vascular Disease under Dr C. M. Fisher.

14. Laboratory for Study of Children's Neurological Diseases. Dr Philip Dodge. Technical assistants 3.

15. Cortical Testing laboratory.

The expansion of our research program has been proceeding somewhat unevenly but we are gratified with how much has been possible. There still remains the problem of more firmly establishing neuropathology as one of the areas of scientific work in the Medical School itself. The opening of Pediatric Neurology Laboratories, which will take place this coming winter, brings to a realization a long cherished hope for a strong unit of Pediatric Neurology. The financing of these laboratories is still in a highly unstable condition and we hope that some way will be found to provide more adequately for this in the near future.

The greatest strength of our specialty unit is its close association with the various divisions of the Medical and Surgical and Pediatric Services at the Massachusetts General Hospital.

RDA: tw

1/18/62

Appendix H: Selected Dedications and Tributes

It is said that comparisons are odious, but I would say that he was the greatest neurologist of his time. I knew all the Canadians, many Queen Square people, the modern Parisian group and many of the leaders of American neurology. They couldn't even carry his bags; he was that superior.

C. Miller Fisher

In clinical skills and in pathological skills nobody could compare with Ray Adams... He had enormous intellectual integrity ...

Joseph Foley

If one looks at the 20th century he was the single most important figure in American neurology.

Joseph Martin

I thought that he was a truly exceptional human being. I had a great deal of respect for his manner. He was a proud man. He took a great deal of pride in being right; he was uncomfortable if confronted with being wrong. A gentleman, soft spoken. I have nothing but the greatest respect for him as a person and a scientist.

George Collins

I had enormous heart-splitting pride to be one of Ray's guys. We idolized him so.

Jay Angevine

his breadth of understanding of diseases of the nervous system was unparalleled.

Darryl DeVivo

a great hero to me ... central to the development of my career.

Richard Sidman

I revere Ray as the most brilliant person I have encountered in my long medical career. In his time he had an unmatched grasp of the fundamentals of all the clinical, physiological, and neuropathological facets of nervous system disorders. He was simultaneously the best neurologist I ever met and the best neuropathologist. The Tuesday night sessions with him were just incredible. Even Bob Terry said he was the best neuropathologist he had ever seen. (Bob Terry is a very critical guy.) Ray was just a remarkable man in an era, where one person could really and singly master all.

Herbert Schaumburg

I have nothing but respect and admiration for the work of Raymond D. Adams. And also I value his friendship very, very much. He is a very fine friend, a great man to talk to when you have a problem. He's one of the perfect people I have known in the field of medicine.

Betty Banker

We offered our best inducements not long ago, to your brilliant neurologist and neuropathologist, Raymond Adams, hoping he would move to Montreal. Our plan of abduction failed, alas.

Dr Wilder Penfield
On the dedication of the new Warren Building
At Massachusetts General Hospital, Dec. 3, 1956
in the Massachusetts General
Hospital News, No 163, January 1957

father figure, teacher, mentor, friend.

Henry def. Webster

a giant of a man, a great oak.

Robert Delong

I want to say that everything I've done in my life came through Ray Adams. And what I'm doing now, specifically, is setting up controlled trials for new treatments. All of that, everything I do, was Ray Adams' mentorship's creation.

He is the greatest neurologist, as far as I know, who has existed.

Hugo Moser

Ray Adams left an indelible mark on the textbook with his first contributions. He advocated what was to become the chief feature of the book, namely, the use of the introductory chapters to discuss symptoms and signs—the "Cardinal Manifestations of Disease." He argued forcefully for including disease of the nervous system as a major component.

A salute to Raymond D. Adams
by the editors of Harrison's
Harrison's *Principles of Internal Medicine*
Twelfth Edition 1991

I am grateful to Raymond Adams, who introduced me to neurology and neuropathology and provided a model of scholarship in medicine that I have since striven to achieve.

Joseph T. Volpe
Acknowledgements
Neurology of the Newborn
WB Saunders, Philadelphia, 2001

Ray was the dominant person in the development of pediatric neurology.

Robert Cook

Appendix I: Family Information

MATERNAL SIDE

Great Grandfather

Philemon Delacy Morriss[1] of Kentucky moved to New Salem, Illinois, in 1831. He split rails with Abraham Lincoln, who made a family chart in the Morriss family bible. Philemon was a private in the Blackhawk Wars and the Mexican War. He became a cabinetmaker. In 1852 he left Iowa with his family including Philemon Delacy Morriss, Jr (age 6), to cross the Great Plains to settle in the Oregon territory.

From the flyleaf of his diary:

> A certain cure for a sur pain in the head. Shave a plais on top of your head. And take and cut around peas of thin leather as big as a dollar. Spread some beefs gall on the lather and stick it on your head and it will affect a cure. Let it stic till it comes off. Perhaps it will bee 2 or 3 weeks.

Note

1. Mentioned in Sandburg, Carl Abraham Lincoln. *The Prairie Years, and The War Years* (One Volume Edition). Harcourt Bruce and Co., New York, 1954.

Mother's Parents

Philemon Delacy Morriss, Jr, was a private in the civil war in the 1st Regiment, Oregon Volunteer Infantry. He served as a drummer boy and was involved in action against hostile Indians. He married Sarah Ellen Tarplay, who had been born in Oregon.

Mother of Raymond Adams

Eva Mabel Morriss born in Oregon. She married William Henry Adams. She lived into her eighties.

PATERNAL SIDE

Father's Parents

Henry Adams of Kent England married Elizabeth Maurer of Bern, Switzerland. They resided in Churchville, New York, near Rochester.

Father of Raymond Adams

William Henry Adams left New York State, migrated west, and settled in Oregon, where he married Eva Morriss. He lived into his eighties.

SIBLING

Ray Adams' only sibling was Dorothy Ellen, known to the Adams children as Aunt Dodo. She married a pediatrician, who practiced in Maine. A social worker, she displayed, like her brother, leadership qualities, organizational abilities, and an interest in patients with mental disorders.

CHILDREN OF RAYMOND DELACY ADAMS AND MARGARET ELINOR CLARK ADAMS:

1. Mary Elinor, a retired biochemist.
2. John William is Headmaster of Morgan Park Academy, a preparatory school. Previously he was headmaster of two schools for dyslexic boys, one of which he founded.
3. Carol Ann, a retired schoolteacher.
4. Sarah Ellen, a housewife.

Appendix J: Correspondence About the Origin of the Term "Asterixis"

Dr Charles Davidson at Boston City Hospital had consulted Ray Adams and colleagues about many of his patients with liver disease. From these patients Adams et al. made extensive clinical observation on hepatic encephalopathy. For the characteristic movement disorder of liver failure, Foley and Adams coined the term, "asterixis." Ten years later Davidson inquired about it; he had apparently forgotten that his neurology consultants had created this new term. In fact, Davidson did not know how to spell it! The term had been so well accepted in internal medicine that Davidson seemed irritated by its frequent use at Boston City Hospital. His scatological reference also suggests his annoyance.

Foley recalls his meeting with a classics professor from Boston College to seek advice about terminology. Beyond what he describes in his letter, Foley recalls that the first idea was to use the term "anisosterixis." When Foley reported back to Ray Adams, they abbreviated the term to "asterixis."

July 31, 1963

Dr. Joseph Foley
Department of Neurology
Western Reserve University
Medical School
Cleveland, Ohio

Dear Joe:

It was good to see your face at the BCH, but I did forget to ask you a question.

House Officers and students are continually referring to asterexis. The simple four-letter word "flap" has been forgotten. I suppose the elegance of the word "intercourse" and "bowel movement" for their simpler 4-letter components may have influenced them. At any rate, they tell me you invented the word. Did you? If so, why and what does it mean?

Best regards.

Sincerely yours,

Charles S. Davidson, M.D.
CSD/ach

August 4, 1963

Charles S. Davidson, M.D.
Department of Medicine
Boston City Hospital
818 Harrison Avenue
Boston 18, Massachusetts

Dear Charlie:

I know that Ray Adams and I must plead guilty to initiating the term "asterixis." We did it with some reluctance, and also with tongue in cheek, but it seemed unreasonable for two people who had stopped using the word "adiadokokinesis" to start using the word "asterixis." Although I have rarely used the word, I still must defend the necessity to find some term that will define the movement disorder. Flap is very good and very descriptive but hardly describes what one sees in the feet, the neck, or the face and tongue. Furthermore, the blunt fact is that the movement is quite different from the tremor which underlies it. Therefore, the unknown pundit who wrote the enclosed squib in MEDICAL TRIBUNE clearly doesn't understand the full nature of the movement disorder. (There is an unwarranted implication in that last sentence that I do. This is still not true.)

In regard to the origin of the word itself, you may not be aware that in my background I have a small undistinguished career of Greek scholarship. By the time I was studying the liver with intensity I had forgotten most of my Greek—but I had not forgotten that any Greek scholar is a good man to sit down and have a drink with. It seems to me that on one winey evening we coined the term from a combination of a-privative plus the noun-forming suffix of stereo, infinitive sterein, meaning roughly to place or to make a thing assume a fixed position. On a non-winey evening I presented the possibility to Ray, and we decided to go along with this.

It was good to see you even for so briefly last week. I look forward to the pleasure again.

With best regards.

Sincerely yours,

Joseph M. Foley, M.D.

JMF/dss
Enclosure

Appendix K: The Long Shadow of Cerebral Localization

This article,[1] published in 2005, caught the attention of Raymond Adams. Over ninety years of age, he continued to receive and read many medical journals. The author of the piece reminisces about the "late Raymond Adams." He remembers presenting a case to Dr Adams. "Despite my best efforts, I could not remove the look of displeasure from his face. I defended myself, invoking time efficiency and what not, but Dr Adams was unforgiving." "You can't rush a neurologic examination," he said. "A proper one takes three days." The author goes on to state that, subsequent to his residency, CT and MRI scanning have liberated neurology from the "shackles" of clinical localization exercises and patient demonstrations in the teaching of neurology, i.e. from the thought process and method of Raymond Adams.

About this article Adams wrote, "Surely I would not have restricted the neurologic exam to 3 days." Adams also noted that the author "overlooks the fact that a sizeable proportion of neurologic diseases are not identifiable by MRI. Also, without clinical evidence of localization of lesions, laboratory methods may be misdirected." One must suspect that the author of the paper once again caused a look of displeasure on the face of Raymond Adams. (see Figure 65.)

Note

1. Shafqat S. The Long Shadow of Cerebral Localization. *J R Soc Med* V98, p 549, 2006.

Appendix L: Concerning Certain Psychological Principles

This essay by Adams illustrates his sense of history and his deep understanding of the relationships of neurology psychiatry, psychology, and neuropathology.(Reproduced from the Transactions and Studies of the College of Physicians of Philadelphia, 1959, by permission of the College of Physicians of Philadelphia.)

(For a more detailed treatment of this subject see: Adams RD. Important Contributions to an Understanding of the Mind and Nervous Function Which Have Emanated From the Clinic. In Beecher HK (ed.), *Disease and the Advancement of Basic Science*. Harvard University Press, Cambridge, pp 265–314, 1960.)

TRANSACTIONS & STUDIES

of the

College of Physicians of Philadelphia

Volume 27

(Fourth Series)

Number 1

(July 1959)

Concerning Certain Psychological Principles which have been Derived from Clinico-pathologic Study[1]

By RAYMOND D. ADAMS, M.D.[2]

PRESIDENT RHOADS, Fellows of the College of Physicians and Guests: Permit me first to tender my thanks for the invitation to appear before you as Weir Mitchell Orator, a post around which are clustered so many pleasant and honorable associations. I am fully sensible to the duty which this selection places upon me and to the special difficulties which it imposes. This Society constitutes an audience of the widest professional competence with interests in all branches of medical science. By long established custom it has come to expect from each of its orators the report of a new discovery or the expression of the seasoned views of a physician or scientist on some topic of general medical interest. In this reasonable expectation I fear I may disappoint you, for much of what I have to say is familiar, and undoubtedly many of the members of your society could expound the ideas I am about to present far more eloquently than I.

That a neurological physician from Boston

should address this Society in a lecture which commemorates the life and works of Silas Weir Mitchell has a degree of propriety which deserves passing comment. You may know that one of my predecessors at the Massachusetts General Hospital, Professor James Jackson Putnam, was a contemporary of Weir Mitchell and expressed his admiration for the clinical and scientific work of this great physician on several occasions. Moreover, Dr. Mitchell was a member of that select and intimate circle of versatile American physicians, so well represented in Boston in the nineteenth century, whose talents ranged broadly in medicine, science and literature. He was a close friend and frequent correspondent of our Professor Oliver Wendell Holmes.

Before choosing a topic for this occasion, I refreshed my memory of some of Dr. Weir Mitchell's work. It covers such a broad field of medicine that it leaves the present and any future orators much latitude, if they essay, as the stipulation of this lectureship enjoins them to do, some topic consonant with the interests of this distinguished physician. Two aspects of his work attracted my attention—1) his interest in psychic phenomena as revealed in his clinical studies and novels; 2) his acknowledged

[1] Weir Mitchell Oration XV, College of Physicians of Philadelphia, 4 February 1959.

[2] Bullard Professor of Neuropathology, Harvard University, Chief, Neurology Service, Massachusetts General Hospital, Boston 12, Massachusetts.

skill in clinical observation and in drawing cogent inferences, some of no little scientific merit, from the study of the sick. The thesis which I intend here to submit and to document in a limited way—that the clinico-pathologic method of case study represents a valid approach both in the investigation of disease and in the acquisition of knowledge of the natural functions of the mind, would meet with his approval, I am sure. And it may serve to remind us that not all of the problems of medical science, particularly those relating to the human nervous system, need find their immediate solution through the techniques of biochemistry and biophysics which are presently so widely extolled in the American and Russian press.

But before proceeding to the main topic of my discourse, a brief discussion of the *method* of *medical observation*, also called the *clinico-pathologic method*, may be of some value. Probably the method is as old as medicine itself but it first became fruitful during the nineteenth century when clinical medicine began to feel the guiding influence of pathology. Its application to problems of human nervous function will forever be associated with the name of Charcot and his followers at the Salpêtrière in Paris.

Essentially the method consists of "accurate and unbiased observation of organ (here nervous) function deranged by disease". It involves a series of steps as follows:

1). The detailed history of an illness, including both the patient's statement as to what is wrong and the observations of family and friends as to behavioral changes.

2). The systematic examination of the patient's nervous function.

3). The gross and microscopic examination of the central nervous system of those so unfortunate as to succumb to disease.

4). The correlation of the manifestations of disturbed nervous function, both the subjective and objective, with one another and with morbid anatomy.

5). The drawing of inferences as to the function of the nervous system and of mind.

6). The testing of these tentative hypotheses in other clinical situations or in animals and man in the experimental laboratory.

Many difficulties are encountered in the effective application of the clinico-pathologic method some of which are not fully appreciated even by clinical investigators. However, time does not permit further elaboration upon these matters.

I would like now to invite your attention to certain features of mind and its nervous arrangements which have been learned by the application of the clinico-pathologic method. At the very outset it would seem desirable, however, to fix the limits of our discussion lest I become too diffuse and am forced to speak and speculate on matters about which little or nothing is known. I propose to exclude the large category of psychoneuroses, schizophrenia and manic depressive psychoses from the orbit of this discourse and to refer only to those diseases of established pathology which induce predictable changes in psychic function.

Limits of time prohibit an examination of all the psychic derangements which result from disease of the brain, and we must concentrate on a few which are of current interest or which may be profitably studied in the clinic and pathology laboratory in the near future.

I. CONSCIOUSNESS AND ITS NEUROLOGICAL SUBSTRATUM

Consciousness, which is the very core and nucleus of our psychic life, has been investigated in a number of physiology laboratories in recent years and several interesting hypotheses concerning its relation to other mental functions have been formulated. Some of these facts and hypotheses demand our contemplation for they have application to the practice of medicine.

When the word consciousness is brought up for general medical discussion, all informed physicians in the audience will at once think of the interesting recent publications of Bremer, Ranson, Magoun, Lindlsey, Jasper and many other contemporary anatomists, physiologists and psychologists. And the two excellent volumes, one the "Symposium on Brain Mechanisms and Consciousness", the other "Reticular Formation of the Brain", which have recently been published, present well the existing state of our knowledge as gained from recent investigations. But it would only be fair to say it was the clinical neurologist and neurosurgeon who, confronted daily with the concomitance of brain lesion and derangement of the mind, were the first to appreciate that small lesions in the upper part of the brain stem and thalamus produce prolonged disturbances of consciousness. Moreover, it has been possible to discern two clinical entities in diseases of this part of the neuraxis, one *true coma* with its characteristic unreceptiveness of external stimulus and inner need and unresponsiveness, and *pseudocoma* with retained receptiveness but nearly total unresponsiveness owing to virtual paralysis of all four extremities and all bulbar musculature (face, tongue, jaw, pharynx and larynx). Doubtless other syndromes representing partial derangements of consciousness will later be defined.

Two cases are presented which exemplify these clinical conditions. It is to be noted that in true coma, represented in the first case, the lesion was located in the tegmentum of the midbrain and subthalamus, whereas in pseudocoma, the second case, the morbid change was in the base and tegmentum of the upper pons and lower midbrain leaving the diencephalon and upper midbrain unaffected. In other words, the difference between the two cases was the involvement of the reticular formation of the upper brain stem in one but not the other. This fact appears to be in harmony with recent physiologic experiments which demonstrate that in animals the destruction of this loose array of neurones in the upper brain stem produces a prolonged coma with slowing of the electroencephalogram, and the stimulation of this same region arouses the sleeping animal and desynchronizes the brain waves. Further, the clinical state obtains some clarification from the experimental findings that sensory stimuli not only initiate volleys of impulses which traverse the specific sensory tracts to the thalamus and cortex but also extend, via collaterals, to activate this reticular formation; and it in turn sends and receives fibers from all parts of the cerebral cortex. Alcohol, barbiturates and some anesthetic agents act by suppressing this part of the reticular formation. Penfield has attempted to subsume this entire system under the term *centrencephalon* and has postulated that it is the highest center of the brain, the integrating mechanism of the entire cerebral cortex.

However attractive and provocative this hypothesis may be, it is open to certain criticisms, one of which is that it equates consciousness with the mere appreciation of "sensory impulses which reach the cerebrum" or with the capacity to react to stimuli. There is an inherent danger in this oversimplification and with the assumption that consciousness is a unitary state which can be localized within the upper brain stem. It requires but little reflection to appreciate that our own states of consciousness, which are the foremost facts of our existence, are not easily reducible to a series of sensory events. A remarkable and important feature of our consciousness is its continuity throughout every instant of waking life. From a vague, inchoate beginning in infancy until the termination of life there is never an unrecoverable hiatus in this continuum, except in sleep and in the instance of certain diseases of the central nervous system. A second quality is that of incessant change which takes place from minute to minute, aptly likened by William James to the flowing of a stream. Another essential attribute is its personal character; always it is "I" who is having the experience —a person with a finite spatial-temporal existence, separable from other parts of the physical world. This self consciousness requires at all times a clear perceptual and conceptual distinction between ourselves and the world about us. It is more than a succession of sensory events; in fact our own introspection informs us that it is the medium of coherence between separate experiences, whether excited by external stimuli or within ourselves by ideas or thoughts in the form of word symbols. Moreover, consciousness always maintains a focal or central point and a periphery, which is called the process of attention. All of this and more is embodied in our personal concept of consciousness and the thoughtful clinical investigator senses a vague remoteness from reality when he observes the experimentalist, in the interest of expediency, reducing consciousness to a mere awareness of stimuli, a process which may go on and off like an incandescent light. This is not to deny that consciousness is a separable quality of mind with its concomitant behavioral manifestations but merely that the study of it in animals in which it is equated with responsiveness to stimuli can do no more than elucidate one manifestation of it.

On the anatomical side the conclusion that there is an "awake" or "consciousness center" in the upper brain stem merely because lesions here in humans produce coma exemplifies our inveterate tendency to "hypostasize and anatomize abstractions". The important fact which has been established is that the reticular formation in the upper brain stem is in intimate relationship to specific sensory fiber systems and to the cerebral cortex and that the latter as an integrative mechanism depends more on these central connections than with intercortical ones. To say, however, that the reticular formation is "higher" or is the "pace maker" or "integrating mechanism" because it is the site where the smallest lesion may have the most widespread effect is illogical. The further study of these problems should turn to the analysis of the many partial disorders of consciousness which result from focal lesions of man's brain; and the subjective phenomena should be granted the same primacy of value as the behavioral change.

II. The Intellectual (Cognitive) Processes and the Cerebrum

Let us turn now to some of the observed alterations in perceiving and thinking which attend brain disease, and for which modern psychology uses the word *cognition*. In commenting on these cognitive processes apart from the conscious state of which they are an essential ingredient one must answer critics who argue that cognition cannot be treated separately from conation and affection, the other two Kantian divisions of mind. The importance of dissecting them, I believe, even though it may seem artificial is that scientific study must begin by analyzing its subject matter.

The idea that mental ability, cognition or intelligence is a highly individual quality with a range from feebleminded to genius, that heredity is an important determining factor in its development though education and environment are not without their effects; and that individual differences in this quality of mind are expressions of fundamental differences in the organization and function of the brain— all these have a long and interesting history, but time does not permit me to review it with you. Only in the last half of the 19th century, however, did the study of clinical and pathological manifestations of brain disease persuade us of the necessity of investigating the cognitive functions per se. And, of course, scientific advance entailed measurement, which was undertaken on a large scale in the early part of this century.

The possibility of subjecting the separate components of mind to specific test suggested itself to several leading scientists in the period 1880–1890. Francis Galton began testing sensory functions in his laboratory at this time, and in 1889 Oehrn, working under the direction of Kraepelin, published the results of the first actual measurements of mental capacities, in an effort to show in what manner patients with mental disease differed from normal. Binet, a student of Charcot in Paris, Munsterberg, Jastrow, Cattell and Terman in this country, extended these observations into the classroom. Since then the whole field of psychometry has developed.

The nature of intelligence or intellectual functions and their relationship to the anatomy and physiology of the brain continue to be fundamental problems in neurological medicine. The physician in this field is often confronted by individuals who have failed to develop mentally—to be amented in the language of Esquirol; and then there are the unfortunate individuals who have lost their mental powers through age or disease, a state known as dementia. Thus the initial impulse for the scientific study of the intellect came from the clinic and it continues to be prompted by the needs and daily problems of the clinic.

The subject of brain structure and its relation to intellectual ability has been studied only in its more general aspects. The human brain is extremely variable in weight and size and only at the extreme limits of largeness and smallness is there a rising incidence of enfeebled mentality or exceptional ability. Lassek in his recent monograph on The Human Brain reports that the smallest human brain on record weighed only 289 gms. and belonged to a mental defective, whereas the largest, weighing 2012 gms., was that of Turgenev, the celebrated Russian writer. The average weight is about 1450 gms., the female brain being lighter by 50 gms. Brains below 1000 and above 1600 gms. are exceptional and more often than not belong to mental defectives. Brain mass correlates better with height than with intellect, within the more normal range. Brain weight-body weight ratio is not overly informative; for humans it is about 44-1, in comparison to the marmoset which has a ratio of 27-1 and the whale 8500-1. Age is also a major factor. The brain doubles its weight from birth to the first year and thereafter its mass increases at a diminishing rate to the age of 20–25 years. From the age of 30–80 years there is a 10 per cent loss in weight. Inasmuch as the human brain contains 14,000,000,000 nerve cells Burns, in his discussion of the Mammalian Cortex, has calculated that this would mean a loss of several thousand cells during each day of adult life. Presumably 1,000,000 nerve cells have disintegrated, like meteorites, in this audience since I began to speak—a most alarming thought! Intelligence test scores parallel brain weight closely during early life but not in late life and senility, according to most recent reports.

In reviewing the literature on intellectual impairment in special types of human brain disease two hypotheses suggest themselves for study. These have recently been examined by McFie and Percy.

a) Is intelligence a single or unitary trait or is it composed of more or less independent abilities?

b) Does this trait or group of abilities depend on the normal function of some particular part or parts of the brain?

It is not possible, in this brief time to review all of the arguments for and against intelligence being a single monarchic mental power or a pleurality of separate powers. Spearman, Lashley and many others offer evidence in favor of both theories. One's view of this problem depends somewhat on one's definition of intelligence, whether a sum total of those qualities possessed by the most gifted members of our society (Galton) or "the innate ability to learn", "educability", "problem solving ability" and capacity for clear thinking especially along abstract lines. The tests most commonly employed require the subject to be alert, willing to take the test and to try to excel in it and to be able to understand and use language. Perception, learning, memory, ability to calculate, discriminative judgment, all these and more are exercised in successful mental performance.

General intelligence tests have been administered to patients with brain injury of known type and location and a number of interesting results have been obtained. One finding is clear enough, that disease of the brain does not interfere with the performance on each of these tests to the same degree. Retentive memory correlates poorly with verbal ability, visual-spatial discrimination, calculation and arithmetic ability and capacity for abstract thinking. The latter do cross-correlate with one another but not to a high degree. Similarly the process of attention may be affected separately, as shown by the fact that the patient may be incapable of maintaining attention, which in turn may impair his performance on all tests of mental function; or the achievement of good results may be hampered on these tests even though the patient appears to be fully attentive. Unfortunately attention itself as a unitary process has not been subjected to careful measurement in brain disease but one would expect derangements in this sphere to be related to the more fundamental process of consciousness.

In searching for the anatomical substratum of dementia several facts have emerged. The thalamus itself has been identified as playing an important role in mentation, as illustrated in the case of Stern where there was a widespread degenerative disease limited to the thalamus. Lesions of the dominant hemisphere impair verbal functions out of proportion to nonverbal ones, even when there is no true evidence of aphasic disorder. Arithmetic calculation suffers disproportionately in lesions of the dominant parietal lobe, indicating a relationship to the clinical state known as acalculia. Visual-spatial discriminations suffer the greatest reduction in abnormalities of the nondominant parietal lobe. Abstract reasoning is said to be reduced most in frontal lobe disease although there is still much uncertainty as to the accuracy of this statement.

Further study and more exact definition and measurement of these special brain functions is necessary before we can begin to understand their anatomical relationships; and anatomical studies must become more systematic and quantitative. The data at hand seem to support Spearman's theory of general as well as several special factors which are crucial to normal intellectual activity.

III. Perception and its Disorders

Our notions of sensation and perception have undergone many modifications in recent years in part because patients with diseases of the brain have revealed sensory findings incompatible with older theories. The conventional dichotomy of sensation and perception has been challenged for the reason that lesions which interrupt sensory nerves and tracts are observed to interfere with both functions, whereas cerebral lesions, which impair perception, are now believed to have a definite though variable influence on the most elementary forms of sensation. This latter effect has been difficult to define because the patient exhibits a peculiar indifference to his defect (we say he lacks insight or denies his disease) and is inattentive to stimuli applied to or arising within the affected parts. Anatomical study suggests not separate loci for sensation and perception but edifies the entire posterior temporal, parietal, occipital parts of each cerebral hemisphere as a vast suprasensory integrative area. Destructive lesions here cause to become manifest a remarkable array of gnostic defects; and stimulation of these parts, naturally as in a convulsion or by the surgeon on the operating table, evokes complicated hallucinatory phenomena (i.e. perceptions in the absence of observed stimulation). The integrative action of these parts of the brain and the thalamus and brain stem is poorly understood but there is much anatomical evidence which indicates that the whole system functions as a unit. Complex visual hallucinations, known to arise upon stimulation of the cerebral cortex, may also be associated with thalamic and mesencephalic lesions (the so-called *peduncular visual hallucinosis of Lhermitte*) and Fisher and I have observed a number of cases of *pontine auditory hallucinosis*. In the latter the patient reports a repertoire of chimes, chants, fragmentary harmonic sounds like an orchestra tuning up, whistles, sirens and other noises and even a voice calling one's own name (the nearest to audition of words). There is no measurable loss of hearing and the hallucinations do not interfere with the reception of ordinary auditory stimuli. The anatomical pathology of these cases has never been studied thoroughly, nor have the clinical anatomical relationships of other sensory phenomena been worked out in detail, except where the interruption of peripheral nerve fibers and spinal cord tracts has occurred. Moreover, the prominent role of hallucinations and the derangements of attention and sleep in delirium emphasize the possibility of a brain stem or diencephalic pathology as yet unfathomed. Here the experimentalist needs to delineate more clearly the fundamental nature of the psychic changes, for the disease state is but a syndrome.

IV. Memory

All investigations of intelligence, to which I have alluded, indicate that retentive memory is a process closely related to, yet qualitatively different from that of intellection. Profound disturbances of memory, to the degree that new material cannot be retained for more than a few seconds, is incompatible with all forms of intellectual activity, as would be expected. It is, in this respect, as widespread in its effects and as devastating to tasks requiring intellection as are inattentiveness, drowsiness, stupor and coma. Yet the opposite state may prevail in which the memory span for newly presented material is greatly reduced, to as brief a period as two to three minutes, without impairment of the ability to solve any problem that can be finished within that span of time. One may infer that the mechanisms which subserve memory function have an anatomy and a physiology different from those of intellectual functions.

Memory involves many things—the making of an impression, the retention of some record of that experience, the subsequent recall and reproduction of it. Excluded from serious consideration here are single parts of this process, such as the more or less permanent modification of the physical state of any object or cell by some previous activity. In this broader psychological sense, memory is but one side of perception and learning; and the relation of the object or rather its memory image epitomizes the whole problem of mind and matter.

A number of clinico-pathological observations have recently shed some light on the anatomy of memory mechanisms. The most consistent lesion in the remarkable disease known as Korsakow's psychosis has been in the mammillary bodies and medial parts of the diencephalon. Dr. Victor and I have endeavored to show that this special psychosis is but the mental component of Wernicke's disease and is due to a critical degree of thiamine chloride deficiency. Patients so afflicted, after an acute onset of pronounced mental confusion with paralysis of eye muscles and ataxia of gait, rapidly improve when given thiamine chloride alone or in an adequate diet. They then exhibit a state of reasonable alertness with minimal perceptive defect but with a total inability to recall and reproduce events of the past few weeks, months or years (events which occurred before onset of illness) and an equally striking inability to memorize, i.e. to learn. This improvement may continue for a time but much of the damage is often irreversible and leaves the patient permanently handicapped solely because of this inability to learn new experiences and to recall past ones. As the memory span lengthens to 3 or 4 minutes it may allow the patient to achieve a normal or superior score on a Wechsler-Bellevue intelligence test, and 5 minutes later not remember having taken the test or having seen the examiner. Tumors, aneurysms and other diseases affecting the mammillary bodies and walls of the third ventricles are known to have similar effects on learning and memory.

A case is presented which illustrates the lesions in Korsakow's psychosis. The fine anatomical details of this disease have never been elucidated but are now under study in several laboratories including our own. Progress here has been slow and halting because of a lack of knowledge of the normal human thalamus for which satisfactory reference material has not been available. The subtle qualities of the lesion in vitamin B deficiency recommend it for study, especially if the disease has existed for some months prior to death and the full range of functional deficit has been determined.

Equally exciting and provocative has been the confirmation of a poorly documented observation by Glees and Griffith of severe retentive memory defect following upon bilateral infarction of the hippocampal convolutions. Scoville made the accidental discovery that surgical excision of these parts as a therapeutic procedure in psychotic patients has a similar effect, and Penfield and Milner produced a clinical picture much like Korsakow's psychosis by excising one temporal lobe in patients believed to have preexistent disease in the other one.

A case is presented, a patient observed by C. Miller Fisher and myself, who was noted to have suffered a permanent loss of retentive memory and capacity to learn after occlusion of branches of the posterior cerebral arteries and infarction of medial and posterior parts of each temporal lobe.

The significance of these new findings is at once evident when it is recalled that the hippocampus is connected with the mammillary bodies and tegmental fields of diencephalon and midbrain which are the site of the abnormality in Wernicke's disease. One may postulate then that the hippocampi, fornices, mammillary bodies and medial thalamic nuclei, the mammillo-thalamic tracts of Vicq d'Azyr, the thalamo-cingulate tracts, constitute a system of great biological importance which in conjunction with all parts of the cerebral cortex represent a mechanism for learning and memory, whether of a relatively simple variety as in the elicitation of a conditioned reflex or the memorizing of nonsense-syllables or complex, meaningful material. The detailed workings of this mechanism demand penetrating anatomical, physiological and psychological investigation.

We have the impression that this basic memory mechanism may be temporarily abrogated by disease with complete recovery of function. Fisher and I have collected notes on more than 15 patients in the last few years, all middle-aged or elderly and without sign of psychiatric illness, in whom there has been a sudden onset of global amnesia which lasted some hours. Without change in color, or any overt manifestation of seizure, the patient suddenly betrays, by a bewildered expression or a remark, that he does not know where he is or what he has been doing. Throughout the attack, while conscious and apparently in contact with his environment and able to move gracefully, to speak coherently, to read and understand spoken words, to calculate (in one instance), to recognize common objects, to drive a car, or to prepare a salad, the patient is unable to orientate himself or to hold in mind any new information given him concerning his orientation. During the attack there is retrograde amnesia for hours or days; and, after it is over, the amnesic period shrinks to the length of the period represented by the attack itself. The attack passes off leaving no residual abnormality, and, except in one instance, has not recurred. Suspected usually of being a stroke or a seizure, clinical study, x-rays, electroencephalography and lumbar puncture have provided no clue as to its nature. We believe this to be a unique clinical state involving these regions which are critical to memory. The condition awaits pathological verification.

V. WILL, VOLITION, CONATION; IMPULSIVITY AND PURPOSEFUL MENTAL ACTIVITY

If you will permit me to speak for a few more minutes, I would like to remark upon two other features of mind which at the present time are largely beyond the orbit of scientific study but which merit thorough investigation. One of these is will or volition, also called conation, the other is affection or emotion.

It is apparent when one reflects on the matter, that volition or conation shows its influence in all perceptive and cognitive processes. In test procedures the whole efficiency of an intellectual process may in a large measure depend on the effort the patient puts into it, that is to say, how hard he tries. Weakness of motive or lack of desire to succeed hampers action and may prevent the attainment of ends well within the reach of the subject. Strong effort, contrariwise, often permits excellence of performance beyond that which would be expected of the individual.

The neurologically-minded physician, pondering the various derangements of mind by disease, must take cognizance of this quality and inquire as to whether it constitutes an essential and measurable attribute of psychic function. Does disease of the brain reveal something of the nature of impulse to action and volition?

In seeking further information on these matters we have found textbooks of neurology and psychiatry to be strangely silent. By traditional usage the term will or volition has both a narrow and a broad psychological meaning. In its broad sense it is more or less synonymous with all the psychic activity which arises from an idea or mental stimulus (in contrast to a physiological one) and accomplishes some result. In its more restricted sense it refers to action arising from an idea and ending in the realization of that idea. The basis of will is said to be an impulse which has its origin in a physiological state and leads to mental unrest. The impulse expresses itself in producing some physical change. In the more precise language of Dewey volition is defined as "regularized, harmonized impulse ... consciously directed towards the attainment of a recognized end which is held desirable". He points out that the elements of volition or act of will involve, over and above the impulse, knowledge and feeling.

In evaluating this complex attribute of mind the clinical investigator has recourse to two sources of information. He may inquire of the patient as to his state of mind, his conscious awareness of his impulse to action, of the persistence in his mind of a certain idea or of a goal. Or, behavior itself may be taken as an expression of whether the patient is capable of volition i.e. evidence by act or verbal report of sustained attention, of persistent and self-directed activity, of restless, aimless movements of an apprehensive mental state, or merely continuous psychic activity of a particular type.

In comparison to the incessant psychic activity, the press of speech and movement of the average normally motivated urban individual with only brief periods of idleness from morning until night, patients with brain disease are frequently inactive for long periods of time. There is a poverty of both psychic and motor activity. An English teacher on one of our wards, with an aneurysm of the anterior cerebral artery, uttered not a single word for a period of several weeks and was judged to be aphasic until one day when two of her room mates were reciting a poem and found themselves unable to remember the fourth line of the third stanza, she supplied the missing line, speaking clearly, and then lapsed into her mute state for several weeks more. These patients are likely to react only to their immediate situation, making no effort to plan for the future, and their demeanor provides no hint of anxiety. In all diseases which cause profound confusion or stupor this apathy, hebetude, silence and paucity of movement are characteristic. The most extreme degree of it was noted by Hugh Cairns in a patient with a third ventricular tumor and for this state the term *akinetic mutism* was proposed, with the implication that the morbid anatomy was diencephalic in location. However, we have seen this psychic peculiarity most often with a variety of diseases located in the posterior parts of one or both frontal lobes. A similar state has occasionally attended a frontal lobotomy which has been inadvertently extended too far posteriorly.

The full significance of this extreme lack of impulse to thought and action, so-called abulia in older psychological terminology, cannot be assessed from available data. Nor can we state its frequency as a manifestation of disease of different parts of the cerebral hemispheres for the reason that a suitable index or measure of impulsivity to action and of voluntary attention has not been developed. Nor has the converse of abulia, an uncontrollable uninhibitable impulse to action, the so-called "organic driveness" of Eugene Kahn, been subjected to careful study. Only the extreme degrees of it, manifest in the wild, senseless, uncontrolled, destructive actions of children with brain disease, have even been mentioned in the medical literature; and the morbid anatomy of this condition has yet to be divulged.

VI. Affect and Emotion

Disorders of the affective or emotional life are conceded to be the central abnormality in all the major psychiatric illnesses. Considering their importance, it is surprising that so little attention has been given to the nervous derangements upon which the emotional states depend. But this neglect is probably due to the fact that contemporary psychiatry has concerned itself more with expected emotional reactions to the thought content of mind and its psychological origins in past experience than with general biological processes.

At the present time it is impossible to do more than summarize a few of the changes in emotional life that have been observed during the course of established diseases of the human nervous system.

To turn directly to the neurology of emotion it should be noted that the term implies two conditions—"a way of feeling and a way of acting" (Papez). The former denotes the subjective experience, the latter, the outward expression. A complete analysis would require consideration of the stimulus situations (their nature, threshold, etc.), the adequacy, appropriateness and duration of the emotional experience or feeling and the form and duration of the emotional response.

Clinical study of diseases of the brain has revealed more information concerning the expression of emotion than of the subjective experience itself, which is regrettable. Numerous patients come to the attention of the medical profession in which disease of the brain has rendered them incapable of controlling their emotions or of expressing them in the usual manner. A notable example of the former is pathological laughter or crying. Here the slightest stimulus will cause uncontrollable laughter or crying which may persist for minutes. One of our patients with amyotrophic lateral sclerosis was so convulsed with laughter whenever he saw the house physician, who had told him a joke at the time of their first meeting, that it was necessary to transfer him to the care of another physician. And another patient with "lacunar" vascular disease of the brain wept disconsolately for minutes every time he attempted to relate the history of his illness. Lesser degrees of this phenomenon present themselves as excessive emotional lability or weakness of the mechanism for the normal inhibition of the emotional reactions, e.g. weeping upon hearing the national anthem or upon greeting a friend.

The question naturally arises as to whether these emotional outbursts are accompanied by the appropriate, subjective emotional experience or are pure sham. The stimuli themselves are usually appropriate for the excitation of the emotional reaction though one cannot always be certain on this point. Merely speaking to the patient may initiate the emotional response; or, as in the report of Giannuli (cited by Wilson) the patient was forced to keep his eyes glued to the ground because if he raised them to meet anyone's gaze he would immediately be seized by laughter. The stimulus may be one which for a normal person would be relatively ineffective. Further, the reaction, once initiated, cannot be checked. Brissaud's patient, upon being told by a lady that her little dog was dead, adopted a mournful countenance which was followed by "tears, tears by sobs and sobs by a Rabelaisian effect on the sphincters". Concerning the subjective experience it does not always correspond to the outward emotional display. The patient may laugh against his will, even when his mood is one of sorrow or annoyance. Brissaud made the amusing observation of a patient with marked pathological crying in bed next a patient with pathological laughter. The latter would roar with laughter at the weeping of the former and occasionally it would cause the one who was crying to begin to laugh while retaining some of the facial expressions of weeping. The emotional display itself is unquestionably genuine though sometimes not well differentiated.

The best known lesions in these cases of pathological emotionality are in the corticobulbar tracts, which would suggest a release-effect on the emotional mechanisms. The latter are believed to extend from the frontal lobes through the hypothalamus to the autonomic nervous system and the facial-respiratory centers in the lower brain stem. The anatomical studies of these central regulatory arrangements by Bard and his associates indicate that lesions of the limbic portions of the macaque and cat are the cortical areas which have a pronounced effect on emotional reactions. Papez from purely anatomical studies of the human brain, but doubtless influenced by animal experiments, postulated the existence of a complicated nervous arrangement involving the inferior orbital, cingulate and insular parts of the cerebral cortex, the amygdaloid nuclei, hippocampi, fornical systems and hypothalamus with their various connections as the mechanism for emotion. The details of this neuronal system and its physiology are being studied by many medical scientists at the present time but our understanding of it is far from complete.

The anatomy of persistent nervous syndromes dominated by uncontrollable anxiety and worry has not been investigated systematically in patients with focal brain lesions. So far the most impressive fact to emerge has been the remarkable loss of these symptoms in diseases which damage the inferior parts of the frontal lobes and the fronto-thalamic and thalamo-frontal pathways through the anterior limb of the internal capsule (Freeman and Watts). One may speculate that this fronto-thalamic neuronal system may be the one which is liberated in pathological laughter and crying.

The systematic study of the feelings and emotions in patients with brain disease, of the altered reactions of these patients to drugs such as chlorpromazine, reserpine, mescaline and lysergic acid which are known to inhibit or facilitate emotionality, and of the morbid anatomy of the lesions which underlie these states is almost certain to yield important insights into the major symptoms of psychiatric disease. Already the anatomical studies of lobotomized brains by Yakovlev have provided us with a new conception of the general plan of the nervous system and particularly of the cerebral cortex. Reference is made here to his major division of the brain into the *entopallium*, which includes all the central matrix of the brain stem and spinal cord, the *mesopallium*, which now extends to include all of the limbic system as well as the insular and sensori-motor cortex, and the *ectopallium*, which comprises the association areas of the cortex. This is a welcome substitute for the archaic lobar anatomy.

A final case illustrates the tranquilizing effect of an orbital frontal lesion, changing the whole emotional pattern of a previously tense, sensitive, energetic woman.

Conclusion: From these remarks it should be evident that there is great need of further clinico-pathologic study of well established, stable, focal lesions of the brain. Definition of clinical phenomena, their accurate measurement and complete and systematic studies of the anatomy of the nervous system, all are sorely needed. The careful observation of the action of drugs which affect the nervous system in these patients with focal brain disease is another worthy scientific undertaking and could form the basis of neuropharmacology. Medical neurology will be enriched by studies of these types and should attain a degree of precision never before reached. I trust that some future orator on this celebrated occasion may be able to speak with more authority on these matters.

INDEX